ANESTHESIA
Drug Manual

WHITE

ANESTHESIA
Drug Manual

Paul F. White, Ph.D., M.D.
Professor and McDermott Chair of Anesthesiology
University of Texas Southwestern Medical Center
Dallas, Texas

W.B. SAUNDERS COMPANY
A Division of Harcourt Brace & Company
PHILADELPHIA LONDON TORONTO
MONTREAL SYDNEY TOKYO

W.B. SAUNDERS COMPANY
A Division of Harcourt Brace & Company

The Curtis Center
Independence Square West
Philadelphia, Pennsylvania 19106

Library of Congress Cataloging-in-Publication Data

Anesthesia drug manual / [edited by] Paul F. White.

   p.   cm.

ISBN 0–7216–6221–8

1. Drug interactions—Handbooks, manuals, etc.   2. Anesthesiology—Handbooks,
   manuals, etc.   3. Drugs—Handbooks, manuals, etc.
   4. Anesthesia—Handbooks, manuals, etc.   I. White, Paul F.
   [DNLM: 1. Anesthesia—handbooks. 2. Anesthetics—handbooks.
   QV 39 A578 1996]

RD82.7.D78A54   1996

617.9′6—dc20

DNLM/DLC   95–46940

ANESTHESIA DRUG MANUAL   ISBN 0–7216–6221–8

Printed in the United States of America.

Last digit is the print number: 9   8   7   6   5   4   3   2   1

To Trev
for stimulating my interest
in pharmacology as a graduate
student at UCSF.

To Skip
for his ongoing support and
encouragement during my medical
and postgraduate training.

To Linda
for tolerating me for
the last 25 years!

Contributors

Michail N. Avramov, M.D., Ph.D.
Assistant Instructor, Department of
Anesthesiology and Pain Management,
University of Texas Southwestern
Medical Center, Dallas, Texas.

Anticonvulsants

Michael A. Campagni, M.D.
Assistant Professor, Department of
Anesthesiology, The Ohio State
University, Columbus, Ohio.

Adrenergic Agonists and Antagonists

Yifeng Ding, M.D.
Clinical Research Fellow, Department of
Anesthesiology, Washington University
School of Medicine, St. Louis, Missouri.

Antineoplastics and Immunosuppressants

Ralph A. Farina, M.D.
Assistant Professor, Department of
Anesthesiology, The Ohio State
University, Columbus, Ohio.

Cholinesterase Inhibitors

Arnold S. Friedman, M.D.
Staff Anesthesiologist, Department of
Anesthesiology, Cedars-Sinai Medical
Center, Los Angeles, California.

Diuretics

Noor M. Gajraj, M.B.B.S., F.R.C.A.
Senior Registrar, Queen's Medical
Centre, Nottingham, United Kingdom.

Local Anesthetics

Ahmed F. Ghouri, M.D.
Senior Resident, Department of
Anesthesiology, University of California
at Irvine, Irvine, California.

*Bronchodilators and Antiasthmatics;
Metabolic (Nonhormonal) Therapies*

Julian A. Gold, M.D.
Co-Chairman, Department of
Anesthesiology, Cedars-Sinai Medical
Center, Los Angeles, California.

Antihistamines

Michele E. Gold, C.R.N.A., Ph.D.
Assistant Professor of Clinical
Anesthesiology, Department of
Anesthesiology, University of California
School of Medicine, Los Angeles,
California.

Antihistamines

Naomi M. Gonzales, Pharm.D.
Acute Pain Service Pharmacist, Cedars-
Sinai Medical Center, Los Angeles,
California.

Hormones

Michael Guertin, M.D.
Assistant Professor, Department of
Anesthesiology, The Ohio State
University. Director, Orthopedic
Anesthesia, The Ohio State University
Medical Center, Columbus, Ohio.

Beta Blockers

Ronald L. Harter, M.D.
Assistant Professor, Department of
Anesthesiology, The Ohio State
University, Columbus, Ohio.

Intravenous Anesthetics

Thomas Heiman, M.D.
Associate Clinical Professor, Department
of Anesthesiology, University of
California at Irvine, Irvine, California.
Staff Anesthesiologist, San Bernardino
County Medical Center, San Bernardino,
California.

Diuretics

Henry Huey, M.D.
Staff Anesthesiologist, Western Medical
Center, Anaheim, California.

Hormones

Michael W. Jopling, M.D.
Assistant Professor, Department of
Anesthesiology, The Ohio State
University, Columbus, Ohio.

Miscellaneous Compounds

**Girish P. Joshi, M.B.B.S., M.D.,
F.F.A.R.C.S.I.**
Assistant Professor, Department of
Anesthesiology and Pain Management,
The University of Texas Southwestern
Medical Center, Dallas, Texas.

Vasodilator Drugs

Marshal B. Kaplan, A.B., M.S., M.D.
Associate Clinical Professor, Department
of Anesthesiology, University of
California School of Medicine, Los
Angeles. Attending Anesthesiologist,
Cedars-Sinai Medical Center, Los
Angeles, California.

Anticoagulants and Thrombolytics

William B. Kelly, M.D.
Assistant Professor, Department of
Anesthesiology, The Ohio State
University, Columbus, Ohio.

Calcium Channel Blockers

Ana Diez R.-Labajo, M.D.
Anesthesiologist, Anesthesia,
Reanimacion y Dolor, Madrid, Spain.

Vitamins and Nutritional Supplements

Eugene Y. Lai, M.D.
Senior Resident, Department of
Anesthesiology, University of California
at Irvine, Irvine, California.

*Bronchodilators and Antiasthmatics;
Metabolic (Nonhormonal) Therapies*

Charles Louy, Ph.D., M.D.
Attending Anesthesiologist, Department
of Anesthesiology, Cedars-Sinai Medical
Center, Los Angeles, California.

Hormones

Steven J. Luke, M.D.
Instructor, Department of Anesthesiology
and Pain Management, The University
of Texas Southwestern Medical Center,
Dallas, Texas.

Central Stimulants

Dori Ann McCulloch, M.D.
Consultant Anesthetist, Stafford District
General Hospital, Stafford, United
Kingdom.

Muscle Relaxants

Robert T. Naruse, M.D.
Assistant Clinical Professor, Department
of Anesthesiology, University of
California School of Medicine, Los
Angeles. Staff Anesthesiologist, Cedars-
Sinai Medical Center, Los Angeles,
California.

Anticholinergics

**Michael H. Nathanson, M.R.C.P.,
F.R.C.A.**
Consultant Anesthetist, University
Hospital, Queen's Medical Centre,
Nottingham, United Kingdom.

Antihypertensive Drugs

Carl E. Noe, M.D.
Attending Physician, Department of
Anesthesia, Baylor Medical Center,
Dallas, Texas.

Antimicrobial Agents

Anthony M. Nyerges, M.D.
Associate Professor, Department of
Anesthesiology, University of California
School of Medicine, Los Angeles,
California.

Psychotropic Drugs

Vincent A. Romanelli, M.D.
Clinical Assistant Professor, Department
of Anesthesiology, The Ohio State
University, Columbus, Ohio.

Opioid Agonists and Antagonists

**Shiv K. Sharma, M.B.B.S., M.D.,
F.R.C.A.**
Assistant Professor, Department of
Anesthesiology and Pain Management,
The University of Texas Southwestern
Medical Center, Dallas, Texas.

Antacids

Harbhej Singh, M.D.
Assistant Instructor, Department of
Anesthesiology and Pain Management,
The University of Texas Southwestern
Medical Center, Dallas, Texas.

*Blood Substitutes; Cutaneous-Topical
Drugs*

Ian Smith, B.Sc., M.B.B.S., F.R.C.A.
Senior Lecturer in Anaesthetics, Keele
University, North Staffordshire
Hospitals, Stoke-on-Trent, United
Kingdom.

Inhalation Anesthetics

**Andrew J. Souter, M.B., Ch.B.,
F.R.C.A.**
Senior Registrar in Anaesthesia, Oxford
Radcliffe Hospital, Oxford, United
Kingdom.

Nonsteroidal Anti-inflammatory Drugs

Rui Sun, M.D., Ph.D.
Research Fellow, Department of
Anesthesiology and Pain Management,
The University of Texas Southwestern
Medical Center, Dallas, Texas.

Dermatologic Drugs

Jun Tang, M.D.
Research Fellow, Department of
Anesthesiology and Pain Management,
The University of Texas Southwestern
Medical Center, Dallas, Texas.

Gastrointestinal Drugs

Mehernoor F. Watcha, M.D., D.Ch.
Associate Professor, Department of
Anesthesiology and Pain Management,
The University of Texas Southwestern
Medical Center, Dallas, Texas.

Antiemetics

Paul E. Wender, M.D.
Staff Anesthesiologist, Cedars-Sinai
Medical Center, Los Angeles,
California.

Benzodiazepines and Antagonists

Ronald H. Wender, M.D.
Assistant Professor, Department of
Anesthesiology, University of California
School of Medicine, Los Angeles. Co-
Director, Department of Anesthesiology,
Cedars-Sinai Medical Center, Los
Angeles, California.

Benzodiazepines and Antagonists

**Paul F. White, M.D., Ph.D.,
F.A.N.Z.C.A.**
Professor and McDermott Chair of
Anesthesiology, University of Texas
Southwestern Medical Center, Dallas,
Texas.

*Vitamins and Nutritional Supplements;
Appendix: Immunizing Agents*

Russell P. Woda, D.O.
Assistant Professor, Department of
Anesthesiology, The Ohio State
University, Columbus, Ohio.

Antiarrhythmics

It is a familiar truth that "the practice of anesthesiology is the practice of clinical pharmacology." The development of new anesthetic drugs and of novel uses for old drugs is critically important for the advancement of our specialty in the future. The clinician attempting to keep pace in the 1990s and beyond must contend not only with many new anesthetic drugs but also with an ever increasing number of chronic or adjuvant medications that have now become an essential part of our routine anesthetic practices.

In early 1994, Paul White and I spoke with Avé McCracken of W.B. Saunders Company, who was interested in having us jointly publish a comprehensive textbook of anesthesia pharmacology. Since Paul and I felt that the specialty did not need another huge textbook to sit on our bookshelves, we recommended that the publisher consider an up-to-date drug compendium for quick reference in the preoperative assessment clinic, operating room, recovery room, pain clinic, and intensive care unit. Most of the currently available drug references are not specifically targeted to anesthesia practitioners and the perioperative setting, and even fewer of them would be considered portable! We agreed that most practitioners would appreciate a relatively complete drug data base having a simple, intuitive format that allows rapid access to essential information—minus the unnecessary verbiage. Just as important, the text should make it easy for the reader to tell when a particular fact is *not* available. Other commitments ultimately kept me from participating in the creation of this book, but Paul brought his customary energy to the task, and I am delighted with the result.

The *Anesthesia Drug Manual* appears to have succeeded on all counts. I am sure that it will join the select group of books that become dog-eared from daily use by anesthesia residents as well as by nurse and physician practitioners of our specialty.

CARL E. ROSOW, M.D., Ph.D.
Associate Professor of Anesthesia and Pharmacology
Massachusetts General Hospital
Harvard Medical School
Boston, Massachusetts

As the number of drugs that our patients receive continues to increase at a rapid rate, it has become more difficult for busy practitioners to keep abreast of the pharmacologic properties of the new compounds and their potential interactions with existing drugs. From the clinician's perspective, the problem has been compounded by the dramatic shift in health care delivery from the hospital to the ambulatory setting. Currently, more than 90% of all patients undergoing elective surgery are admitted on the day of the operation. The difficulty in assessing the potential implications of chronic medications on their perioperative course is further complicated by the fact that many more elderly patients with complex medical problems are now routinely undergoing surgery on an ambulatory basis.

The inability to casually evaluate patients awaiting surgery in a hospital setting has necessitated a more efficient process for identifying potential adverse drug interactions during the perioperative period and for having more rapid access to key pharmacologic and drug dosage information. The availability of a pocket-size drug reference manual would allow the practitioner to quickly review essential pharmacokinetics, pharmacodynamics, drug dosage, and interactions. The concept in writing the *Anesthesia Drug Manual* was to develop a concise template containing key information on the pharmacology of virtually all drugs in the *Physicians' Desk Reference (PDR)*.

The drugs in this book are grouped according to the pharmacologic classification system utilized by the *PDR* and the *United States Pharmacopeia (USP)*. Within each specific drug group, the drugs are alphabetically arranged according to their generic name. The properties listed include the generic and trade names, clinical indications, primary pharmacokinetics and dynamic features, dosages and concentrations, and adverse drug interactions. The concept was to allow the busy practitioner to quickly identify the salient pharmacologic properties of an unfamiliar drug without having to wade through pages of text material or locate one of the large reference sources.

The *Anesthesia Drug Manual* was originally conceived by Carl Rosow, M.D., Ph.D., and myself at the encouragement of Avé McCracken (formerly at W.B. Saunders Company). Although Carl was unable to collaborate on the project because of his other commitments, many of my current (and former) research associates assisted in organizing the material for this manual. Given the large number of new drugs that are introduced into clinical practice each year, it is our intention to update the book on a biennial basis.

In acknowledging the individuals who made substantial contributions to this manual, I would like to start with my secretary, Joyce Mandujano. Joyce had the oftentimes onerous task of putting rather diverse material into a proper format. Second, Carol Robins at W.B. Saunders Company had the equally challenging task of trying to achieve a standardized style for drugs with widely differing pharmacologic profiles. Although we had to go through two other editors before she finally took over the project, Lesley Day was extremely helpful in getting the manual published! I would also like to express my sincere appreciation to my current and former colleagues at the University of California–San Francisco, Stanford University, Washington University, and the University of Texas Southwestern Medical Center at Dallas. Finally, I would like to thank my family—Linda, Kristine, and Lisa—and friends for their strong support and encouragement throughout my career in academic medicine.

PAUL F. WHITE

Contents

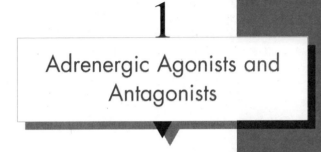

1

Adrenergic Agonists and Antagonists

Michael A. Campagni, M.D.

AMRINONE

Trade Name:	Inocor
Indications:	Congestive heart failure.
Pharmacokinetics:	Onset: IV effects begin within 2–5 min. Peak effect: 10 min; persists for 0.5–2 hr. Vd: 1.2 L/kg. $T_{1/2}$: α, 4.6 min; β, 3.6 hr; β, 5.8 hr in congestive heart failure. Metabolized in liver. Excreted in urine.
Pharmacodynamics:	Inhibits phosphodiesterase and $\uparrow$ cAMP
CVS:	Positive inotrope vasodilator, $\downarrow$ LVEDP, $\downarrow$ SVR, $\downarrow$ MAP, $\downarrow$ PCWP.
Hepatic:	Can be hepatotoxic.
GI:	Nausea, vomiting, diarrhea, anorexia, abdominal pain.
Dosage/ Concentrations:	Parenteral: 5 mg/ml. Initial injection of 0.75 mg/kg IV (may repeat in 30 min), then maintenance infusion 5–10 µg/kg/min. Total dose not to exceed 10 mg/kg/ day. Continue infusion as needed. Store at room temperature, and protect from light.
Contraindications:	Liver disease, severe thrombocytopenia, and debilitating adverse GI effects; obstructive cardiomyopathy.
Drug Interactions/ Allergy:	Hypersensitivity reactions, sulfite allergy, additive inotropic effects with cardiac glycosides, and excessive hypotension with disopyramide. Incompatible with dextrose; mix with saline. Incompatible with furosemide (precipitate).

CLONIDINE

See Chapter 9
(Antihypertensive
Drugs)

DEXMEDETOMIDINE

Trade Name:	N/A
Indications:	Prevention of perioperative tachycardia and hypertension and anesthetic and analgesic sparing effects.
Pharmacokinetics:	Onset: 3–5 min; $\downarrow$ HR/systolic BP 20–30 min. $T_{1/2}$: α, <5 min; Vd at steady state: $\sim$ 2.2 L/kg; β, $\sim$2 hr. Clearance: $\sim$ 0.75 L/kg/hr.

Pharmacodynamics
CNS: Sedation-hypnosis, analgesia, anxiolysis.
CVS: Sympatholysis (↓ catecholamines), bradycardia (even sinus arrest), hypotension.
GI: Dry mouth.
Musculoskeletal: ↓ Shivering.
Other: ↓ ACTH, ↓ ADH, ↓ insulin, ↑ growth hormone.

Dosage/
Concentration:
Adult: 0.25–1.0 μg/kg IV, or 0.5–2.5 μg/kg IM.

Contraindications: Sinus node disease, AV conduction abnormalities, or acute hypovolemia.

Drug Interactions/ None known.
Allergy:

DOBUTAMINE

Trade Name: Dobutrex

Indications: Cardiac decompensation after cardiac surgery, congestive heart failure, and acute MI.

Pharmacokinetics: Onset 1–2 min; duration <10 min.
$T_{1/2}$: 2.4 min. Vd: 0.25 L/kg. Clearance: 2.35 L/min/m^2. Metabolized in liver. Excreted in urine.

Pharmacodynamics:
CNS: ↑ CBF.
CVS: ↑ Contractility, ↑ SV (↑ cardiac output), ↑ HR, ↓ SVR (pressure may be unchanged), ↓ atrial filling pressure.
Pulmonary: ↓ pulmonary vascular resistance.
Renal: ↑ RBF.
GI: Nausea and vomiting.

Dosage/ Supplied in 20-ml bottle (250 mg), 12.5 mg/ml.
Concentrations:
Adult and Pediatric: IV, 2–20 μg/kg/min infusion (do not mix with alkaline solutions).

Contraindications: Idiopathic hypertrophic subaortic stenosis, known hypersensitivity, and pregnancy.

Drug Interactions/ Unopposed alpha-adrenergic effects when beta blockers are used (↑ peripheral resistance).
Allergy: ↑ Arrhythmia with halothane (commercial solution may contain sulfites).

DOPAMINE

Trade Name:	Intropin
Indications:	Shock or hypotensive emergency, acute renal failure.
Pharmacokinetics:	$T_{1/2}$: 2 min. Vd: 0.25 L/kg. Onset of action: following IV administration, within 5 min; duration 10 minutes. Does not cross blood-brain barrier. Metabolized in kidney and plasma by MAO and COMT. Excreted in urine.
Pharmacodynamics:	Endogenous catecholamine.
CNS:	Vasodilation of intracerebral vascular bed; headache.
CVS:	↑ Cardiac output, ↑ HR and SBP, coronary dilation, vasoconstriction with ↑ dose; arrhythmias.
Pulmonary:	↑ Pulmonary artery occlusion pressure.
Renal:	Renal vasodilation, ↑ RBF; ↑ GFR, ↑ Na excretion.
GI:	Nausea and vomiting, mesenteric vasodilation.
Musculoskeletal:	Extravasation may cause sloughing and necrosis in surrounding tissue.
Dosage/ Concentrations:	80 mg/ml, 5-ml vial. IV: Renal effects, 0.5–2 µg/kg/min. Cardiac effects, 2–10 µg/kg/min. Vascular effects, 10–20 µg/kg/min.
Contraindications:	Pheochromocytoma, uncorrected tachyarrhythmia, and known hypersensitivity.
Drug Interactions/ Allergy:	Effects prolonged and intensified by MAOIs, arrhythmia with halothane, hyperglycemia; concomitant use with phenytoin may cause seizures, hypotension, and bradycardia.

EPHEDRINE

Trade Name:	N/A
Indications:	Bronchospasm and hypotension (shock, during anesthesia).
Pharmacokinetics:	Completely absorbed after oral, IM, or SC dose. Onset: <1 min; duration: 10–60 min. Peak effect: single IV dose (10–25 mg), 1 hour. Crosses placenta. $T_{1/2}$: 3–6 hr. Metabolized in liver. Excreted in urine.
Pharmacodynamics:	Noncatecholamine sympathomimetic.
CNS:	Stimulation (nervousness, restlessness, insomnia); tremor.
CVS:	↑ Cardiac output, ↑ BP, ↑ HR, ↑ contractility; arrhythmias.

Pulmonary:	Bronchodilation, pulmonary edema.
Hepatic:	Glycogenolysis, hyperglycemia.
Renal:	↓ RBF (secondary to vasoconstriction).
GI:	Relaxes smooth muscle of GI tract.
GU:	↑ Uterine blood flow when hypotension is treated after spinal anesthesia.
Musculoskeletal:	Constricts arterioles in skin and mucous membrane; dilates arterioles in skeletal muscle.

Dosage/ Concentrations:	Parenteral: Ephedrine sulfate available (25 or 50 mg/ ml) for IM or IV.
Adult:	10–25 mg IV q 5–10 min (not to exceed 150 mg in 24 hr). SC/IM 25–50 mg.
Pediatric:	3 mg/kg IV q day (divided into 4–6 doses).

Contraindications:	Angle-closure glaucoma, heart disease, hypertension, diabetes, hyperthyroidism, and benign prostatic hypertrophy.
Drug Interactions/ Allergy:	Additive effects with other sympathomimetics. Arrhythmia when drug is used with halogenated hydrocarbon anesthetics. MAOIs potentiate pressor effects. α and β blockers negate effects.

EPINEPHRINE

Trade Name:	Adrenalin
Indications:	Bronchospasm, anaphylaxis, use in CPR and cardiac arrhythmia, ↑ myocardial contractility, prolongs local anesthetic action, and allergic reactions.
Pharmacokinetics:	Absorption: SC or IM dose well absorbed. Onset: rapid and of short duration; parenteral. SC for bronchodilation, effects within 5–10 min; maximal effects in 20 min. $T_{1/2}$: ~ 2 min. Clearance: 35–89 ml/kg/min. Crosses blood-brain barrier but not placenta. Terminated by uptake and metabolism in sympathetic nerve ending. Metabolized in liver by COMT and MAO. Excreted in urine.
Pharmacodynamics:	Endogenous catecholamine.
CNS:	Stimulation (restlessness, tremor, anxiety, headache).
CVS:	Positive inotrope/chronotrope, ↑ cardiac output, ↑ MVO_2, ↑ SV, ↑ HR, ↑ MAP, ↑ arrhythmia, ↑ coronary blood flow, vasoconstriction, angina.
Pulmonary:	Bronchodilation, ↑ pulmonary artery pressure, pulmonary edema.
Hepatic:	↑ Hepatic blood flow, glycogenolysis, hyperglycemia.
Renal:	↓ RBF, ↑ renin secretion.

EPINEPHRINE   *(continued)*

GI:	↑ Splanchnic blood flow, relaxes GI smooth muscle.
Musculoskeletal:	Vasoconstriction of skin and mucosa and of skeletal muscle vessels.
GU:	Uterine relaxant.
Other:	Inhibited insulin release, lipolysis, hypokalemia, ↑ body temperature.

Dosage/
Concentrations: Solution, 1/1000 or 1/10,000.
   For bronchospasm:
Adult: 0.1–0.5 mg SC/IM q 0.5–4 hr (0.1–0.5 ml of 1:1,000 solution). 0.1–1 μg/kg/min infusion (for inotropic support).
Pediatric: 0.01 mg/kg SC q 0.5–4 hr.
   For anaphylaxis:
Adult: 0.1–0.25 mg IV q 5–15 min.
Pediatric: 0.1 mg IV, then infuse 0.1 μg/kg/min.
   For CPR:
Adult: 0.5–1 mg IV q 3–5 min (5–10 ml of 1:1000 solution).
Pediatric: 0.01 mg/kg IV q 3–5 min.
Neonate: 0.01–0.03 mg/kg IV q 3–5 min.

Contraindications: Known hypersensitivity and angle-closure glaucoma; patients taking β blockers; hyperthyroidism.

Drug Interactions/
Allergy: Additive with other sympathomimetics. Arrhythmia with inhalational agents. Antagonized by α and β blockers. ↑ Insulin requirements in diabetics. Unstable in alkaline solution. TCAs, antihistamine, and thyroid hormones potentiate effects.

ISOPROTERENOL

Trade Name:	Isuprel
Indications:	Bronchodilation (IV or aerosol), bradyarrhythmias, AV heart block, and shock.
Pharmacokinetics:	Rapidly absorbed following parenteral administration or oral inhalation. Bronchodilation occurs promptly after oral inhalation and persists for up to 1 hr. Onset: <1 min and persists for a few minutes after IV dose, up to 2 hr after SC or sublingual dose.
Pharmacodynamics:	Synthetic sympathomimetic amine.
CNS:	Nervousness, tremor, insomnia, dizziness.
CVS:	↑ HR, ↑ contractility, ↑ cardiac output, ↑ automaticity, ↓ SVR, ↓ diastolic BP.
Pulmonary:	Bronchodilation, ↓ pulmonary vascular resistance, pulmonary edema.

Hepatic:	Metabolized in liver.
Renal:	Excreted in urine, slight ↓ RBF in healthy people, ↑ RBF in shock.
GI:	Nausea, vomiting, ↑ mesenteric blood flow.
Musculoskeletal:	Vasodilation in skeletal muscle.

Dosage/ Concentrations:
0.2 mg/ml, 5-ml ampule.

Other preparations: Aerosol, 0.25%; nebulization, 0.5 or 1%; sublingual, 10 mg.

For bronchospasm: 0.25% aerosol metered dose inhaler; 1–2 inhalations 4–6 times/day; 0.5% solution for nebulization; 5–15 deep inhalations up to 5 times/day.

For shock: IM/SC 0.2 mg; IV 0.5–5 μg/min adult dose; 0.05–0.1 μg/kg/min pediatric dose.

For heart block: 0.02–0.06 mg IV bolus (adult); 0.01–0.03 mg IV bolus (pediatric) (↑ heart rate persists for 15–20 min).

Infusion: 0.02–0.15 μg/kg/min.

Contraindications:
Preexisting cardiac arrhythmia, angina pectoris, known hypersensitivity (sulfite), and AV block or tachycardia caused by glycoside intoxication.

Drug Interactions/ Allergy:
Arrhythmia with halothane. Cardiotoxicity when used with other sympathomimetics or theophylline derivatives. Effects antagonized by beta blockers.

↑ Arrhythmia with cardiac glycosides. ↑ Arrhythmia in potassium-depleting diuretic. Potentiation of pressor response with TCAs, bretylium, oxytocics, and guanethidine.

MEPHENTERMINE

Trade Name:	Wyamine
Indications:	Hypotension (shock, spinal anesthesia, ganglionic blockade).
Pharmacokinetics:	Onset: After IV dose, pressor response immediate, persists for 15–30 min. After IM dose, pressor response within 5–15 min, persists for 1–4 hr. Metabolized in liver. Excreted in urine.

Pharmacodynamics:

CNS:	↑ CBF, stimulation (restlessness, nervousness).
CVS:	↑ Cardiac contractility, ↑ MAP, variable change in HR.
GI:	Dilated splanchnic arteries.
Musculoskeletal:	Dilated skeletal muscle arteries.

MEPHENTERMINE *(continued)*

Dosage/ Concentrations:	Parenteral: 15 mg/kg and 30 mg/ml.
Adult:	0.5 mg/kg IM. IV: 20–60 mg initially, then titrate with infusion (1.2 mg/ml) at 1–5 mg/min.
Pediatric:	0.4 mg/kg IM.
Contraindications:	Sensitivity to drug.
Drug Interactions/ Allergy:	↑ Arrhythmia with halogenated hydrocarbon general anesthetic. Digitalis sensitizes myocardium to effects (arrhythmia). MAOIs may potentiate effects. Phenothiazine, reserpine, and guanethidine may reduce the pressor response of mephentermine.

METARAMINOL

Trade Name:	Aramine
Indications:	Hypotension (shock during anesthesia) and paroxysmal atrial tachycardia.
Pharmacokinetics:	Onset: pressor response within 1–2 min after start of IV infusion, within 10 min after IM dose and within 5–20 min after SC dose. Peak effect: 20–90 min. Does not cross blood-brain barrier. Is terminated by uptake of drug into tissues. Not metabolized. Excreted in urine.
Pharmacodynamics:	
CNS:	↓ CBF, ↓ $CMRO_2$ possible.
CVS:	↑ MAP, reflex bradycardia, positive inotrope, ± cardiac output.
Hepatic:	↓ Blood flow.
Renal:	↓ RBF.
GI:	↓ Blood flow.
GU:	Contraction of uterus; ↓ uterine blood flow.
Musculoskeletal:	↓ Blood flow to skin and skeletal muscle.
Other:	Glycogenolysis, inhibits insulin release, lipolysis, ↑ body temperature.
Dosage/ Concentrations:	Parenteral: 10 mg/ml.
Adult:	2–10 mg IM/SC q 10 min if needed; 0.5–5 mg IV followed by infusion if needed.
Pediatric:	1 mg/kg SC/IM q 10 min as needed; 0.01 mg/kg IV, then infusion of 0.4 mg/kg as needed.
Contraindications:	Sulfite allergy and peripheral/mesenteric thrombosis.

Drug Interactions/ Allergy:	α and β blockers negate effects. Arrhythmia with halogenated hydrocarbon general anesthetic. MAOIs, TCAs, guanethidine, and ergot alkaloids may potentiate pressor effects.

METHOXAMINE

Trade Name:	Vasoxyl
Indications:	Hypotension (shock, during anesthesia) and PSVT.
Pharmacokinetics:	Onset: after IV of 2–4 mg, immediate response lasting 5–15 min. Peak effect: after IM of 10–40 mg, peak pressor effect within 15–20 min and persisting for 60–90 min; hepatic elimination.
Pharmacodynamics:	Selective α_1-agonist.
CNS:	Nervousness, anxiety, restlessness, $\uparrow$ CBF, secondary to $\uparrow$ MAP.
CVS:	$\uparrow$ MAP, $\downarrow$ HR (reflex bradycardia).
Pulmonary:	$\uparrow$ In pulmonary artery pressure.
Hepatic:	$\downarrow$ Blood flow.
GI:	Projectile vomiting.
Renal:	$\downarrow$ RBF.
GU:	Contraction, $\downarrow$ uterine blood flow.
Musculoskeletal:	$\downarrow$ Blood flow to skin and muscle.
Dosage/ Concentrations:	Parenteral: 20 mg/ml.
Adult:	5–20 mg IM; may be repeated in 15 min; 2–5 mg IV. For PSVT: 10 mg IV over 3–5 min or 10–20 mg IM.
Pediatric:	0.25 mg/kg IV; 0.08 mg/kg IV.
Contraindications:	Sulfite allergy and severe hypertension.
Drug Interactions/ Allergy:	Extravasation may cause sloughing. Alpha blockers negate effect. Phenothiazine may reduce pressor effect. Pressor effect potentiated if used with MAOIs, TCAs, vasopressin, or ergot alkaloid. Furosemide and other diuretic may decrease response to methoxamine.

NOREPINEPHRINE

Trade Name:	Levophed
Indications:	Hypotension (shock, anesthesia) and prolonged duration of local anesthetics.

NOREPINEPHRINE *(continued)*

Pharmacokinetics:	Poorly absorbed after SC dose. $T_{1/2}$: 2 min. Onset: After IV dose, rapid; action stops 1–2 min after injection. Localizes mainly in sympathetic tissue. Crosses placenta but not blood-brain barrier. Uptake and metabolism in nerve ending. Metabolized in liver by COMT and MAO. Excreted in urine.

Pharmacodynamics: Endogenous catecholamine.
CNS: ↓ CBF, headache, restlessness, tremor.
CVS: ↑ SVR, ↑ BP, positive inotrope, ↓ HR
Pulmonary: ↑ Pulmonary artery pressure.
Hepatic: ↓ Hepatic blood flow.
Renal: ↓ RBF, ↓ GFR.
Metabolic: ↑ Glycogenolysis, inhibits insulin release, ↑ lipolysis, ↑ body temperature.
GI: ↓ Splanchnic blood flow.
Musculoskeletal: ↓ Blood flow to skin and skeletal muscle; extravasation may cause necrosis and sloughing.

Dosage/ Concentrations: 1 mg/ml, 4-ml vial. Mix infusion in 5% dextrose.
Adult: 8–12 μg/min IV.
Pediatric: 2 μg/min IV.

Contraindications: Pregnancy (contracts uterus), sulfite allergy, and mesenteric or peripheral vascular thrombosis.

Drug Interactions/ Allergy: α- and β-Adrenergic blocking agents inhibit effects of norepinephrine. Halogenated hydrocarbon general anesthetics predispose to arrhythmia. Use of TCAs, MAOIs, antihistamines, guanethidine, or methyldopa may result in severe hypertension.

PHENOXYBENZAMINE

Trade Name: Dibenzyline

Indications: Hypertension in pheochromocytoma and vasospastic disorders (Raynaud's syndrome).

Pharmacokinetics: Variably absorbed from GI tract. Onset: gradual over several hours; persists for 3–4 days; highly lipid-soluble. $T_{1/2}$: 24 hr. Metabolized in liver; excreted in urine and bile.

Pharmacodynamics:
CNS: Sedation.

CVS:	↓ MAP, reflex tachycardia, possibly ↑ cardiac output.
Renal:	↑ RBF.
GI:	↑ Splanchnic blood flow, rarely nausea and vomiting, diarrhea.
Musculoskeletal:	↑ Cutaneous blood flow.
Dosage/ Concentrations:	Capsule: 10 mg.
Adult:	Oral 10 mg b.i.d. dosage ↑ every other day to 20–40 mg b.i.d./t.i.d.
Pediatric:	0.2 g/kg q day; ↑ dose until adequate response not to exceed 10 mg; maintenance, 0.4–1.2 mg/kg q day.
Contraindications:	Shock or severe hypotension.
Drug Interactions/ Allergy:	α-Adrenergic stimulating agents are antagonized by phenoxybenzamine. When used with agents that stimulate α and β receptors (e.g., epinephrine), can cause hypotension and tachycardia.

PHENTOLAMINE

Trade Name:	Regitine
Indications:	Hypertension in pheochromocytoma and autonomic hyperreflexia, dermal necrosis and sloughing following extravasation of norepinephrine or dopamine, and controlled hypotension.
Pharmacokinetics:	Onset: IV dose produces effects within 2 min and lasts 10–15 min; 10% of IV dose recovered in urine; fate of remainder unknown; hepatic metabolism.
Pharmacodynamics:	
CNS:	Dizziness, CBF maintained.
CVS:	↓ MAP, positive inotrope and chronotrope, ↑ cardiac output; ↑ HR; arrhythmias; angina.
Pulmonary:	↓ Pulmonary artery pressure, bronchodilation.
GI:	Hyperperistalsis, abdominal pain, diarrhea, ↑ gastric secretion of acid and pepsin; nausea and vomiting.
GU:	Relaxation of uterus.
Dosage/ Concentrations:	Parenteral: 5 mg/ml. For dermal necrosis, 5–10 mg in 10 ml of 0.9% NaCl injected into area of extravasation.
Adult:	5 mg IM/IV 1–2 hr preoperatively. Infusion 0.1–1 mg/min (10–20 μg/kg/min).
Pediatric:	0.1 mg/kg IM/IV preoperatively.
Contraindications:	Gastritis, peptic ulcer, and severe hypotension.

PHENTOLAMINE   *(continued)*

Drug Interactions/ Allergy:	The vasoconstricting and hypertensive effects of epinephrine and ephedrine are antagonized (potentiates β_2-adrenergic vasodilatation).

PHENYLEPHRINE

Trade Name:	Neo-Synephrine
Indications:	Hypotension, shock, to slow heart rate in SVT, and prolonged duration of local anesthetic action.
Pharmacokinetics:	Onset: After IV, pressor effect immediate, persists for 15–20 min. After IM, pressor effect within 10–15 min, persists for 30 min to 1–2 hr. After SC, pressor effect in 10–15 min, lasts for 1 hr. Effects terminated by uptake of drug into tissues. Metabolized in liver and intestine by MAOIs.

Pharmacodynamics:
CNS:	Headache, restlessness.
CVS:	Vasoconstriction, ↑ MAP, ↓ HR (reflex); ↑ coronary blood flow.
Pulmonary:	↑ Pulmonary artery pressure.
Hepatic:	↓ Blood flow.
Renal:	↓ RBF.
GI:	↓ Splanchnic blood flow.
Musculoskeletal:	↓ Blood flow to skin and skeletal muscle.
GU:	Contraction of uterus, ↓ uterine artery blood flow.

Dosage/ Concentrations:	1-ml ampule (10 mg/ml).
	For hypotension:
Adult:	0.2–0.5 mg IV (titrate up); 2–5 mg IM.
	For PSVT: 0.5–1 mg IV, subsequent doses; ↑ 0.1–0.2 mg increments.
Pediatric:	0.1–0.4 mg/kg IM and SC.
Contraindications:	Hypersensitivity, severe hypertension or ventricular tachycardia, mesenteric vascular thrombosis, and injections into fingers, toes, ears, nose, and genitalia.
Drug Interactions/ Allergy:	Pressor effects potentiated by oxytocin, MAOIs, TCAs, and guanethidine; arrhythmias with volatile anesthetics.

RITODRINE

Trade Name:	Yutopar

Indications: Preterm labor (inhibits uterine contractions).

Pharmacokinetics: Bioavailability: 30% of oral 10-mg dose. Peak effect: IV dose: Peak plasma concentration in 50 min with 150 μg/min. Oral dose: Peak plasma concentration in 30–60 min with 10 mg. Crosses placenta and blood-brain barrier. For IV dose, 150 μg/min for 1 hr. $T_{1/2}$: α, 6–9 min; β, 10 hr; for oral 10-mg dose, $T_{1/2}$: α, 1.3 hr; β, 20 hr. Metabolized in liver. Excreted in urine.

Pharmacodynamics:
CNS: Headache, anxiety, tremor.
CVS: $\uparrow$ HR, $\uparrow$ cardiac output, $\uparrow$ MAP in mother and fetus.
Pulmonary: Bronchodilation, pulmonary edema possible.
GI: Nausea, vomiting.
GU: Uterine relaxation.
Metabolic: $\uparrow$ Maternal/fetal glucose, $\uparrow$ maternal insulin, maternal hypokalemia.

Dosage/ Concentrations: Tablets: 10 mg.
Parenteral: 10 mg/ml or 15 mg/ml. IV: 50–100 μg/min; continue infusion for 12 hr following cessation of uterine contractions.
Oral therapy after IV infusion: 10 mg q 2 hr for 24 hr, then 10–20 mg q 4–6 hr.

Contraindications: Pulmonary edema, sulfite allergy, prior to 20 weeks' gestation, conditions of mother in which continuation of pregnancy would be hazardous (eclampsia, hemorrhage, fetal death, abruptio placentae, placenta previa), and certain diseases (e.g., cardiac, arrhythmia, pulmonary hypertension, pheochromocytoma, hyperthyroidism, uncontrolled diabetes/hypertension).

Drug Interactions/ Allergy: With corticosteroids, pulmonary edema. Additive effects with sympathomimetics. Ritodrine antagonized by β-adrenergic blockers. Adverse cardiovascular effects with meperidine, anticholinergics, and $MgSO_4$; potentiates CVS depression produced by volatile anesthetics.

2

Antacids

Shiv K. Sharma, M.B.B.S., M.D.

ALUMINUM HYDROXIDE, MAGNESIUM HYDROXIDE, MAGNESIUM TRISILICATE, CALCIUM CARBONATE

Trade Names:	Amphojel, Milk of Magnesia, Alamag, Maalox, Almacone, Gelusil, Aludrox, Mylanta, Magnatril, Calcilac
Indications:	Hyperacidity, gastric or duodenal ulcer, gastroesophageal reflux disease, and prophylaxis against gastric acid aspiration.
Pharmacokinetics:	Particulate antacids (Mg trisilicate). Onset: rapid ($CaCO_3$, MgOH); slow (AlOH, Mg trisilicate). Duration: empty stomach, 20–60 min; after meal, 2–3 hr. Renal elimination: 15%–30% in salt form. Cross placenta. Excreted in breast milk.

Pharmacodynamics:

CNS:	Neurotoxicity, encephalopathy, to be avoided in patients with Alzheimer's disease.
Pulmonary:	Pulmonary damage if drug is aspirated.
GI:	Gastric acid neutralized, ↑ gastric pH, inhibited proteolytic activity of pepsin, ↑ gastric volume, ↑ lower esophageal sphincter tone, laxative effect (Mg), constipation and intestinal obstruction (Al), and rebound hyperacidity (Ca).
Other:	Metabolic alkalosis, aluminum intoxication, osteomalacia, osteoporosis, hypophosphatemia (aluminum binds phosphate ions in the intestine and reduces serum phosphate levels), inhibited precipitation of calcium oxalate (by Mg OH), hypermagnesemia, milk-alkali syndrome (by $CaCO_3$).

Dosage/ Concentrations:	Liquids, combinations.
Adult:	15–45 ml q 3 to 6 hr.
Pediatric:	5–15 ml q 3 to 6 hr.
Contraindications:	None known.
Drug Interactions/ Allergy:	Increased gastric pH leads to reduced absorption of digoxin, phenytoin, chlorpromazine, isoniazid; increased absorption of pseudoephedrine, levodopa. Reduced bioavailability of tetracycline and cimetidine due to adsorption. Increased urinary pH leads to inhibited excretion of quinidine and amphetamine and enhanced excretion of salicylates. Aluminum and magnesium intoxication with renal function impairment. Renal calculi with prolonged use of calcium antacids.

CIMETIDINE HYDROCHLORIDE

Trade Name:	Tagamet
Indications:	Gastric acid aspiration (parturients and patients with hiatus hernia or esophageal dysfunction).
Pharmacokinetics:	Absorption: rapid. Bioavailability: 60%–70%. Protein binding: 15%–20%. Biotransformation: hepatic, 30%–40%. Peak concentration: plasma/2 hr (oral). $T_{1/2}$: oral, 2.0 hr; parenteral, 1.6–2.1 hr. Duration of action: 4–5 hr. Renal elimination: oral—48% unchanged; parenteral—75% unchanged. Crosses placenta. Excreted in breast milk.

Pharmacodynamics:	H2 receptor antagonist.
CNS:	Dizziness, mental confusion, agitation, headache.
CVS:	Bradycardia, hypotension.
Pulmonary:	Bronchospasm.
Hepatic:	↓ Blood flow, ↑ AST, ↑ ALT.
Renal:	↑ Creatinine.
GI:	↓ Gastric and acid secretion and volume, mild diarrhea.
Musculoskeletal:	Myalgia.
Other:	Gynecomastia, impotence, neutropenia.

Dosage/ Concentrations:	Tablets: 200, 300, 400, or 800 mg. Liquid: 300 mg/ 5 ml. Injection: 300 mg/2 ml. Oral: 400 mg 60–90 min before induction. IV: 200 mg 60–90 min before induction.
Contraindications:	None known.
Drug Interactions/ Allergy:	↓ Hepatic metabolism of lidocaine, theophylline, phenytoin, metronidazole, triamterene, quinidine, propranolol, coumarin, TCAs, alcohol, and diazepam. ↓ Elimination of procainamide. Antacids may reduce absorption of cimetidine. Causes skin rash with burning and itching.

FAMOTIDINE HYDROCHLORIDE

Trade Name:	Pepcid
Indications:	Prophylaxis against gastric acid aspiration during anesthesia.
Pharmacokinetics:	Absorption: rapid. Bioavailability: 40%–45%. Protein binding: low (15%). Biotransformation: hepatic. $T_{1/2}$: 2.5–3.5 hr. Peak effect: oral, 1–3 hr; parenteral, ½ hr. Duration: 10–12 hr. Elimination: primarily renal (70%). Crosses placenta. Excreted in breast milk.

Pharmacodynamics:	Gastric histamine H2 receptor antagonist.
CNS:	Dizziness, headache, mental confusion, ringing in ears.
CVS:	Cardiac arrhythmias.
GI:	Constipation, nausea, vomiting, loss of appetite, ↓ gastric acidity and volume.
Musculoskeletal:	Arthralgia.
Other:	Skin rash, dry skin, thrombocytopenia.
Dosage/ Concentrations:	Injection: 10 mg/ml. Syrup: 40 mg/5 ml. Tablet: 20 and 40 mg.
Adult:	40 mg p.o. in evening prior to surgery. Reduce dosage in patients with renal disease.
Contraindications:	None known.
Drug Interactions/ Allergy:	Weak inhibitor of hepatic drug metabolism. Antacids may decrease famotidine absorption. ↑ Serum transaminase.

NIZATIDINE HYDROCHLORIDE

Trade Name:	Axid
Indications:	Prophylaxis against gastric acid aspiration during anesthesia.
Pharmacokinetics:	Absorption: rapid. Bioavailability: >90%. Protein binding: moderate (35%). Biotransformation: hepatic. $T_{1/2}$: oral, 1–2 hr. Peak effect: ½–3 hr. Duration: 6–8 hr. Elimination: primarily renal (60%). Crosses placenta. Excreted in breast milk.
Pharmacodynamics:	Gastric histamine H2 receptor antagonist.
CNS:	Dizziness, sedation, malaise, mental confusion.
CVS:	Bradycardia, tachycardia.
Hepatic:	Hepatitis.
GI:	Constipation, nausea, and vomiting, ↓ gastric acidity and volume.
Endocrine:	Gynecomastia.
Other:	Rash, sweating, thrombocytopenia.
Dosage/ Concentrations:	Capsules: 150 and 300 mg.
Adult:	300 mg p.o. evening prior to surgery.
Pediatric:	1.5–2 mg/kg p.o. before surgery. Reduce dosage in patients with renal disease.
Contraindications:	None known.
Drug Interactions/ Allergy:	Weak inhibitor of hepatic drug metabolism. Antacids may decrease nazatidine absorption. ↑ Serum ALT, AST, and alkaline phosphatase.

RANITIDINE HYDROCHLORIDE

Trade Name:	Zantac
Indications:	Gastric acid aspiration during anesthesia (parturients, patients with hiatus hernia or esophageal dysfunction).
Pharmacokinetics:	Absorption: rapid. Bioavailability: 40%–90%. Protein binding: low (15%). Biotransformation: hepatic. $T_{1/2}$: 2–2.5 hr. Peak effect: 1–3 hr. Renal elimination (70%). Crosses placenta. Excreted in breast milk.

Pharmacodynamics:	H2 receptor antagonist.
CNS:	Dizziness, sedation, malaise, mental confusion.
CVS:	Bradycardia, tachycardia, arrhythmias.
Hepatic:	Hepatitis.
Renal:	↑ Serum creatinine.
GI:	↓ Gastric acidity and volume, constipation, nausea, vomiting.
Musculoskeletal:	Arthralgia.
Other:	Gynecomastia, skin rash, thrombocytopenia.

Dosage/ Concentrations:	Injection: 25 mg/ml; syrup 15 mg/ml. Tablet: 150, 300 mg.
Adult:	150 mg p.o. evening prior to surgery, or 150 mg p.o. or 50 mg IV 60–90 min before anesthesia.
Pediatric:	1.5–2 mg/kg p.o. before surgery; reduce dosage with renal disease.
Contraindications:	None known.
Drug Interactions/ Allergy:	Weak inhibitor of hepatic drug metabolism. May ↓ clearance of coumarin, nifedipine, phenytoin and theophylline, midazolam, alcohol, and metaprolol. Antacids may ↓ ranitidine absorption. Renal elimination of procainamide may be reduced.

SODIUM CITRATE

Trade Names:	Bicitra, Polycitra, Alka-Seltzer Gold (effervescent tablet)
Indications:	Parturients, emergencies prior to induction of anesthesia.
Pharmacokinetics:	Nonparticulate antacid (pH 8.4) with an unpleasant taste. Onset: rapid. Complete mixing with gastric acid. Minimal foreign body reaction after pulmonary aspiration. Duration: 1–3 hr. Metabolized to bicarbonate.

Pharmacodynamics:

CVS: Congestive heart failure in patients with heart disease.
Pulmonary: Minimal pulmonary damage if drug is aspirated.
GI: Neutralized gastric acid, ↑ gastric volume, ↑ gastric distention, ↑ flatulence.
Endocrine/Metabolic: Metabolic alkalosis, hypernatremia, hypocalcemia, hyperkalemia.

Dosage/   Oral: 0.3 mol/L solution.
Concentrations:
Adult: 15–30 ml.
Pediatric: 10–15 ml within 30 min prior to anesthesia.
Elderly: 10–15 ml.

Contraindications: None known.

Drug Interactions/   ↑ Toxicity with potassium-containing medications and
Allergy: potassium-sparing diuretics.

3

Antiarrhythmics

Russell P. Woda, D.O.

ACEBUTOLOL

Trade Name:	Sectral
Indications:	Supraventricular tachycardia.
Pharmacokinetics:	Selective β_1-adrenergic reception blockade. Absorption: <50% bioavailability; 26% plasma protein bound. Clearance: 6.8 ml/min/kg. Vd: 1.2 L/kg. $T_{1/2}$: β, 3 hr.
Pharmacodynamics:	Class II.
CNS:	Lightheadedness, mental depression, insomnia, lassitude, weakness, fatigue.
CVS:	Selective blockade of β receptors, slowed sinus heart rate, inhibited automaticity in Purkinje fibers, ↑ ERP of AV node, ↑ AV nodal refractoriness, PR interval, blocked β_1 and β_2 receptors, ↓ cardiac output.
Dosage/ Concentrations:	Capsules: 200 and 400 mg. Oral Dose: 200 mg b.i.d. up to 1200 mg daily.
Contraindications:	Uncontrolled congestive heart failure and bronchospastic disease. Use with caution in diabetes and hypoglycemia.
Drug Interactions/ Allergy:	None known.

ADENOSINE

Trade Name:	Adenocard
Indications:	PSVT and Wolff-Parkinson-White syndrome.
Pharmacokinetics:	Onset: immediate; duration 3–7 sec. $T_{1/2}$: β, 10 sec. Biotransformation: very rapid; deamination, phosphorylation, and cellular uptake.
Pharmacodynamics:	
CNS:	Lightheadedness, dizziness, tingling in arms, numbness, blurred vision, headaches.
CVS:	Slowed conduction time through AV node blockade, bradycardia, ↓ PVR, arrhythmias, angina, hypotension and palpitations, depressed LV function.
Pulmonary:	Shortness of breath; bronchoconstriction (in asthmatic patients).
GI:	Nausea; metallic taste.
Other:	Flushing.

ADENOSINE   *(continued)*

Dosage/ Concentrations:	Injection: 3 mg/ml. Adult: IV: 6 mg over 1–2 min; second dose, 12 mg over 1–2 min. Pediatric: IV: 0.05–0.25 mg/kg
Contraindications:	Second- or third-degree AV block, sick sinus syndrome, and known hypersensitivity to adenosine.
Drug Interactions/ Allergy:	Adenosine is antagonized by methylxanthines and potentiated by dipyridamole.

AMIODARONE

Trade Name:	Cordarone
Indications:	Life-threatening ventricular and supraventricular tachyarrhythmias and sustained ventricular tachycardia.
Pharmacokinetics:	Clearance: 1.9 ml/min/kg. Vd: 66 L/kg. $T_{1/2}$: β, 25 days. Onset: 2–4 days; duration: 45 days. Oral bioavailability: 46%. 99% plasma protein bound. Effective plasma concentration: 0.5–2.5 μg/ml.
Pharmacodynamics: *CNS:* *CVS:*	Class III. Peripheral neuropathy, ataxia, tremor. Actions of classes I, II, III, and IV antiarrhythmics; prolonged action potential duration and refractoriness in all cardiac tissue; ↑ PR, RR, and QT intervals; prolonged antegrade and retrograde atrioventricular nodal refractoriness; T-wave abnormalities and U waves; ↑ QRS duration by 10%–20%; weak α- and β-adrenergic receptor antagonist; proarrhythmic state.
Pulmonary: *GI:* *Musculoskeletal:* *Other:*	Fibrosis. Nausea/vomiting, elevated liver enzymes. Muscle necrosis from IM injection. Parotitis, hyperthermia, hyperthyroidism, hypothyroidism.
Dosage/ Concentrations:	Tablets: 200 mg. Loading dose: 800–1600 mg/day in 2–3 divided doses for 10–14 days, then 600–800 mg/day for 4–8 wk, followed by 200–600 mg/day.
Contraindications:	Sinus node dysfunction with marked bradycardia, second- and third-degree AV blockade.
Drug Interactions/ Allergy:	Quinidine (antagonism of antiarrhythmic effect). Digitalis (catecholamine release aggravates arrhythmias). ↑ Plasma concentration and effects of digoxin, warfa-

rin, quinidine, procainamide, phenytoin, encainide, precainide and diltiazem. ↑ Likelihood of bradycardia, sinus arrest, and AV block when given concurrently with β-adrenergic antagonists and Ca^{2+} channel blockers and halothane.

BRETYLIUM

Trade Name:	Bretylol
Indications:	↑ Fibrillation threshold and suppresses life-threatening ventricular arrhythmias.
Pharmacokinetics:	Onset 1–3 min. Clearance: 10 ml/min/kg. Vd: 8 L/kg. $T_{1/2}$: β, 6–10 hr. Excretion: unchanged in urine. Protein binding: negligible.
Pharmacodynamics:	Class III.
CNS:	Dizziness, syncope.
CVS:	Antiadrenergic effect, initial transient tachycardia and hypertension, ↓ HR, ↓ BP, ↓ vascular resistance, ↑ APD.
GI:	Nausea, vomiting.
Other:	Rash
Dosage/ Concentrations:	Injection: 50 mg/ml. IV: 5–10 mg/kg over 10–30 min. Subsequent dosing intervals of 1–2 hr. Max: 30 mg/kg. Infusion: 1–2 mg/min (therapeutic level 0.5–1.0 μg/ml)
Contraindications:	Use with caution in patients with pheochromocytoma, aortic stenosis, and pulmonary hypertension.
Drug Interactions/ Allergy:	TCAs can prevent uptake of bretylium by adrenergic nerve terminals.

DIGOXIN

Trade Name:	Lanoxin
Indications:	Congestive heart failure and slow ventricular rate in atrial fibrillation or flutter.
Pharmacokinetics:	Clearance: 0.88 ml/min/kg. Vd: 3.12 L/kg. $T_{1/2}$: β, 39 hr. Oral absorption: variable (45%–100%). Peak plasma concentration: 2–3 hr. Maximal effect: 4–6 hr. Plasma protein binding: 25%. Effective plasma concentration: >0.8 mg/ml. Elimination: primarily by kidney.

DIGOXIN   *(continued)*

Pharmacodynamics:
CNS: Headache, fatigue, malaise, psychosis, confusion.
CVS: Inhibition of membrane-bound Na^+, K^+-activated
                       ATP, slow inward Ca^{2+} current during action potential,
                       positive inotropic effect, ↑ rate of phase 4 depolariza-
                       tion, enhancement of automaticity, ↓ rate of phase 0
                       depolarization, ↓ conduction velocity through AV
                       node.
GI: Anorexia, nausea, vomiting, diarrhea.
Other: Blurred vision, "halos," gynecomastia.

Dosage/   Tablets: 0.125, 0.25, or 0.5 mg.
Concentrations: IV: 0.1 mg/ml or 0.25 mg/ml. Digoxin must first be
                       loaded with a digitalizing dose (oral, 0.75–1.25 mg;
                       IV, 0.5–1.0 mg) and a subsequent maintenance dose
                       (oral, 0.215–0.5 mg; IV, 0.25 mg).

Contraindications: None known.

Drug Interactions/ ↑ Plasma concentration of digoxin. Diuretics and am-
Allergy: photericin B may potentiate the effect of digoxin.

DISOPYRAMIDE

Trade Names: Norpace, Napamide

Indications: Atrial flutter, atrial fibrillation, PSVT, VPD, unsus-
                       tained ventricular tachycardia.

Pharmacokinetics: Oral absorption: 90% of dose. Clearance: 1.2
                       ml/min/kg. Vd: 0.6 L/kg. $T_{1/2}$: β, 5–7 hr; prolonged
                       with renal insufficiency. Peak concentrations in plas-
                       ma: 1–2 hr. 70% plasma protein bound. Excretion:
                       50% of dose excreted by kidneys unchanged.

Pharmacodynamics: Class Ia.
CVS: Prolonged refractoriness in the atria, ventricles, His-
                       Purkinje system, and accessory bypass tracts; widened
                       QRS and QT; vasolytic properties similar to those of
                       quinidine; ↑ baseline HR; shortened AV nodal refrac-
                       toriness; enhanced direct depression left ventricular per-
                       formance with decreased cardiac output;
                       anticholinergic action; ↑ peripheral vascular resis-
                       tance.
Renal: Urinary hesitancy, retention.
GI: Dry mouth, constipation, nausea, abdominal pain, vom-
                       iting, diarrhea.
Other: Blurred vision.

Dosage/ Concentrations:	Capsules: 100 and 150 mg. Usual total daily dose is 400–800 mg divided in 4 doses.
Contraindications:	None known.
Drug Interactions/ Allergy:	None known.

ENCAINIDE

Trade Name:	Enkaid
Indications:	Wolff-Parkinson-White syndrome and life-threatening ventricular arrhythmias.
Pharmacokinetics:	70% protein bound. Clearance: 4–13 ml/min/kg. Vd: 1.3–2.6 L/kg. $T_{1/2}$: β, <2 hr. Oral absorption: 85% bioavailability. Peak serum concentrations: 1–2 hr after administration. Metabolized 80% in liver with an active metabolite.
Pharmacodynamics:	Class Ic.
CNS:	Headache, dizziness, tinnitus, diplopia, vertigo.
CVS:	Proarrhythmic state; profound conduction depression of AV node or His bundle; ↓ phase 4 automaticity and depressed phase 0 of action potential; ↑ APD and ERPs of all cardiac tissue; slowed conduction in atrial, AV nodal, His-Purkinje, and ventricular tissue, lengthened PR, QRS, and QT duration, prolonged ERP of atria, AV node, ventricles, and accessory pathways.
Musculoskeletal:	Leg cramps.
Dosage/ Concentrations:	Capsules: 25, 35, and 50 mg; 25 mg 3 times a day to maximum of 50 mg 4 times a day.
Contraindications:	Cardiogenic shock, second- or third-degree AV block, ↑ QT.
Drug Interactions/ Allergy:	↑ Plasma concentration during concurrent ingestions of cimetidine.

ESMOLOL

Trade Name:	Brevibloc
Indications:	Supraventricular tachycardia and perioperative hypertension.
Pharmacokinetics:	Clearance: 170 ± 70 ml/min/kg. Vd: 2 L/kg. 55% plasma protein bound. $T_{1/2}$: β, 8 min. Onset: ≤ 1 min.

ESMOLOL   *(continued)*

Pharmacodynamics:	Class II. Cardioselective β blocker.
CNS:	Lightheadedness, mental depression, insomnia, lassitude, weakness, fatigue.
CVS:	↓ Effect of β-adrenergic stimulation, ↓ phase 4 depolarization, slowed sinus HR, inhibited automaticity in Purkinje fibers, ↑ ERP of AV node, ↑ AV nodal refractoriness, ↑ PR interval, blocked $β_1$ and $β_2$ receptors, ↓ cardiac output, bradycardia, hypotension.
Hepatic:	↓ Hepatic blood flow.
Pulmonary:	Bronchospasm.
Dosage/ Concentrations:	Injection: 250 mg/ml, 10 mg/ml; IV: loading dose, 500 µg/kg over 1 min, then 50–200 µg/kg/min.
Contraindications:	Uncontrolled congestive heart failure and bronchospastic disease. Use with caution in diabetes and hypoglycemia.
Drug Interactions/ Allergy:	Pharyngitis, agranulocytosis, erythematous rash, fever, laryngospasm. Hypotension, marked bradycardia, vertigo, syncopal episodes, or orthostatic hypotension when combined with catecholamine-depleting drugs. Severely depressed myocardial contractility and atrioventricular conduction when used with calcium channel blockers. Hypotension and cardiac arrest when used with haloperidol. Theophylline clearance reduced with concomitant use. Phenytoin, phenobarbital, and rifampin accelerate esmolol clearance.

FLECAINIDE

Trade Name:	Tambocor
Indications:	Life-threatening ventricular arrhythmias.
Pharmacokinetics:	40% protein bound. Clearance: 5.6 ml/min/kg. Vd: 4.9 L/kg. $T_{1/2}$: β, 14–20 hr. Therapeutic serum concentration: 0.4–0.8 µg/ml. Oral absorption: 95% bioavailability. Peak serum concentration: 2–4 hr. 70% metabolized by liver.
Pharmacodynamics:	Class Ic. Fluorinated analog of procainamide.
CNS:	Dizziness, visual disturbances, headache, tremor, tinnitus.
CVS:	Proarrhythmic state; ↑ phase 4 automaticity; ↑ ERP in ventricular and His-Purkinje tissues; depressed phase 0 of action potential; ↑ APD; slowed conduction in all cardiac tissue; lengthened PR, QRS, and QT

duration; prolonged ERP of atria, ventricles, His-Purkinje tissue, and accessory pathway tissue, depressed LV function.

Pulmonary: Bronchospasm.
GI: Nausea, vomiting.

Dosage/ Concentrations: Tablets: 50, 100, and 150 mg; 100 mg twice daily up to 400–600 mg/day.

Contraindications: None known.

Drug Interactions/ Allergy: Concentrations of flecainide in serum increase with concurrent ingestion of cimetidine, additive with negative atropinic effective beta blockers.

LIDOCAINE

Trade Name: Xylocaine

Indications: Ventricular arrhythmias.

Pharmacokinetics: pKa 7.9. 50%–70% protein bound. Clearance: 9.2 ml/min/kg. Vd: 1 L/kg. $T_{1/2}$: β, 1–2 hr. Oral absorption: poor (20% bioavailability). Metabolism: 90% by liver into 2 active metabolites. Serum therapeutic concentration: 1–5 μg/ml. Onset: 45–90 sec.

Pharmacodynamics: Class Ib.
CNS: Dissociated sensorium, perioral paresthesias, drowsiness, agitation, decreased hearing, disorientation, muscle twitching, convulsions, respiratory arrest.
CVS: Shortened APD, ↓ conduction in His-Purkinje tissue and ventricular muscle, ↓ automaticity in Purkinje fibers, depressed phase 0 of action potential in a use-dependent fashion, affinity for inactivated sodium channels, ↓ slope of phase 4 depolarization, ↑ threshold for ventricular fibrillation.

Dosage/ Concentrations: IV: Infusion, 2, 4, 8 mg/ml. Direct administration, 10, 20 mg/ml. Dilution into admixtures, 40, 100, 200 mg/ml.
IM: 100 mg/ml; 0.7–1.4 mg/kg IV body weight for effective concentration; maximal dose is 200–300 mg in 1 hr.
Infusions: 1–4 mg/min; 4–5 mg/kg body weight IM for effective concentration within 15 min; maintain for 90 min.

Contraindications: Hypotension, amide-type local anesthetic.

LIDOCAINE   *(continued)*

Drug Interactions/ Allergy:	With β-adrenergic antagonists, ↓ rate of lidocaine metabolism and ↑ serum concentration. Plasma concentrations are higher in patients taking cimetidine. Lidocaine can potentiate effects of succinylcholine and beta blockers.

MEXILETINE

Trade Name:	Mexitine
Indications:	Ventricular arrhythmias.
Pharmacokinetics:	Oral congener of lidocaine. Clearance: 6.3 ml/min/kg. Vd: 4.9 L/kg. $T_{1/2}$: β, 10 hr. Oral absorption: 90% bioavailability. Strongly protein bound (50%). Therapeutic serum concentration: 0.5–2 μg/ml. Hepatic metabolism: route of elimination (85%) with 10% peak action in 2 hr.
Pharmacodynamics:	Class Ib.
CNS:	Dizziness, lightheadedness, tremor, ataxia.
CVS:	Effects similar to those of lidocaine.
GI:	Nausea, vomiting, anorexia, upper gastric distress.
Dosage/ Concentrations:	Capsules: 150, 200, 250 mg; 200–300 mg p.o. up to 400 mg every 8 hr.
Contraindications:	None.
Drug Interactions/ Allergy:	Hepatic metabolism accelerated by concurrent administration of phenytoin or rifampin.

MORICIZINE

Trade Name:	Ethmozine
Indications:	Ventricular arrhythmias, sustained ventricular tachycardia.
Pharmacokinetics:	Phenothiazine derivative. 95% protein bound. $T_{1/2}$: β, 6–14 hr. Oral absorption: 35%–40% bioavailability. Peak serum concentrations: ½ to 2 hr after administration.
Pharmacodynamics:	Class Ib.
CNS:	Headache, dizziness, vertigo, paresthesias, fatigue.
CVS:	Shortened repolarization, ↓ V_{max} in Purkinje fiber preparations, ↓ conduction through AV node, pro-

	longed PR and QRS duration, prolonged AV nodal and accessory pathway refractoriness, proarrhythmic state.
GI:	Dry mouth, nausea, vomiting, diarrhea, dyspepsia.
Dosage/ Concentrations:	Tablets: 200, 250, or 300 mg; 600–900 mg/day divided q 8 hr.
Contraindications:	Pre-existing second- or third-degree AV block, RBBB with associated left hemiblock, and cardiogenic shock.
Drug Interactions/ Allergy:	Concomitant administration of cimetidine decreases clearance of moricizine and increases plasma level. Theophylline clearance is increased, and plasma half-life is decreased when given with moricizine.

PHENYTOIN

Trade Names:	Dilantin, Diphenylan
Indications:	Ventricular arrhythmias, paroxysmal atrial flutter or fibrillation, supraventricular arrhythmias caused by digitalis, and long QT syndrome.
Pharmacokinetics:	pKa 10.1. Oral absorption: slow, 90% bioavailability. Clearance: 5.9 ml/min/kg. Vd: 0.64 L/kg. $T_{1/2}$: β, 18–30 hr. 90% protein bound. Therapeutic serum concentration: 10–20 μg/ml. Metabolism: 85% by liver via hydroxylation. Inactive metabolites are excreted in urine.
Pharmacodynamics:	Class IB.
CNS:	Drowsiness, nystagmus, vertigo, ataxia.
CVS:	Slowed phase 4 depolarization, depressed conduction, $\downarrow$ resting membrane potential, shortened APD and ERP, enhanced AV nodal conduction, shortened QT interval.
GI:	Nausea.
Dosage/ Concentrations:	Tablets: 50 mg. Capsules: 30 and 100 mg. Injection: 50 mg/ml. IV: 100 mg q 5 min until arrhythmia is controlled, up to 700 mg total. Oral: 15 mg/kg first day, 7.5 mg/kg second day, 4–6 mg/kg third day and thereafter.
Contraindications:	None known.
Drug Interactions/ Allergy:	Concurrent administration of chloramphenicol, dicumarol, disulfiram, isoniazid, cimetidine, or certain sulfonamides increases the concentration of phenytoin in plasma. $\uparrow$ Clearance of theophylline. Multiple interactions with other antiseizure medication.

PROCAINAMIDE

Trade Names:	Procan SR, Pronestyl
Indications:	Atrial flutter, atrial fibrillation, PSVT, VPD, and unsustained ventricular tachycardia.
Pharmacokinetics:	pKa 8.9. Bioavailability: 80%–90% after oral indigestion. $T_{1/2}$: β, 2–4 hr. 20% protein bound. Peak serum concentration: 15 min to 2 hr after oral ingestion. Metabolism: acetylation in liver. Metabolite is *N*-acetyl-procainamide. Elimination: 4–8 hr. Therapeutic concentration: 3–10 µg/ml.
Pharmacodynamics:	Class Ia
CNS:	Giddiness, psychosis, hallucinations, mental depression.
CVS:	↓ Purkinje fiber automaticity; ↓ rate of rise of phase 4 depolarization; depressed phase 0 of action potential; prolonged atrial and ventricular ERPs and APD; much less "vagolytic" effect than with quinidine; shortened AV nodal refractoriness; enhanced AV nodal conduction; prolonged ERP of atria, ventricles, His-Purkinje system, and accessory pathways; slowed conduction in ventricular muscle; widened PR interval and QRS complex; less QT prolongation and torsades de pointes; hypotension if dose administered rapidly.
GI:	Anorexia, nausea, vomiting, diarrhea.
Musculoskeletal:	Myalgias, angioedema.
Other:	Drug fever, agranulocytosis, digital vasculitis, Raynaud's phenomenon.
Dosage/ Concentrations:	Capsules and tablets: 250–500 mg. Oral, IV, IM sustained-release tabs: 250–1000 mg. Injection: 100, 500 mg/ml. IV: 1000 mg as loading dose in 100-mg increments over 2–4 min.
Contraindications:	Prolonged QT syndrome.
Drug Interactions/ Allergy:	Arthralgias, hepatomegaly, pericarditis, fever, pleuropneumonic involvement. Hemorrhagic pericardial effusion with tamponade. ANAs after 1 to 12 months of therapy. Rash.

PROPAFENONE

Trade Name:	Rythmol
Indications:	Life-threatening ventricular arrhythmias.
Pharmacokinetics:	95% protein bound. $T_{1/2}$: β, 6–13 hr. Oral absorption: 95% bioavailability. Peak serum concentrations: 1–3 hr after administration.

Pharmacodynamics:	Class Ic. Weak β-adrenergic blockade.
CNS:	Dizziness, tinnitus, bitter metallic taste, fatigue, tiredness, sluggishness.
CVS:	Proarrhythmic effect, calcium channel blockade at high doses; lengthened PR, QRS, and QT duration; ↑ ERP of atria, ventricles, His-Purkinje tissue, and accessory pathway tissue; depressed LV function.
Other:	Granulocytopenia, SLE-like syndrome.
GI:	Nausea, vomiting, constipation.
Dosage/ Concentrations:	Tablets: 150, 225, 300 mg. Start at 150 mg 3 times/ day up to a total of no more than 900 mg/day.
Contraindications:	Known hypersensitivity to propafenone; uncontrolled congestive heart failure; cardiogenic shock; and sino-atrial, atrioventricular, and intraventricular conduction abnormalities.
Drug Interactions/ Allergy:	Rash. Increased concentrations of propafenone in plasma during concurrent ingestion of cimetidine.

PROPRANOLOL

Trade Name:	Inderal
Indications:	Supraventricular arrhythmias, atrial fibrillation, atrial flutter or PSVT, hypertension, angina pectoris due to coronary arteriosclerosis, migraine, essential tremor, hypertrophic subaortic stenosis, and pheochromocytoma.
Pharmacokinetics:	Oral absorption: extensive first-pass metabolism with resulting bioavailability of 25%. Clearance: 16 ml/min/kg. Vd: 43 L/kg. $T_{1/2}$: β, 4 hr. Therapeutic effect: 20 to 1000 mg/ml.
Pharmacodynamics:	Class II.
CNS:	Lightheadedness, mental depression, insomnia, lassitude, weakness, fatigue.
CVS:	Selective blockade of β receptors, slowed sinus HR, inhibited automaticity in Purkinje fibers, ↑ ERP of AV node, ↑ AV nodal refractoriness, ↑ PR interval, blocked $β_1$ and $β_2$ receptors, ↓ cardiac output.
Hepatic:	Hepatic blood flow.
GI:	Nausea, vomiting, diarrhea, constipation.
Dosage/ Concentrations:	Tablets: 10, 20, 40, 60, and 80 mg. Injection: 1 mg/ml. Oral: Up to 120–240 mg b.i.d. IV: 1–3 mg at no more than 1 mg/min.
Contraindications:	Uncontrolled congestive heart failure and bronchospas-

PROPRANOLOL   *(continued)*

	tic disease. Use with caution in diabetes and hypoglycemia.
Drug Interactions/ Allergy:	Pharyngitis, agranulocytosis, erythematous rash, fever, and laryngospasm. Hypotension, marked bradycardia, vertigo, syncopal episodes or orthostatic hypotension when combined with catecholamine-depleting drugs. Severely depressed myocardial contractility and atrioventricular conduction when used with calcium channel blockers. Hypotension and cardiac arrest when used continuously with haloperidol. Aluminum hydroxide gel and ethanol greatly reduce absorption of propranolol. ↓ Theophylline clearance when used concomitantly with propranolol. Phenytoin, phenobarbital and rifampin accelerate propranolol clearance.

QUINIDINE

Trade Names:	Quinaglute, Quinidex, Cardioquin
Indications:	Atrial flutter, atrial fibrillation, PSVT, VPD, and unsustained ventricular tachycardia.
Pharmacokinetics:	pKa 8.0. 90% protein bound. Clearance: 4.7 ml/min/kg. Vd: 2–3 L/kg. $T_{1/2}$: β, 4–7 hr. Binding: constant 1–3 sec. Recovery time (unbinding): constant 4–5 sec. Oral absorption: 70%–90% bioavailability. Peak concentration: 1–3 hr after administration. Metabolism: hydroxylation in the liver. Excreted in urine. Therapeutic serum concentration: 1.5–4 μg/ml. Has active metabolites.
Pharmacodynamics: *CVS:*	Class Ia. ↓ Purkinje fiber automaticity, ↓ rate of rise of phase 4 depolarization, depressed phase 0 of action potential, prolonged atrial and ventricular ERPs and APD, "vagolytic" effect, ↑ baseline HR, shortened AV nodal refractoriness, enhanced AV nodal conduction, α-adrenergic blockade properties, hypotension, widened QRS complex and QT interval.
GI:	Nausea, vomiting, diarrhea.
Other:	Drug fever, rash, tinnitus, blurred vision, headache, diplopia, drug-induced thrombocytopenia.
Dosage/ Concentrations:	200–300 mg three or four times a day. For PSVT, larger doses. Tablets: 100–300 mg. Capsules: 200, 300 mg.

Sustained-release tabs: 300 mg.
Parenteral: 200 mg/ml.

Contraindications: Long QT syndrome.

Drug Interactions/   Digoxin dosages should be halved with quinidine.
Allergy: Quinidine dosages should be halved with amiodarone.
Possible proarrhythmia properties.

SOTALOL

Trade Name: Betapace

Indications: Life-threatening ventricular arrhythmias, sustained ventricular tachycardia, PSVT, and atrial fibrillation.

Pharmacokinetics: Vd: 1.5 L/kg. $T_{1/2}$: β, 7–18 hr. Oral absorption: 90%–100% bioavailability; minimal plasma protein binding.

Pharmacodynamics: Class III.
CNS: Fatigue, impotence, dizziness, weakness.
CVS: Noncardioselective β-adrenoceptor blocker; prolonged APD and refractory period of atrial, ventricular, Purkinje fiber, and sinoatrial node tissues; ↑ PR and QT intervals; ↓ accessory pathway refractoriness; ↓ in sinus HR; proarrhythmic state; congestive heart failure; hypotension.
Pulmonary: Bronchospasm.

Dosage/   80 mg twice daily up to about 600 mg/day.
Concentrations:

Contraindications: Long QT syndrome.

Drug Interactions/   Albuterol is antagonized by sotalol. Bradycardia and
Allergy: hypotension when given concurrently with amiodarone. QT prolongation and a proarrhythmic state when given with TCAs.

TOCAINIDE

Trade Name: Tonocard

Indications: Ventricular arrhythmias.

Pharmacokinetics: Absorption: complete. Bioavailability after oral injection: 95%. Clearance: 2.6 ml/min/kg. Vd: 3.0 L/kg. $T_{1/2}$: β, 10–15 hr. 50% protein bound. Therapeutic serum concentration: 6–12 μg/ml. Elimination: hepatic and renal routes. Onset: 2 hr after oral injection.

TOCAINIDE   *(continued)*

Pharmacodynamics:	Class Ib.
CNS:	Dizziness, lightheadedness, tremor.
CVS:	Similar to effects of lidocaine, shortened ADP and ERP, minor effect on atrial and ventricular ERP, possibly shortened QT interval.
GI:	Nausea, vomiting, anorexia.
Other:	Agranulocytosis, bone marrow depression, thrombocytopenia.
Dosage/ Concentrations:	Tablets: 400 or 600 mg q 8 hr up to 2400 mg/day; no more than 1200 mg/day with renal or hepatic impairment.

VERAPAMIL

Trade Names:	Calan, Isoptin
Indications:	PSVT, AV nodal re-entry, and anomalous AV connections.
Pharmacokinetics:	Clearance: 15 ml/min/kg. Vd: 5 L/kg. $T_{1/2}$: β, 4 hr. Bioavailability after oral injection: 22%. 90% protein bound. Effective concentration in plasma: 120 ng/ml.
Pharmacodynamics: *CVS:*	Class IV. Ca^{2+} channel blocker, slowed conduction through AV node, slowed spontaneous firing of pacemaker cells in sinus node, ↓ rate of phase 4 spontaneous depolarization in cardiac Purkinje fibers, ↓ functional refractory period of AV node, ↓ PR interval, hypotension and bradycardia.
Dosage/ Concentrations:	Tablets: 40, 80, 120, 240 mg. Injection: 2.5 mg/ml. IV: 5–10 mg IV (75–150 μg/kg) over 2 min. Oral: 80–120 mg 3 times/day up to 480 mg daily.
Contraindications:	Hypotension, severe heart failure, sick sinus syndrome.
Drug Interactions/ Allergy:	Concurrent use with β-adrenergic blocking agents or digitalis can cause significant bradycardia or AV block.

4

Anticholinergics

Robert T. Naruse, M.D.

ATROPINE SULFATE

Trade Name: Atropine

Indications: Reversal of neuromuscular blockade in conjunction with an anticholinesterase (edrophonium or neostigmine), presurgical premedicant/antisialagogue, bradyarrhythmias, bronchoconstriction (administered aerosolized), visceral spasms, peptic ulcer disease (although H$_2$ blockers, carafate, and antacids are more effective), and organophosphate poisoning.

Pharmacokinetics: Tertiary amine; competitive antagonist of acetylcholine at muscarinic receptors. Absorption: from GI tract and other mucosal surfaces. Total absorption: 10%–25% of administered dose. T$_{1/2}$: α, 1 min; β, 2.3 hr (prolonged in the elderly and young children). Vd: 210 L (larger in the very young→prolonged elimination). Atropine undergoes hepatic enzymatic hydrolysis→tropine + tropic acid. 50% urinary excretion of unchanged drug. 50% plasma protein bound.

Pharmacodynamics:
CNS: Sedation, excitement, agitation, confusion, mild antiemetic effects, ↓ tremor of parkinsonism.
CVS: ↑ HR (dominant effect), ↓ HR (small dose), atrial arrhythmias, AV dissociation, ↑ velocity of AV conduction, shortened PR interval.
Pulmonary: Mucous plug formation, bronchodilator effect secondary to relaxation of bronchial smooth muscle, ↑ airway dead space.
GI: ↓ secretions, ↓ lower esophageal sphincter tone, ↓ motility/gastric emptying, gastroesophageal reflux, ↓ tone of biliary tract and ureteral smooth muscle.
Other: Pupillary dilation and cycloplegia, ↓ lacrimal secretions, abolished HR variability in fetus.

Dosage/ Concentrations: IV, SC, IM: 0.05, 0.1, 0.3, 0.4, 0.5, 1.0, 1.2 mg/ml.
Adult: For bradyarrhythmias/asystole: 0.5–1.0 mg IV q 5–10 min to a maximum of 2 mg (AHA-ACLS guidelines).

As antisialagogue/premedicant: 0.2–0.6 mg IM 30–60 min before surgery.

As adjunct in reversal of neuromuscular blockade: 0.01 mg/kg IV before or with edrophonium or neostigmine.

As bronchodilator, inhalation of 0.025–0.05 mg/kg q 4–6 hr (max. dose 2.5 mg)

As antidote to organophosphate poisoning: 1–2 mg IV/IM q 20–30 min as soon as cyanosis clears.

Pediatric:	10–20 μg/kg IV/IM. 30 μg/kg p.o.
Contraindications:	Narrow-angle glaucoma, tachycardia, prostatic enlargement, paralytic ileus, and pyloric stenosis. Use with caution in elderly, Down's syndrome, cardiovascular disease, and fever.
Drug Interactions/ Allergy:	Sedative/hypnotics may potentiate CNS depressant effects. Haloperidol may increase intraocular pressure. Urinary alkalinizers may delay urinary elimination. MAOIs may potentiate effects, because of their own intrinsic anticholinergic activity, and may decrease metabolism. Opioids increase risk of constipation and urinary retention. Allergic reactions rare.

GLYCOPYRROLATE

Trade Name:	Robinul
Indications:	Reversal of neuromuscular blockade in conjunction with an anticholinesterase (neostigmine or pyridostigmine), presurgical premedicant/antisialagogue, bradyarrhythmias, peptic ulcer disease, and organophosphate poisoning.
Pharmacokinetics:	Semi-synthetic quaternary ammonium compound; competitive antagonist of acetylcholine at muscarinic receptors. Absorption: from GI tract and other mucosal surfaces. Total absorption: 10%–25% of administered dose. Onset: IV, 1 min; IM, 15–30 min. Duration: 6–8 hr; vagal block, 2–3 hr. $T_{1/2}$: β, 1.25 hr (prolonged in the elderly and young children). 60% urinary excretion of unchanged drug in 6 hr.
Pharmacodynamics: CVS:	↑ HR (dominant effect), ↓ HR (small dose), atrial arrhythmias, AV dissociation, ↑ velocity of AV conduction, shortened PR interval.
Pulmonary:	Mucous plug formation, bronchodilator effect secondary to relaxation of bronchial smooth muscle, ↑ airway dead space.
GI/GU:	↓ Secretions, ↓ lower esophageal sphincter tone, ↓ motility/gastric emptying; urinary retention.
Other:	Lacrimal secretions; pupillary dilatation.
Dosage/ Concentrations:	IV, SC, IM: 0.2 mg/ml.
Adult:	For bradyarrhythmias: 0.005 mg/kg IV q 2–3 min.

GLYCOPYRROLATE *(continued)*

As antisialagogue/premedicant: 0.005 mg/kg IM 30–60 min before surgery (0.1–0.2 mg IV/IM/SC).

As adjunct in the reversal of neuromuscular blockade: 0.2 mg IV for each 1 mg of neostigmine or 5 mg of pyridostigmine.

For peptic ulcer disease: 0.1–0.2 mg IV/IM q 4 hr to q.i.d.

Contraindications: Tachycardia, prostatic enlargement, paralytic ileus, and pyloric stenosis. Use with caution in elderly with glaucoma, Down syndrome, cardiovascular disease, and fever.

Drug Interactions/ Allergy: Sedative/hypnotics may potentiate CNS depressant effects. Urinary alkalinizers may delay urinary elimination. MAOIs may potentiate effects, because of their own intrinsic anticholinergic activity, and may decrease metabolism. Opioids increase risk of constipation and urinary retention. Allergic reactions rare.

IPRATROPIUM BROMIDE

Trade Name: Atrovent

Indications: Chronic bronchitis and emphysema and chronic bronchospasm associated with COPD. Bronchial asthma.

Pharmacokinetics: Quaternary amine; competitive antagonist of acetylcholine at muscarinic receptors. Systemic absorption: minimal after inhalation. Absorbed poorly from GI tract and other mucosal surfaces. Onset: 5–15 min after inhalation. Duration: 3–4 hr, up to 6 hr in some patients. $T_{1/2}$: β, 2 hr. Metabolism: hepatic for the small amount absorbed systemically. Elimination: primarily fecal; 90% excreted as unchanged drug.

Pharmacodynamics:
Pulmonary: Bronchodilator effect, ↑ airway dead space.
Other: Pupillary dilatation and cycloplegia.

Dosage/ Concentrations: Metered dose inhaler, 18 μg/puff.
Adult: 2 puffs (36 μg) every 4–6 hr; not to exceed 12 puffs in 24 hr.
Pediatric: Dosage not established for children under 12 yr.

Contraindications: Narrow-angle glaucoma, prostatic enlargement, and obstructive uropathy.

Drug Interactions/ Allergy:	With other aerosols, raises risk of fluorocarbon toxicity, therefore, allow 5 min between inhalations when given with other aerosolized drugs. With other anticholinergics, results may be additive. May cause skin rash, oral ulcers, headache, nervousness, nausea, dry mouth, blurred vision, tachycardia, insomnia, or difficult urination.

SCOPOLAMINE (HYOSCINE) HYDROBROMIDE

Trade Names:	Transderm Scōp
Indications:	Presurgical premedicant/antisialagogue/sedative, motion sickness and vertigo, and parkinsonism.
Pharmacokinetics:	Tertiary amine; competitive antagonist of acetylcholine at muscarinic receptors. Absorption: from GI tract and other mucosal surfaces. Bioavailability: 21%–26% of administered dose. Onset: ≤ 30 min IV/IM, 30–60 minutes p.o. Duration: 4 hr. $T_{1/2}$: β, 1.6–3.3 hr (prolonged in the elderly and young children). Scopolamine undergoes enzymatic hydrolysis→scopine + tropic acid. 1.7%–5.9% urinary excretion of unchanged drug.
Pharmacodynamics:	
CNS:	Sedation, euphoria, amnesia, excitement, agitation, confusion, antiemetic effect, "anti-vertigo" effect, reduced tremor of parkinsonism; CNS depression and hemorrhage in neonates.
CVS:	↓ HR (small dose), ↑ HR (large dose).
Pulmonary:	Inspissation, bronchodilator effect, ↑ airway dead space (~ 30%).
GI:	↓ Secretions, ↓ lower esophageal sphincter tone, ↓ GI motility/gastric emptying.
Other:	Pupillary dilatation and cycloplegia, ↓ lacrimal secretions, ↓ respiratory secretions, ↓ GI secretions, ↓ perspiration (↑ risk of hyperthermia).
Dosage/ Concentrations:	IV, SC, IM: 0.3, 0.4, 0.5, 0.6 mg/ml; scopolamine transdermal system, 1.5-mg patch; 0.4–0.8 mg p.o.
Adult:	As antisialagogue/sedative premedicant: 0.2–0.6 mg IM 30–60 min before surgery.
Pediatric:	0.006 mg/kg IM (max.: 0.3 mg). For motion sickness/antiemetic: scopolamine transdermal system, 1.5-mg patch for 72 hr (applied before exposure to noxious stimulus).
Contraindications:	Narrow-angle glaucoma, altered mentation, prostatic

SCOPOLAMINE (HYOSCINE) HYDROBROMIDE   *(continued)*

enlargement, paralytic ileus, and pyloric stenosis. Use with caution in elderly, Down's syndrome, and fever.

Drug Interactions/ Allergy:

Sedative/hypnotics may potentiate CNS depressant effects. Haloperidol may increase intraocular pressure. Urinary alkalinizers may delay urinary elimination. MAOIs may potentiate effects, because of their own intrinsic anticholinergic activity, and may decrease metabolism. Opioids increase risk of constipation and urinary retention. Allergic reactions rare.

5

Anticoagulants and Thrombolytics

Marshal B. Kaplan, A.B., M.S., M.D.

HEPARIN

Trade Name:	N/A
Indications:	Acute MI, DVT, venous thromboembolism, pulmonary embolism, cardiopulmonary bypass, and adjunct to thrombolytic regimen.
Pharmacokinetics:	Vd: Adult: 40–60 ml/kg. Clearance: 10 min. $T_{1/2}$: α, not directly measurable; β, dose dependent (1 to 5 hr).

Pharmacodynamics:

Hepatic:	Altered hepatic function tests.
Musculoskeletal:	Osteoporosis.
Endocrine:	Hypoaldosteronism.
Other:	Hemorrhage (major effect), thrombocytopenia, thrombosis ("white clot syndrome"), urticaria, skin necrosis.

Dosage/ Concentrations: Adult:	IV: Initial bolus of 5000 U, followed by infusion of 700 to 2000 U/hr monitored by aPTT. SC: 5000 U q 8–12 hr.
Contraindications:	Severe thrombocytopenia, uncontrollable active bleeding.
Drug Interactions/ Allergy:	Heparin may be partially inhibited by digitalis, tetracyclines, antihistamines, and nicotine. Heparin effect is antagonized by protamine. Aspirin and other drugs with platelet-inhibiting effects may increase likelihood of bleeding.

ANISTREPLASE, ANISOYLATED PLASMINOGEN-STREPTOKINASE ACTIVATOR COMPLEX (APSAC)

Trade Name:	Eminase
Indications:	Lysis of thrombi in acute MI.
Pharmacokinetics:	Some binding to fibrin prior to activation, which may confer increased specificity over streptokinase for clots. $T_{1/2}$: $\sim$ 94 min.

Pharmacodynamics:

CNS:	Cerebral hemorrhage.
CVS:	Hypotension.
Dosage/ Concentrations:	Lyophilized powder in 30-unit vials. 30 U IV over 5 min.
Contraindications:	Hypersensitivity to the drug.

| Drug Interactions/ Allergy: | Concurrent therapy with anticoagulants or antiplatelet agents increases risk of bleeding. Hypersensitivity reactions mild to severe. |

ASPIRIN (ACETYLSALICYLIC ACID)

Trade Name:	Many proprietary preparations
Indications:	Prophylaxis for thrombosis in atherosclerotic vascular disease; ↓ risk of TIA, stroke, MI, aortocoronary graft occlusion, thromboembolism in atrial fibrillation.
Pharmacokinetics:	Vd: ~ 170 ml/kg for usual doses. $T_{1/2}$: ~ 15 min. Acetylates platelet cyclooxygenase and blocks production of thromboxane A_2. The latter induces platelet aggregation and is a vasoconstrictor. Absorption: Good after oral ingestion. Highly protein bound.
Pharmacodynamics: *CNS:*	Tinnitus.
Hepatic:	Reye's syndrome in children; hepatotoxicity with high sustained plasma concentrations.
Renal:	At low doses, ↓ urate excretion.
GI:	Stomach pain, nausea, vomiting, exacerbation of gastric or duodenal ulcer, ↑ bleeding.
Dosage/ Concentrations:	Antithrombotic dose: 160–320 mg/day.
Contraindications:	Hypersensitivity to salicylates.
Drug Interactions/ Allergy:	Hypersensitivity is well documented. ↑ bleeding with anticoagulants. Alcohol, corticosteroids, and phenylbutazone increase risk of GI ulceration. ↓ Diuretic effect of spironolactone.

STREPTOKINASE

Trade Name:	Streptase
Indications:	Acute MI, pulmonary embolism, and acute arterial thrombosis.
Pharmacokinetics:	No intrinsic activity. Forms complex with plasminogen to form free plasmin. Circulating antibodies, the result of previous streptococcal infection, must be depleted by the initial IV loading dose; thereafter, $T_{1/2}$: ~ 80 min.

STREPTOKINASE   *(continued)*

Pharmacodynamics:	
CNS:	Cerebral hemorrhage.
CVS:	Hypotension (risk <10%).
Other:	Major bleeding due to systemic fibrinolysis.
Dosage/ Concentrations:	For acute MI: 1.5 million units IV or 20,000 U directly into coronary artery, followed by infusion of 2000 U/min for 1 hr. For pulmonary embolism, DVT, or arterial thrombus: Loading dose, 250,000 U, followed by infusion of 100,000 U/hr.
Contraindications:	Hypersensitivity to the drug, history of hemorrhagic stroke, embolic or thrombotic stroke within 6 months, intracranial surgery or trauma within 6 months, uncontrolled hypertension, active internal bleeding within 2 weeks, surgery trauma or organ biopsy within 2 weeks, bleeding diathesis, active pancreatitis, diabetic retinopathy.
Drug Interactions/ Allergy:	Concurrent therapy with anticoagulants or antiplatelet agents increases risk of bleeding. Hypersensitivity reactions mild to severe. Streptokinase is antigenic.

TISSUE PLASMINOGEN ACTIVATOR (ALTEPLASE)

Trade Name:	Activase
Indications:	Coronary thrombolysis in acute MI, massive pulmonary embolism.
Pharmacokinetics:	Clearance: hepatic. Preferentially binds to fibrin associated with hemostatic plugs or thrombi. Activates bound plasminogen to plasmin. $T_{1/2}$: ~ 4 min.
Pharmacodynamics:	
CVS:	Reperfusion $\rightarrow$ arrhythmias.
Other:	Bleeding.
Dosage/ Concentrations:	Vials of 20, 50, 100 mg.
Adult:	>65 kg: 100 mg with 6%–10% given as IV bolus over 1–2 min with remainder given over 2 hr.
Elderly:	<65 kg: 1.25 mg/kg administered proportionally as above.
Contraindications:	Active internal bleeding, history of CVA, severe hyper-

tension, bleeding diathesis, recent surgery or organ biopsy, intracranial neoplasm, AVM, and aneurysm.

Drug Interactions/ Allergy: Heparin, vitamin K antagonists, and antiplatelet agents increase risk of bleeding. Allergic reactions rare.

UROKINASE

Trade Name: Abbokinase

Indications: Lysis of acute pulmonary emboli, lysis of deep venous thrombus, clearing of IV catheters, and lysis of arterial thrombus.

Pharmacokinetics: Activates plasminogen to plasmin. $T_{1/2}$: 14 min.

Pharmacodynamics:
CVS: Rapid lysis of coronary thrombus → reperfusion arrhythmias, stroke.
Other: Hypotension, bleeding at injection and surgical sites.

Dosage/ Concentrations: Vials of 250,000 U. For coronary thrombolysis: 1 million U bolus, then 1 million U over 1 hr.

Contraindications: History of hemorrhagic stroke, embolic or thrombotic stroke within 6 months, intracranial surgery or trauma within 6 months, uncontrolled hypertension, active internal bleeding within 2 weeks, surgery trauma or organ biopsy within 2 weeks, bleeding diathesis, active pancreatitis, and diabetic retinopathy.

Drug Interactions/ Allergy: ↑ Bleeding risk with concomitant use of antiplatelet agents or anticoagulants. Mild reactions, such as skin rash.

WARFARIN SODIUM

Trade Name: Coumadin

Indications: Atrial fibrillation; prosthetic heart valves, DVT, MI, and peripheral vascular disease.

Pharmacokinetics: Vd: 0.14 L/kg (albumin space). Clearance: 0.045 ml/min/kg. $T_{1/2}$: 20–60 hr (avg. 36–42 hr). 99% protein bound.

Pharmacodynamics: Anticoagulation effect from inhibition of vitamin K epoxide reductase, limiting carboxylation of vitamin K–dependent coagulation factors (II, VII, IX, X, and prothrombin).

WARFARIN SODIUM   *(continued)*

Hepatic:	Anticoagulant effect potentiated in liver disease.
Endocrine:	Hypermetabolic states (hyperthyroidism increases catabolism of vitamin K–dependent factors, potentiating response to warfarin).
Other:	Hemorrhage, hereditary resistance.
Dosage/ Concentrations:	Tablets.
Adult:	2–15 mg/day; monitor PT.
Contraindications:	Hemorrhage.
Drug Interactions/ Allergy:	Variations in effect may be due to changes in dietary vitamin K. Interactions include: (1) drugs that inhibit warfarin clearance (trimethoprim-sulfamethoxazole, cimetidine); (2) drugs that influence absorption (cholestyramine); (3) drugs inhibiting platelet function (aspirin, nonsteroidal anti-inflammatory drugs; (4) drugs inhibiting cyclic interconversion of vitamin K (cephalosporins); and (5) erythromycin and other antibiotics (unclear mechanism).

6

Anticonvulsants

Michail N. Avramov, M.D., Ph.D.

CARBAMAZEPINE

Trade Names:	Tegretol, Epitol
Indications:	Partial seizures, generalized tonic-clonic seizures, and trigeminal and glossopharyngeal neuralgia.
Pharmacokinetics:	Protein binding: 70%–80%. Vd: 0.8–1.8 L/kg. Clearance: 0.025–0.096 L/kg/hr. $T_{1/2}$: β, 20–48 hr (↓ with chronic administration). Metabolism: extensive (95%) by liver. Therapeutic plasma concentration: 4–12 μg/ml. Toxicity: >14 μg/ml.
Pharmacodynamics:	Nonsedating and antineuralgic action.
CNS:	Blurred vision, nystagmus, dysarthria, drowsiness, lethargy.
Pulmonary:	Dyspnea, pneumonitis, respiratory depression.
Hepatic:	Jaundice, hepatitis
Renal:	Volume expansion, dilutional hyponatremia.
GI:	Diarrhea, nausea, vomiting.
Musculoskeletal:	Muscle twitching and tremor.
Other:	Bone marrow depression, aplastic anemia, leukopenia, eosinophilia, thrombocytopenia, fever.
Dosage/ Concentrations:	Oral: 200-mg tablets; 100-mg chewable tablets; 100 mg/5 ml suspension.
Adult:	Up to 1.2 g daily.
Pediatric:	10–20 mg/kg, up to 1 g daily.
Contraindications:	History of bone marrow depression, hypersensitivity to TCAs, and concomitant use of MAOIs.
Drug Interactions/ Allergy:	Resistance to neuromuscular blocking drugs. With haloperidol, ↓ serum levels and efficacy. With acetaminophen, ↑ metabolism, risk of acetaminophen-induced hepatotoxicity and decreased analgesic or antipyretic effects. With oral anticoagulants: ↑ metabolism and ↓ hypoprothrombinemic effect. With primidone, phenytoin, ethosuximide, valproic acid, and clonazepam, ↓ plasma levels. With concurrent use of TCAs, haloperidol, and phenothiazines, ↑ CNS depressant effects of carbamazepine, ↓ seizure threshold, and ↓ anticonvulsant effects. Risk of hepatotoxicity after anesthesia with halothane, enflurane, and possibly sevoflurane.

CLONAZEPAM

Trade Name:	Klonopin
Indications:	Absence seizures, myoclonic seizures, and infantile spasms.

Pharmacokinetics:	Elimination: renal. Inactive metabolites excreted in urine. Protein binding: 85%. Vd: 2.0–4.8 L/kg. Clearance: 0.04–0.07 L/kg/hr. $T_{1/2}$: β, 18–50 hr. Therapeutic plasma concentration: 20–70 ng/ml. Toxicity: >60 ng/ml.
Pharmacodynamics:	CNS depressant.
CNS:	Sedative, hypnotic, and amnestic effects; development of tolerance; confusion; drowsiness; ataxia; dysarthria; weakness; withdrawal symptoms with abrupt discontinuation (dysphoria, irritability, restlessness, insomnia, tremor); seizures; status epilepticus.
CVS:	↓ Peripheral vascular resistance, hypotension.
Pulmonary:	Respiratory depression.
GI:	Nausea, vomiting.
Musculoskeletal:	Muscle relaxation; severe weakness.
Dosage/ Concentrations:	Oral: Tablets: 0.5, 1, and 2 mg.
Adult:	Up to 20 mg daily.
Pediatric:	Up to 0.05 mg/kg/day.
Contraindications:	Growing children (adverse effects on physical and mental development).
Drug Interactions/ Allergy:	Potentiates CNS depression with alcohol and other CNS depressants. Potentiates respiratory depression with opiates. Potentiates hypotension during concurrent use with anesthetics and calcium channel blockers. With carbamazepine, ↑ metabolism of clonazepam. Metabolism inhibited and plasma levels increased by concurrent use of cimetidine, contraceptives, disulfiram, and erythromycin.

ETHOSUXIMIDE

Trade Name:	Zarontin
Indications:	Absence (petit mal) seizures.
Pharmacokinetics:	Protein binding: negligible. Vd: 0.6–0.7 L/kg. Clearance: 0.012–0.016 L/kg/hr. $T_{1/2}$: β, 40–60 hr. Therapeutic plasma concentration: 40–120 µg/ml. Toxicity: >100 µg/ml. Excretion: 20% excreted unchanged in urine. Metabolism: extensively (80%) metabolized by hydroxylation and ethylation to inactive metabolites.
Pharmacodynamics:	
CNS:	Confusion, sleepiness, coma.
Pulmonary:	Respiratory depression.
GI:	Nausea, vomiting, stomach cramps, epigastric and abdominal pain, anorexia, diarrhea, weight loss, constipation.

ETHOSUXIMIDE *(continued)*

Musculoskeletal:	Flaccid muscles (acute overdose).
Other:	Agranulocytosis, thrombocytopenia.

Dosage/ Concentrations: Oral: Capsules: 250 mg. Syrup: 250 mg/5 ml.

Adult:	Up to 1.5 g/day p.r.n. and as tolerated.
Pediatric:	20 mg/kg/day (up to 1 g/day).

Contraindications: Severe renal or hepatic disease, intermittent porphyria, and hypersensitivity to succinimides.

Drug Interactions/ Allergy: Coadministration with hepatic microsomal enzyme-inducing anticonvulsants (carbamazepine, phenobarbital, hydantoin) decreases plasma concentration (and β half-life) of ethosuximide.
↑ Hydantoin levels. ↓ Primidone and phenobarbital levels. Combined use of alcohol and CNS depressant medications may enhance CNS depression.

MAGNESIUM SULFATE

Trade Name: N/A

Indications: Seizure prevention, and severe pre-eclampsia or eclampsia, acute nephritis in children, acute hypomagnesemia with signs of tetany, uterine tetany, and atypical ventricular tachycardia.

Pharmacokinetics: Normal plasma Mg levels: 1.5–3 mEq/L. Therapeutic serum levels: 2.5–7.5 mEq/L. Toxicity: >7–10 mEq/L. Excreted in urine.

Pharmacodynamics:	CNS depressant.
CNS:	Loss of deep tendon reflexes, respiratory paralysis.
CVS:	Hypotension, ECG changes (lengthened PR, widened QRS, prolonged QT), dysrhythmias, heart block, asystole.
Renal:	↑ Risk of toxicity in patients with renal impairment.
Other:	Hypotonia, hyporeflexia, hypotension, respiratory depression in neonates.

Dosage/ Concentrations: Individualize dosage; test knee jerk reflexes before each repeated dose; if reflexes absent, do not give Mg.
  IM: 1–5 g 25%–50% solution 6 times a day p.r.n.
  IV: 1–4 g 10%–20% solution (<1.5 ml/min of 10% solution); IV infusion in eclampsia, 1–2 g/hr; monitor Mg plasma concentrations and clinical signs of toxicity.
  Parenteral: 10% (0.8 mEq/ml): 10- and 20-ml ampules, 20-ml vials; 12.5% (1 mEq/L): 8-ml vials; 25%

(2 mEq/L): 150-ml vials; 50% (4 mEq/L): 2- and 10-ml ampules, 5-, 10-, 30-, and 50-ml vials.

Contraindications:	Heart block, myocardial damage, and severe renal impairment.
Drug Interactions/ Allergy:	Potentiates action of neuromuscular relaxants and of CNS depressants (hypnotics, anesthetics, narcotics). Cardiac conduction changes and heart block with digitalis glycosides. Parenteral calcium neutralizes effects of $MgSO_4$.

PHENOBARBITAL

Trade Names:	Barbita, Luminal, Solfoton
Indications:	Partial seizures, generalized clonic-tonic seizures, status epilepticus.
Pharmacokinetics:	Protein binding: 40%–60%. Vd: 0.6 L/kg (1 L/kg in neonates). Clearance: 0.003–0.013 L/kg/hr. $T_{1/2}$: β, 50–160 hr. Elimination: up to 25% excreted unchanged in urine. Therapeutic serum levels: 15–30 μg/ml. Toxicity: >40 μg/ml.
Pharmacodynamics:	CNS depressant.
CNS:	Drowsiness, paradoxical excitement, tolerance development, withdrawal symptoms with abrupt discontinuation, seizures, status epilepticus, sedation, nystagmus, ataxia, learning difficulties.
Pulmonary:	Respiratory depression.
Hepatic:	↑ Acute intermittent porphyria.
GI:	Nausea, vomiting.
Other:	Megaloblastic anemia.
Dosage/ Concentrations:	Oral: Tablets: 8, 16, 32, 65, and 100 mg. Capsules: 16 mg. Elixirs: 20 mg/5 ml. Parenteral: 30, 60, 65, and 130 mg/ml for injection.
Adult:	150–300 mg.
Pediatric:	• Neonate: Loading dose, 20 mg/kg; maintenance, 5 mg/kg daily.
	• Child: Loading dose, 4–8 mg for 2 days; maintenance, 2–5 mg/kg.
Contraindications:	Severe respiratory disease.
Drug Interactions/ Allergy:	Phenobarbital induces the microsomal metabolism of warfarin, phenytoin, phenylbutazone, prednisone, hydrocortisone, and digoxin. Valproic acid and chloramphenicol inhibit phenobarbital metabolism. Hypersensitivity: Skin rash, Stevens-Johnson syndrome.

PHENYTOIN

Trade Names:	Dilantin, Dilantin-125, Dilantin-30 Pediatric, Dilantin Infatabs, Dilantin Kapseals, Diphenylan
Indications:	Tonic-clonic (grand mal), psychomotor, and temporal lobe seizures.
Pharmacokinetics:	Protein binding: 87%–93%. Vd: 0.5–0.8 L/kg. Clearance: 0.008–0.055 L/kg/hr. $T_{1/2}$: β, 15–20 hr. Therapeutic plasma concentration: 8–20 μg/ml. Toxicity: >25 μg/ml. First-order kinetics at low doses and zero-order (capacity-limited) at higher therapeutic doses. Metabolism: Metabolized to inactive hydroxylated metabolites. Excretion: 2% eliminated in urine. 5% excreted unchanged in stool.
Pharmacodynamics:	CNS nonsedating, antineuralgic, and muscle relaxant effects.
CNS:	Nystagmus, ataxia, drowsiness, dysarthria, lethargy.
CVS:	Antiarrhythmic effect, hypotension.
Hepatic:	Hyperglycemia, allergic hepatitis, jaundice.
GI:	Nausea, vomiting, diarrhea, constipation.
Musculoskeletal:	Osteomalacia, gingival hypertrophy.
Other:	Megaloblastic anemia.
Dosage/ Concentrations:	Parenteral: 50 mg/ml; 2- and 5-ml ampules. Oral: Tablets: chewable, 50 mg. Oral suspension: 30 and 125 mg/5 ml. Capsules: 30 and 100 mg.
Adult:	Loading dose: 10–12 mg/kg/12–24 hr. Maintenance dose: 5–6 mg/kg/day (oral and IV, same dosage). For status epilepticus: loading dose, 10–15 mg/kg.
Pediatric:	10 mg/kg/day.
Contraindications:	Sinus bradycardia, sinoatrial block, first- and second-degree AV block, Adam-Stokes syndrome, and pregnancy (twofold to threefold increase in fetal abnormalities).
Drug Interactions/ Allergy:	↑ Effects in presence of drugs that inhibit phenytoin metabolism (benzodiazepines, chloramphenicol, cimetidine, disulfiram, ethanol, isoniazid, succinimides, sulfonamides, valproic acid) or displace from binding proteins (salicylates, TCAs, valproic acid), also with ibuprofen and phenothiazines. ↓ Effects produced by drugs that increase metabolism (barbiturates, carbamazepine, diazoxide, ethanol, rifampin, theophylline), decrease absorption (antacids, charcoal), and by antineoplastics, pyridoxine, folic acid. ↓ Effects of dopamine, furosemide, levodopa, nondepolarizing muscle relaxants.

↑ Metabolism of acetaminophen, amiodarone, carbamazepine, cardiac glycosides, corticosteroids, dicumarol, estrogens, haloperidol, oral contraceptives, quinidine, theophylline, and valproic acid. Hypersensitivity reactions: hepatitis, lymphoma, Stevens-Johnson syndrome, rash, fever, arthralgia, and lymphadenopathy.

PRIMIDONE

Trade Name:	Mysoline
Indications:	Partial seizures, generalized tonic-clonic seizures, benign familial (essential) tremor.
Pharmacokinetics:	Protein binding: <20%. Vd: 0.6 L/kg. Clearance: 0.013–0.041 L/kg/hr. $T_{1/2}$: β, 4–12 hr. Absorption: Readily absorbed from GI tract. Therapeutic plasma concentration: 5–10 μg/ml. Toxicity: >10–15 μg/ml. Elimination: 20%–40%. Eliminated unchanged.

Pharmacodynamics:

CNS:	Drowsiness, ↓ physical dexterity, sedation, nystagmus, ataxia, dizziness, diplopia, learning difficulties, paradoxical excitement, restlessness, status epilepticus (from abrupt withdrawal).
Pulmonary:	Respiratory depression in patients with asthma or emphysema.
Hepatic:	Metabolized to active metabolites: phenobarbital and phenylethylmalonylamide (PEMA). Phenobarbital causes induction of hepatic microsomal enzymes.
Renal:	20%–40% eliminated unchanged.
GI:	Nausea, vomiting, anorexia.
Other:	Megaloblastic anemia, hemorrhage (vitamin K–dependent clotting deficiency) in newborns of mothers receiving primidone.

Dosage/ Concentrations:	Oral: 50- and 250-mg tablets; 250 mg/5 ml suspension.
Adult:	100–750 mg/day (< 2 g/day).
Pediatric:	10–20 mg/kg/day.
Contraindications:	Porphyria and hypersensitivity to phenobarbital.
Drug Interactions/ Allergy:	↓ Effects in combination with acetazolamide, carbamazepine, and succinimides. ↑ Effects by hydantoins, isoniazid, and nicotinamide. Chronic use of primidone prior to anesthesia increases metabolism of enflurane, halothane, and probably sevoflurane.

VALPROIC ACID

Trade Names:	Depakene, Depakote
Indications:	Simple (petit mal) and complex absence seizures.
Pharmacokinetics:	Protein binding: 87%–94%. Vd: 0.14–0.20 L/kg. Clearance: 0.006–0.027 L/kg/hr. $T_{1/2}$: β, 11–20 hr. Therapeutic plasma concentration: 50–100 μg/ml. Toxicity: >150 μg/ml. Metabolism: Metabolized extensively. Excretion: Excreted as glucuronide; partly eliminated as keto-metabolite.

Pharmacodynamics:

CNS:	Sedation, tremor, ataxia, nystagmus, diplopia, dysarthria, incoordination, confusion, dizziness, drowsiness, coma, excitement, restlessness, irritability, seizures or status epilepticus (from abrupt withdrawal).
Hepatic:	↑ Hepatotoxicity in children.
Renal:	Impaired urine test for ketones.
GI:	Nausea, vomiting, abdominal cramps, pancreatitis.
Other:	Inhibited platelet aggregation, prolonged bleeding time, hematoma, leukopenia, thrombocytopenia, eosinophilia, anemia, bone marrow suppression, neural tube defects in fetus of mother receiving valproic acid in first trimester.

Dosage/ Concentrations:	Oral: Capsules: 250 mg. Syrup: 250 mg/5 ml (as sodium valproate). Tablets: 125, 250, and 500 mg (as divalproex sodium).
Adult:	Up to 60 mg/kg/day.
Pediatric:	15–45 mg/kg/day.
Contraindications:	Hepatic dysfunction.
Drug Interactions/ Allergy:	With chlorpromazine and cimetidine; ↓ clearance of valproic acid. With salicylates, ↑ valproic acid levels. ↑ CNS depressant effects of alcohol and other CNS depressants. ↑ Risk of bleeding in patients receiving anticoagulants. ↑ Gastrointestinal ulcerative or hemorrhagic potential of nonsteroidal anti-inflammatory analgesics. Potentiates hepatotoxic effects of concurrent medications. ↑ Serum concentrations of enzyme-inducing anticonvulsants (carbamazepine, phenytoin, primidone, and phenobarbital); their abrupt discontinuation causes an increase in valproic acid serum concentration. Allergic reaction: Skin rash.

7

Antiemetics

Mehernoor F. Watcha, M.D., D.Ch.

Anticholinergics

SCOPOLAMINE (HYOSCINE) HYDROBROMIDE

Trade Names:	Isopto Hyoscine, Transderm Scōp
Indications:	Preoperative sedation, amnesia, decreased salivation, motion sickness, ophthalmic cycloplegia, mydriasis, and postoperative nausea and vomiting.
Pharmacokinetics:	IV: $T_{1/2}$: α, 5.0 $\pm$ 3.2 min; β, 2.4 $\pm$ 1.4 hr. Vd: 1.2 L/kg. Clearance: 15 ml/min/kg. Bioavailability: oral, fair; IM, good.

Pharmacodynamics:

CNS:	Euphoria, drowsiness, amnesia, $\downarrow$ REM sleep during sleep, excitation, restlessness, delirium.
CVS:	Low doses, $\downarrow$ HR; high doses, short-lived $\uparrow$ HR.
GI:	$\downarrow$ Saliva, $\downarrow$ gastric secretion, $\downarrow$ motility.
Other:	Mydriasis, cycloplegia.
Dosage/ Concentrations:	Injection 0.4 mg/ml.
Adult:	0.3–0.6 mg. Transdermal patch: 0.5 mg over 72 hr.
Pediatric:	6 μg/kg. Ophthalmic: 0.25%–1–2 drops b.i.d.
Contraindications:	Narrow-angle glaucoma, intestinal and bladder neck obstruction, infants, children, elderly and those with Down's syndrome.
Drug Interactions/ Allergy:	Additive effects with other anticholinergic agents.

Phenothiazines

CHLORPROMAZINE

Trade Name:	Thorazine
Indications:	Psychosis, nausea and vomiting, intractable hiccups in adults, Tourette's syndrome, and behavioral problems.
Pharmacokinetics:	Adults: $T_{1/2}$: α, 1.8 min; β, 30 hr. Vd: 21 L/kg. Clearance: 9.1 ml/kg/min. Oral bioavailability: $\sim$ 20%. Child: $T_{1/2}$: α, 1.1 min; β, 7.7 hr. Vd: 36.1 L/kg. Clearance: 50.1 ml/kg/min.

Pharmacodynamics:
CNS: Sedative, tranquilizing, and antianxiety effects,
                    ↑ ↑ Prolactin secretion → galactorrhea, ↓ seizure
                    threshold, drowsiness, retinopathy, restlessness,
                    ↑ extrapyramidal signs, photosensitivity.
CVS: Peripheral α-adrenergic blockade, tachycardia, nega-
                    tive inotropic action, prolonged PR and QT intervals,
                    blunted T wave, hypotension.
Metabolic: Temperature fluctuations.
GI: Jaundice, constipation, ↓ gastric secretion and motil-
                    ity.
Other: Urinary retention (rare), inhibited ejaculation (but not
                    erection), dry mouth, galactorrhea, gynecomastia,
                    agranulocytosis.

Dosage/   Concentrate: 30 mg/ml. Oral syrup: 10-mg base/5 ml
Concentrations: in United States and 25 mg/5 ml in Canada. Tablets:
                    10-, 25-, 50-, 100-, and 200-mg base. Suppository:
                    25- and 100-mg base. Injection: 25-mg/ml base.
Adult: For antipsychotic effect, 25–50 mg q 3–12 hr.
                    For anxiety, nausea and vomiting, 12.5–50 mg deep
                    IM q 3–4 hr. Not to exceed 1 mg/min IV.
Pediatric: For antipsychosis, 2.5–6 mg/kg/24 hr in divided
                    doses q 4–6 hr.
                    For anxiety, nausea, and vomiting, 1 mg/kg. Not to
                    exceed 40 mg/day for child <5 yr; 75 mg/day for
                    child 5–12 yr.

Contraindications: Severe cardiovascular disease and coma.

Drug Interactions/   Prolonged and intensified sedative and anticholinergic
Allergy: effects with other CNS depressants. May lower seizure
                    threshold when metrizamide is used. False-positive test
                    for urine bilirubin, pregnancy immunologic tests
                    (false-positive or false-negative). ACTH response to
                    metyrapone. ↑ Serum valproic acid levels. Chlorpro-
                    mazine may precipitate if given with thiopental, atro-
                    pine, or solutions not having a pH of 4–5.

CYCLIZINE

Trade Name: Marezine

Indications: Motion sickness, nausea, and vomiting.

Pharmacodynamics: H1 receptor antagonist.
CNS: ↓ Vestibular stimulation, drowsiness, blurred vision,
                    local anesthetic activity at high doses.
GI: Inhibited histamine effects (but not gastric secretion un-
                    til large doses are used).

CYCLIZINE   *(continued)*

Other:	Inhibited histamine effects on smooth muscle of gut, bronchi, and vascular tree; dry mouth.

Dosage/ Concentrations: Tablets: 50 mg. Injection: 50 mg/ml.

Adult: 50 mg IM.

Pediatric:
- \>6 yr: 25 mg IM
- ≤6 yr: 1 mg/kg.

Contraindications: Bladder neck obstruction, prostatic hypertrophy, severe cardiac failure, narrow-angle glaucoma, and pyloroduodenal obstruction.

Drug Interactions/ Allergy: Concurrent use may potentiate CNS depression effects of other drugs.

DIPHENHYDRAMINE

Trade Name: Benadryl

Indications: Allergy symptoms, vertigo, motion sickness, cough, and parkinsonism (antidyskinetic effect).

Pharmacokinetics: Adults: $T_{1/2}$: β, 9.2 hr. Vd: 17.4 L/kg. Clearance: 23.3 ml/kg/min. Oral bioavailability: ~ 60%. Child: $T_{1/2}$: β, 5.4 hr. Vd: 21.7 L/kg. Clearance: 49.2 ml/kg/min. Elderly: $T_{1/2}$: β, 13.5 hr. Vd: 13.6 L/kg. Clearance: 11.7 ml/kg/min.

Pharmacodynamics: H1 receptor antagonist.

CNS: Pronounced sedative effects, dizziness, fatigue, insomnia.

CVS: Hypotension, palpitations, antimuscarinic effect.

Other: Dry mucous membranes.

Dosage/ Concentrations: Syrup, 12.5 mg/5 ml. Tablets, 25, 50 mg. Injection: 10 and 50 mg/ml.

Adult: 10 mg initially IV, increase to 20–50 mg q 2–4 hr, not to exceed 400 mg/day.

Pediatric: 1–1.25 mg/kg, not to exceed 300 mg/day.

Contraindications: Acute asthma. Use with caution in angle-closure glaucoma, peptic ulcer, urinary obstruction, and hyperthyroidism.

Drug Interactions/ Allergy: Additive effects with alcohol and other CNS depressants. Patients taking drugs that can cause disulfiram reactions (i.e., metronidazole, chlorpropamide) should not take the syrup because of alcohol content.

DROPERIDOL

Trade Name:	Inapsine
Indications:	Nausea and vomiting, adjunct for general anesthesia (tranquilizer).
Pharmacokinetics:	Adults: $T_{1/2}$: α, 10 min; β, 1.73 hr. Vd: 2.4 L/kg. Clearance: 14.1 ml/kg/min. Oral and IM bioavailability: good. Child: $T_{1/2}$: β, 1.69 hr. Vd: 0.58 L/kg. Clearance: 4.66 ml/kg/min.
Pharmacodynamics:	
CNS:	Sedation, dysphoria, extrapyramidal reactions (dystonia, akathisia, oculogyric crisis), apprehension, restlessness, excitation.
CVS:	Hypotension.
Dosage/ Concentrations:	Parenteral: 2.5 mg/ml.
Adult:	0.625–2.5 mg.
Pediatric:	25–75 μg/kg.
Contraindications:	Liver and kidney disease (use with caution).
Drug Interactions/ Allergy:	Additive effects with other CNS depressants; ↓ pressor effect of epinephrine.

GRANISETRON

Trade Name:	Kytril
Indications:	Chemotherapy-induced emesis.
Pharmacokinetics:	Adults: $T_{1/2}$: β, 10.6 hr. Vd: 2.2 L/kg. Clearance: 3.55 ml/min/kg.
Pharmacodynamics:	5-HT3 antagonist.
CNS:	Headache, dizziness, flushing.
GI:	Constipation, warm sensation in epigastrium.
Dosage/ Concentrations:	
Adult:	1–3 mg.
Pediatric:	40 μg/kg.
Contraindications:	None known.
Drug Interactions/ Allergy:	None known.

HYDROXYZINE

Trade Name:	Vistaril
Indications:	Anxiety, sedation-hypnosis, vertigo, nausea, and vomiting.
Pharmacokinetics:	Adult: $T_{1/2}$: β, 20 hr. Vd: 19.5 L/kg. Clearance: 9.8 ml/kg/min. Child: $T_{1/2}$: β, 7.1 hr. Vd: 18.5 L/kg. Clearance: 32.1 ml/kg/min.
Pharmacodynamics:	H1-receptor antagonist.
Dosage/ Concentrations:	Syrup: 10 mg/5 ml. Tablet: 10 and 25 mg. Injection: 25 and 50 mg/ml.
Adult:	50–100 mg q 4–6 hr as anxiolytic or sedative-hypnotic; 25–100 mg IM as antiemetic.
Pediatric:	1 mg/kg.
Contraindications:	Narrow-angle glaucoma, prostatic hypertrophy, and bladder neck obstruction (use with caution).
Drug Interactions/ Allergy:	Potentiates other CNS depressants and anticholinergics. Can antagonize vasopressor effects of epinephrine. May cause false increase in urinary 17-OH steroid concentration.

ONDANSETRON

Trade Name:	Zofran
Indications:	Chemotherapy-induced and postoperative emesis.
Pharmacokinetics:	Adults: $T_{1/2}$: β, 3 hr. Vd: 2.3 L/kg. Clearance: 7.73 ml/kg/min. Oral bioavailability: good (60%). Elderly: $T_{1/2}$: β, 5.4 hr. Clearance: 6.02 ml/kg/min.
Pharmacodynamics:	Selective 5-HT3 receptor antagonist.
CNS:	Headache, dizziness, flushing, extrapyramidal signs (rare).
GI:	Constipation.
Other:	Warm sensation in epigastrium.
Dosage/ Concentrations:	Injection: single-dose (2 ml) and multidose (20 ml) vial, 2 mg/ml. Tablets: 4 and 8 mg.
Adult:	For postoperative nausea and vomiting: 4 mg IV or 8 mg orally. For chemotherapy-induced emesis, 8 mg.
Pediatric:	For postoperative nausea and vomiting: 50–100 μg/kg. For chemotherapy-induced emesis, 150 μg/kg.
Contraindications:	None known.

| Drug Interactions/
Allergy: | Anaphylactic reactions (rare), in cancer patients. |

PERPHENAZINE

Trade Name:	Trilafon
Indications:	Psychosis, nausea, and vomiting.
Pharmacokinetics:	$T_{1/2}$: β, 9.4 hr. Vd: 20.2 L/kg. Clearance: 1.8 ml/kg/min. Oral bioavailability: Poor.
Pharmacodynamics: *CNS:*	Sedative, tranquilizing, and antianxiety effects, ↑ ↑ prolactin secretion causing galactorrhea, ↓ seizure threshold, ↑ extrapyramidal reactions, weak sedative-hypnotic effect, tardive dyskinesia, neuroleptic malignant syndrome.
CVS:	Postural hypotension, peripheral α-adrenergic blockade, tachycardia, negative ionotropic action, prolonged PR and QT intervals, blunted T wave.
GI:	Jaundice, constipation, ↓ gastric secretion and motility.
Other:	Galactorrhea, agranulocytosis.
Dosage/ Concentrations:	Parenteral: 5 mg/ml. Oral solution (United States): 16 mg/5 ml. Syrup (Canada): 2 mg/5 ml. Tablets: 2, 4, 8, and 16 mg.
Adult:	5 mg IM q 6 hr.
Contraindications:	Bladder neck obstruction, prostatic hypertrophy, severe cardiac failure, narrow-angle glaucoma, pyloroduodenal obstruction.
Drug Interactions/ Allergy:	Additive actions with other CNS depressants.

PROCHLORPERAZINE

Trade Name:	Compazine
Indications:	Psychosis, nausea, and vomiting.
Pharmacokinetics:	$T_{1/2}$: β, 7 hr. Vd: 20 L/kg. Clearance: 33 ml/kg/min. Oral bioavailability: ~ 25% (poor).
Pharmacodynamics: *CNS:*	Sedative, tranquilizing, and antianxiety effects, ↑ ↑ prolactin secretion causing galactorrhea, ↓ seizure threshold, ↑ extrapyramidal reactions.

PROCHLORPERAZINE   *(continued)*

CVS:	Peripheral α-adrenergic blockade, tachycardia, negative inotropic action, prolonged PR and QT intervals, blunted T wave.
GI:	Jaundice, constipation, ↓ gastric secretion and motility.
Other:	Urinary retention (rare), inhibited ejaculation (but not erection).
Dosage/ Concentrations:	Oral: syrup, 5 mg/ml; extended-release capsules. Tablets: 5 mg. Rectal suppository: 2.5, 5, and 25 mg. Parenteral: available in Canada.
Adult:	5–10 mg IM q 3–4 hr.
Pediatric:	0.4 mg/kg/24 hr in 3–4 divided doses (0.13 mg/kg/ dose).
Contraindications:	Narrow-angle glaucoma, bone marrow depression, and severe liver or cardiac disease.
Drug Interactions/ Allergy:	Additive effects with other CNS depressants and anticonvulsants.

PROMETHAZINE

Trade Name:	Phenergan
Indications:	Allergy therapy, sedation-hypnosis preoperatively and in early labor, and nausea and vomiting.
Pharmacokinetics:	Adults: $T_{1/2}$: β, 13 hr. Vd: 13 L/kg. Clearance: 16.2 ml/kg/min. Oral bioavailability: ~ 25%. Child: $T_{1/2}$: β, 12.7 hr.
Pharmacodynamics:	H1-receptor antagonist.
CNS:	Dizziness, sedation, confusion, paradoxical excitation, ↑ extrapyramidal signs (in elderly).
Other:	↑ Prolactin secretion.
Dosage/ Concentrations:	Oral: Syrup: 6.25 and 25 mg/5 ml. Tablets: 12.5, 25, and 50 mg. Parenteral: 25 and 50 mg/ml. Suppository: 12.5, 25, and 50 mg.
Adult:	12.5–25 mg.
Pediatric:	>2 yr, 0.25–0.5 mg/kg oral or IM q 6 hr.
Geriatric:	↑ Susceptibility to CNS effects.
Contraindications:	Neonates, premature infants, and children <2 yr; pregnant women, lactating mothers, and geriatric patients.
Drug Interactions/ Allergy:	May potentiate actions of other CNS depressants and anticholinergics. Concurrent use of antithyroid drugs may increase risks of agranulocytosis. May block

α-adrenergic effects of epinephrine. May decrease seizure threshold with the use of metrizamide. May inhibit antiparkinsonian effects of levodopa.

TRIMETHOBENZAMIDE

Trade Name:	Tigan
Indications:	Nausea and vomiting.

Pharmacodynamics:
CNS: Parkinson-like symptoms, drowsiness, dizziness.
CVS: Hypotension.
GI: Potential for dystonic reactions.
Other: ↑ Risk of Reye's syndrome.

Dosage/ Concentrations: Oral (capsule): 100 and 250 mg. Suppository: 100 and 200 mg. Injection: 200-mg ampules.
Adult: 200–250 mg t.i.d.
Pediatric: <15 kg, 100 mg; >15 kg, 200 mg.

Contraindications: Injectable form in children and suppositories in premature and neonates.

Drug Interactions/ Allergy: Adverse reactions with concomitant use of alcohol. May mask symptoms of ototoxicity. Skin reactions.

Gastrokinetic Drugs

CISAPRIDE

Trade Name:	Propulsid

Pharmacokinetics: Adults: $T_{1/2}$: β, 6–12 hr. Vd: 180 L. Clearance: 100 cc/min. Onset: 30–60 min (oral). Elderly: Moderately prolonged $T_{1/2}$ β.

Indications: Nocturnal heartburn caused by gastroesophageal reflux disease.

Pharmacodynamics: 5-HT4 receptor agonist.
CNS: Extrapyramidal effects, fatigue, anxiety.
GI: ↑ Lower esophageal sphincter pressure, ↑ lower esophageal peristalsis, ↑ gastric emptying.

Dosage/ Concentrations:
Adult: 10–20 mg p.o. q.i.d. (15 min a.c. and h.s.)
Geriatric: Similar dose.

CISAPRIDE *(continued)*

Contraindications:	GI obstruction, perforation, or hemorrhage.
Drug Interactions/ Allergy:	Anticholinergics compromise effects of cisapride. $\uparrow$ Gastric emptying can affect rate of absorption of other drugs ($\downarrow$ effect of digoxin; $\downarrow$ effect of atropine). Coagulation times prolonged in patients receiving oral anticoagulants ($\uparrow$ toxicity of warfarin). GI absorption of cimetidine and ranitidine is accelerated by cisapride. Sedative effects of benzodiazepines and alcohol may be accelerated.

METOCLOPRAMIDE

Trade Name:	Reglan
Pharmacokinetics:	$T_{1/2}$: α, 5 min; β, 2.5–6 hr. Vd: 2.2–3.5 L/kg. Excretion: primarily through kidney. Onset: oral, 30–60 min; IM, 10–15 min; IV, 1–3 min. Peak effect: 1–2 hr following a single dose.
Indications:	Gastroesophageal reflux, postoperative and chemotherapy-induced nausea and vomiting; diabetic gastroparesis, small-bowel intubation, radiologic examination, and aspiration prophylaxis (preanesthetic agent).
Pharmacodynamics:	Potent central dopamine receptor antagonist.
CNS:	Sedation and lethargy, $\uparrow$ extrapyramidal reactions, $\uparrow$ parkinsonian symptoms.
CVS:	Antiarrhythmic effects (IV), mild hypertension.
GI:	$\uparrow$ Lower esophageal sphincter pressure, $\uparrow$ gastric emptying and intestinal transit.
Other:	Galactorrhea, amenorrhea, gynecomastia, impotence, $\uparrow$ secretion of prolactin.
Dosage/ Concentrations:	
Adult:	10–20 mg p.o., IM, IV (IV given over 1–2 min).
Pediatric:	0.1–0.25 mg/kg p.o., IM, IV.
Geriatric:	10 mg p.o., IM, IV. If creatinine clearance <40 ml/min, use half the recommended dose.
Contraindications:	Bowel obstruction, perforation, or hemorrhage; pheochromocytoma (may cause hypertensive crises); epilepsy; and concomitant drugs that cause dyskinesia or extrapyramidal reactions.
Drug Interactions/ Allergy:	Additive with other CNS depressants. Effects on GI motility are antagonized by anticholinergic drugs and narcotic analgesics. Use cautiously in patients receiving MAOIs (possible hypertension).

RELATIVE ANTIEMETIC ACTIVITY AND SIDE EFFECT PROFILES

Drug	Antiemetic Activity	Anti-cholinergic	Extra-pyramidal Reactions	Hypo-tension	Sedation
Chlorpromazine	+ + + +	+ + +	+ +	+ + + +	+ + + +
Promethazine	+ + + +			+	+ + + +
Perphenazine	+ + + +	+ +	+ + + +	+	+ +
Prochlorperazine	+ + + +	+	+ + + +	+	+ +
Cyclizine	+ + + +	+ + +	−	+	+
Hydroxyzine	+ + + +	+ +	+	+	+ + +
Diphenhydramine	+ +	+ +			+ +

8

Antihistamines

Julian A. Gold, M.D.
Michele E. Gold, C.R.N.A., Ph.D.

ASTEMIZOLE

Trade Name:	Hismanal
Indications:	Palliative suppression of nasal congestion, rhinitis, urticaria, and conjunctivitis and symptoms of drug allergy (pruritus, urticaria, angioedema).
Pharmacokinetics:	Absorption: Well absorbed from GI tract, reduced 60% when taken with meals. Maximal blood concentration: 2–4 hr. Extensively bound to plasma protein. $T_{1/2}$: 20 hr. Excretion: Metabolized in liver primarily to desmethylastemizole; active H1 compound with a 12-day half-life; eliminated more rapidly in children; eliminated more slowly in those with severe hepatic disease.
Pharmacodynamics:	Highly selective for H1 receptors.
CVS:	Inhibits vasoconstrictor effect of histamine; potential for QT prolongation and ventricular arrhythmias (i.e., torsades de pointes).
Pulmonary:	↓ Response of bronchial smooth muscle to histamine.
Hepatic:	Induced hepatic microsomal enzymes, thereby facilitating their own metabolism.
GI:	Loss of appetite, nausea, vomiting, diarrhea.
Musculoskeletal:	Inhibit most responses of smooth muscle to histamine.
Dosage/ Concentrations:	10 mg p.o. q.d.
Contraindications:	Known hypersensitivity to the drug.
Drug Interactions/ Allergy:	↑ Sedative effects with alcohol and barbiturates. Use cautiously with ketoconazole and erythromycin.

CHLORPHENIRAMINE

Trade Name:	Chlor-Trimeton
Indications:	Palliative suppression of nasal congestion, rhinitis, urticaria, and conjunctivitis; symptoms of drug allergy (pruritus, urticaria, angioedema); and symptoms of anaphylaxis or allergy to blood or plasma.
Pharmacokinetics:	Absorption: Well absorbed from GI tract. Maximal blood concentration: 2–3 hr. Effects last 4–6 hr. $T_{1/2}$: 8 hr. Excretion: Little excreted unchanged in urine, most excreted as metabolites; eliminated more rapidly in children; eliminated more slowly in those with severe hepatic disease.

CHLORPHENIRAMINE   *(continued)*

Pharmacodynamics:	H1 receptor antagonist.
CNS:	Sedation, excitement.
CVS:	Inhibited vasoconstrictor effect of histamine.
Pulmonary:	↓ Response of bronchial smooth muscle to histamine.
Hepatic:	Induced hepatic microsomal enzymes, thereby facilitating their own metabolism.
GI:	Loss of appetite, nausea, vomiting, diarrhea.
Musculoskeletal:	Inhibited responses of smooth muscle to histamine.
Other:	Dry mouth, cough, urinary retention.
Dosage/ Concentrations:	Oral: 4 mg q 4–6 hr; sustained-release formulations available; IV: Same dose.
Contraindications:	Known hypersensitivity to the drug.
Drug Interactions/ Allergy:	↑ Sedative effects of CNS depressants.

CIMETIDINE

Trade Name:	Tagamet
Indications:	Acid hypersecretion (i.e., Zollinger-Ellison syndrome, endocrine adenomas); duodenal, gastric, and stress ulcers; preoperative prophylaxis to reduce risk of acid pneumonitis; and reflux esophagitis.
Pharmacokinetics:	Absorption: Rapid oral absorption. Peak plasma concentrations: 45–90 min. Bioavailability: First-pass hepatic metabolism can limit bioavailability after oral dose. Also given IM or IV. Effects last 4–5 hr. $T_{1/2}$: 2 hr. Excretion: Minimal hepatic metabolism; after oral administration, 35%–60% eliminated unchanged; IM or IV administration 65%–75% eliminated unchanged; renal or hepatic dysfunction prolongs effects.
Pharmacodynamics:	H2 receptor antagonist.
CNS:	Headache, confusion, dizziness, somnolence in severely ill or elderly.
CVS:	Bradycardia, tachycardia, or AV block more likely after rapid IV dose.
Hepatic:	↑ Serum transaminases (dose-related).
Renal:	↑ Plasma concentration in patients with renal dysfunction.
GI:	Inhibited gastric acid secretion, ↓ hydrogen ion concentration, diarrhea.

| *Hematologic:* | Neutropenia, thrombocytopenia, agranulocytosis, aplastic anemia. |
| *Endocrine:* | Gynecomastia. |

| **Dosage/ Concentrations:** | For ulcer: 800 mg p.o. h.s. or 300 mg q.i.d.
 Preoperative prophylaxis:
 • Oral: 300 mg 1–2 hr before surgery, 300 mg h.s. before surgery.
 • IV: 150–300 mg |

| **Contraindications:** | Known hypersensitivity to the drug. |

| **Drug Interactions/ Allergy:** | ↓ Metabolism of β blockers, anticoagulants, cardiac glycosides, benzodiazepines, antiarrhythmics, and barbiturates. |

CLEMASTINE

Trade Name:	Tavist, Tavist-1, Tavist-D
Indications:	Palliative suppression of nasal congestion, rhinitis, urticaria, and conjunctivitis; and symptoms of mild drug allergy (pruritus, urticaria, angioedema).
Pharmacokinetics:	Absorption: Well absorbed after oral dose. Peak concentration: 2–5 hr. Effects last 10–12 hr. Excretion: Hepatic metabolism by methylation and glucuronide conjugation; eliminated in the urine.
Pharmacodynamics:	H1 receptor antagonist and anticholinergic activity.
CNS:	Sedation, headache, dizziness, disturbed coordination.
CVS:	Hypotension, tachycardia.
Pulmonary:	↓ Response of bronchial smooth muscle to histamine, thickened bronchial secretions.
GI:	Epigastric pain, nausea, vomiting, diarrhea.
Musculoskeletal:	Inhibited responses of smooth muscle to histamine.
Other:	Hemolytic anemia, thrombocytopenia, agranulocytosis, dry mouth, cough, urinary retention, dried nasal mucosa.
Dosage/ Concentrations:	Tavist, syrup: 0.5 mg/5 ml, 0.5–1 mg b.i.d. Tavist-1, 1.34 mg, 1–2 tablets t.i.d. Tavist 2.68 mg, 1 tablet t.i.d. Tavist-D with phenylpropanolamine: 1 tablet b.i.d.
Contraindications:	Known hypersensitivity to the drug. Use with caution in patients with bronchial asthma, hypertension, and increased intraocular pressure.
Drug Interactions/ Allergy:	↑ Sedative effects of CNS depressants. MAOIs may prolong anticholinergic effect.

CYPROHEPTADINE

Trade Name:	Periactin

Indications: Palliative suppression of nasal congestion, rhinitis, urticaria, and conjunctivitis; symptoms of mild drug allergy (pruritus, urticaria, angioedema); and symptoms of anaphylaxis and allergy to blood or plasma.

Pharmacokinetics: Absorption: Well absorbed after oral dose. Effects last 8 hr. Excretion: Hepatic metabolism by glucuronide conjugation.

Pharmacodynamics: H1 receptor antagonist.
CNS: Sedation, headache, dizziness, disturbed coordination.
CVS: Hypotension, tachycardia.
Pulmonary: ↓ Response of bronchial smooth muscle to histamine, thickened bronchial secretions.
GI: Epigastric pain, nausea, vomiting, diarrhea.
Musculoskeletal: Inhibited responses of smooth muscle to histamine.
Other: Hemolytic anemia, thrombocytopenia, agranulocytosis, dry mouth, cough, urinary retention.

Dosage/ Concentrations: Syrup, 2 mg/5 ml. Tablets, 4 mg. Dose: 4 mg t.i.d.

Contraindications: Known hypersensitivity to the drug. Use with caution in patients with bronchial asthma, hypertension, and increased intraocular pressure.

Drug Interactions/ Allergy: ↑ Sedative effects of hypnotics, sedatives, tranquilizers, or alcohol. MAOIs prolong anticholinergic effect.

DIPHENHYDRAMINE

Trade Name:	Benadryl

Indications: Palliative suppression of nasal congestion, rhinitis, urticaria, and conjunctivitis; symptoms of drug allergy (pruritus, urticaria, angioedema); symptoms of anaphylaxis and allergy to blood or plasma; and motion sickness.

Pharmacokinetics: Absorption: Well absorbed from GI tract. Maximal blood concentration: 2–3 hr. Effects last 4–6 hr. $T_{1/2}$: 8 hr. Excretion: Little excreted unchanged in urine, most excreted as metabolites; eliminated more rapidly in children; eliminated more slowly in those with severe hepatic disease.

Pharmacodynamics: H1 receptor antagonist.

CNS:	Sedation, excitement.
CVS:	Inhibited vasoconstrictor effect of histamine.
Pulmonary:	↓ Response of bronchial smooth muscle to histamine.
Hepatic:	Induced hepatic microsomal enzymes, thereby facilitating their own metabolism.
GI:	Loss of appetite, nausea, vomiting, diarrhea.
Musculoskeletal:	Inhibited responses of smooth muscle to histamine.
Other:	Significant antimuscarinic effect, dry mouth, cough, urinary retention.

Dosage/ Concentrations: Oral: 25–50 mg orally q 4–6 hr; sustained-release formulations available.
IV: Same dose.

Contraindications: Known hypersensitivity to the drug.

Drug Interactions/ Allergy: ↑ Sedative effects of CNS depressants.

FAMOTIDINE

Trade Name: Pepcid

Indications: Acid hypersecretion (i.e., Zollinger-Ellison syndrome, endocrine adenomas); duodenal and gastric ulcers; preoperative prophylaxis to reduce risk of acid pneumonitis; and reflux esophagitis.

Pharmacokinetics: Absorption: Rapid oral absorption: Peak plasma concentrations: 30–60 min. Bioavailability: First-pass hepatic metabolism can limit bioavailability after oral dose; also administered IM or IV. Effects last 10–12 hr. $T_{1/2}$: 2½–3½ hr. Excretion: 65%–70% excreted unchanged by the kidneys; 30%–35% undergoes hepatic metabolism. Renal dysfunction prolongs effects.

Pharmacodynamics: H2 receptor antagonist (8–10 times as potent as ranitidine).

CNS:	Grand mal seizure (rare), psychic disturbance.
CVS:	Bradycardia, tachycardia, or AV block after following rapid IV administration.
Pulmonary:	Bronchospasm.
Hepatic:	Liver enzyme abnormalities, cholestatic jaundice.
Renal:	↑ Plasma concentration in patients with renal dysfunction.
GI:	Inhibited gastric acid secretion; ↓ hydrogen ion concentration; diarrhea, nausea and vomiting, abdominal discomfort.
Other:	Leukopenia, thrombocytopenia, agranulocytosis, pancytopenia.

FAMOTIDINE   *(continued)*

Dosage/ Concentrations:	For ulcer: 40 mg p.o. h.s. or 20 mg b.i.d. Preoperative prophylaxis: Oral: 20–40 mg 1–2 hr before surgery, 20–40 mg h.s. before surgery. IV: 20 mg.
Contraindications:	Known hypersensitivity to the drug.
Drug Interactions/ Allergy:	None clinically significant.

HYDROXYZINE

Trade Name:	Atarax, Vistaril
Indications:	Anxiety and tension; symptoms of drug allergy (pruritus, urticaria, and dermatitis); and preoperative medication.
Pharmacokinetics:	Absorption: Well absorbed from GI tract. Effects last 4–6 hr. $T_{1/2}$: 20–25 hr. Excretion: Hepatic metabolism to active metabolite.
Pharmacodynamics: *CNS:* *CVS:* *Musculoskeletal:* *Other:*	H1 receptor antagonist. Drowsiness, tremor. Inhibited vasoconstrictor effect of histamine. Inhibited responses of smooth muscle to histamine. Dry mouth.
Dosage/ Concentrations:	25–100 mg q.i.d. Vistaril, oral suspension: 25 mg/5 ml. Vistaril, tablets 25, 50, 100 mg. Vistaril, parenteral solution: 25 mg/ml or 50 mg/ml.
Contraindications:	Known hypersensitivity to the drug.
Drug Interactions/ Allergy:	↑ Sedative effects of barbiturates, narcotics, and alcohol.

LORATADINE

Trade Name:	Claritin
Indications:	Palliative suppression of nasal congestion, rhinitis, urticaria, and conjunctivitis; and secondary treatment of asthma.
Pharmacokinetics:	Absorption: Well absorbed after oral dose. Onset: 27 min. Peak concentration 1–2 hr. Effects last 24 hr.

$T_{1/2}$: 7.8–11 hr. Excretion: Metabolized by cytochrome P_{450} to the active metabolite, descarboethoxyloratadine. Effects may be prolonged in the elderly and patients with hepatic disease.

Pharmacodynamics:	H1 receptor antagonist.
CNS:	Action mainly on peripheral H1 receptors.
Pulmonary:	Bronchodilatory activity with chronic use.
Musculoskeletal:	Inhibited responses of smooth muscle to histamine.
Dosage/ Concentrations:	10 mg q.d.
Contraindications:	Known hypersensitivity to the drug.
Drug Interactions/ Allergy:	Use cautiously with ketoconazole.

NIZATIDINE

Trade Name:	Axid
Indications:	Duodenal ulcers, reflux esophagitis, and preoperative prophylaxis to reduce the risk of acid pneumonitis; and reflux esophagitis.
Pharmacokinetics:	Absorption: Oral, with minimal first-pass effect. Peak plasma concentrations: 30 min–3 hr. Effects last up to 12 hr. $T_{1/2}$: 1–2 hr. Excretion: Minimal hepatic metabolism; 90% renal excretion with 60% excreted unchanged; renal dysfunction prolongs effects.
Pharmacodynamics:	H2 receptor antagonist.
CNS:	Dizziness, anxiety, nervousness, somnolence, mental confusion (rare).
CVS:	Asymptomatic ventricular tachycardia.
GI:	Inhibited gastric acid secretion; ↓ hydrogen ion concentration; diarrhea, nausea and vomiting.
Hepatic:	↑ SGOT, ↑ SGPT, ↑ alkaline phosphatase.
Renal:	↑ Plasma concentration in patients with renal dysfunction.
Other:	Anemia, thrombocytopenia.
Dosage/ Concentrations:	Oral: gelatin capsules For ulcer, 300 mg p.o. h.s. or 150 mg b.i.d.
Contraindications:	Known hypersensitivity to the drug.
Drug Interactions/ Allergy:	None clinically significant.

PROMETHAZINE

Trade Name:	Phenergan
Pharmacokinetics:	Absorption: Well absorbed from GI tract. Effects last 4–6 hr. Excretion: almost entirely hepatic metabolism.
Indications:	Anxiety and tension; symptoms of drug allergy (pruritus, urticaria, and dermatitis); symptoms of anaphylaxis and allergy to blood or plasma; preoperative medication, nausea and vomiting, dizziness.
Pharmacodynamics:	H1 receptor antagonist.
CNS:	Drowsiness and tremor, extrapyramidal symptoms.
CVS:	Tachycardia, bradycardia, hypertension, hypotension.
Hepatic:	Jaundice.
Other:	Thrombocytopenic purpura.
Dosage/ Concentrations:	25–50 mg. Oral suspension: 6.25 mg/5 ml or 25 mg/5 ml. Tablets: 12, 5, 25, and 50 mg. Parenteral solution; 25 mg/ml or 50 mg/ml.
Contraindications:	Known hypersensitivity to the drug.
Drug Interactions/ Allergy:	↑ Sedative effects of barbiturates, narcotics, sedatives, general anesthetics and alcohol. Avoid use with MAOIs. Intra-arterial injections can cause severe chemical irritation, vessel spasm, and gangrene.

RANITIDINE

Trade Name:	Zantac
Indications:	Acid hypersecretion (i.e., Zollinger-Ellison syndrome); duodenal, gastric, and stress ulcers; preoperative prophylaxis to reduce the risk of acid pneumonitis; and reflux esophagitis.
Pharmacokinetics:	Absorption: Rapid oral absorption. Peak plasma concentrations: 30–60 min. Bioavailability: first-pass hepatic metabolism can limit bioavailability after oral dose. Also given IM or IV. Effects last 8–12 hr. $T_{1/2}$: 2–2½ hr. Excretion: 30%–50% hepatic metabolism; 30%–50% eliminated unchanged in urine; renal or hepatic dysfunction prolongs effects.
Pharmacodynamics:	H2 receptor antagonist (5 times more potent than cimetidine).
CNS:	Headache, confusion, dizziness, somnolence; most common in severely ill and the elderly.

CVS:	Bradycardia, tachycardia, or AV block more likely after rapid IV dose.
Hepatic:	↑ Serum transaminases (dose-related)
Renal:	↑ Plasma concentration in patients with renal dysfunction, ↑ serum creatinine.
GI:	Inhibited gastric acid secretion; ↓ hydrogen ion concentration; diarrhea, constipation, nausea and vomiting, abdominal pain.
Other:	Leukopenia, thrombocytopenia, granulocytopenia, agranulocytosis (rare), aplastic anemia.
Dosage/ Concentrations:	For ulcer: 300 mg p.o. h.s. or 300 mg b.i.d. Preoperative prophylaxis: Oral: 150 mg 1–2 hr before surgery, 150 mg h.s. before surgery IV: 50 mg
Contraindications:	Known hypersensitivity to the drug.
Drug Interactions/ Allergy:	None clinically significant.

TERFENADINE

Trade Name:	Seldane, Seldane-D
Indications:	Palliative suppression of nasal congestion, rhinitis, urticaria, and conjunctivitis and secondary treatment of asthma.
Pharmacokinetics:	Absorption: Well absorbed after oral dose. Onset: 72 min. Peak concentration: 2 hr. Effects last 12 hr. Distribution $T_{1/2}$: 2–4 hr; plasma $T_{1/2}$: 17–20 hr. Excretion: First-pass hepatic metabolism by the cytochrome P_{450} system to an active acid metabolite and a dealkylated metabolite; 40% renal excretion, 60% fecal excretion.
Pharmacodynamics:	H1 receptor antagonist.
CNS:	Action mainly on peripheral H1 receptors.
CVS:	Arrhythmias (ventricular tachyarrhythmias, torsades de pointes, ventricular fibrillation), hypotension, palpitations, syncope.
Pulmonary:	Bronchospasm, bronchodilatory activity with chronic use.
Musculoskeletal:	Inhibited responses of smooth muscle to histamine.
Other:	Prolonged effect with hepatic dysfunction.
Dosage/ Concentrations:	Seldane: 60 mg b.i.d. Seldane-D (with pseudoephedrine): 60 mg b.i.d.

TERFENADINE   *(continued)*

Contraindications: Known hypersensitivity to the drug.

Drug Interactions/   Possible cardiotoxic effects with ketoconazole, trolean-
Allergy: domycin, or erythromycin therapy.

9

Antihypertensive Drugs

Michael H. Nathanson, F.R.C.A.

CAPTOPRIL

Trade Name:	Capoten
Indications:	Hypertension (alone or in combination with a diuretic); severe, refractory hypertension; and congestive heart failure.
Pharmacokinetics:	Peak plasma levels: 0.5–1.5 hr. Bioavailability: 65%. Protein binding: 30%. Vd: 0.7 L/kg. Clearance: 13 ml/min/kg. $T_{1/2}$: β, 1.9 hr. 95% urinary excretion.
Pharmacodynamics:	ACE inhibitor.
CNS:	Headache, fatigue.
CVS:	↓ BP, ↓ SVR, ↓ ↓ BP if sodium-depleted, angioedema.
Pulmonary:	Dry cough.
Renal:	Renal impairment, proteinuria.
GI:	Loss of taste.
Other:	Skin rash, blood dyscrasias.
Dosage/ Concentrations:	6.25–12.5 mg initially, then 25–100 mg/day p.o. in 2 to 3 doses. Reduce dose if sodium-depleted (e.g. diuretics), in renal impairment and in elderly.
Contraindications:	Porphyria, bilateral renovascular disease, and pregnancy.
Drug Interactions/ Allergy:	Enhanced hypotensive effects of anesthetic agents.

CLONIDINE

Trade Name:	Catapres
Indications:	Mild to moderate hypertension (combined with a diuretic), analgesia, and anesthesia.
Pharmacokinetics:	Peak plasma levels: 1–3 hr. Bioavailability: 100%. Protein binding: 20%–40%. Vd: 2.1 L/kg. Clearance: 3.1 ml/min/kg. $T_{1/2}$: β: 20–25 hr. 60% urinary excretion. 40% oxidative metabolism.
Pharmacodynamics:	Centrally acting α_2-adrenergic receptor agonist.
CNS:	Drowsiness, up to 50% ↓ MAC of inhalational agents, analgesia (epidural).
CVS:	↓ BP, ↓ SVR, ↓ HR, fluid retention.
GI:	Dry mouth, constipation.
Dosage/ Concentrations:	Oral: 0.2–0.8 mg/day in 2 to 3 doses. IV: 3–5 μg/kg. Epidural: 150 μg.

Contraindications:	Porphyria and Raynaud's syndrome.
Drug Interactions/ Allergy:	Withdrawal syndrome and rebound increased BP. Action antagonized by TCAs.

ENALAPRIL

Trade Name:	Vasotec
Indications:	Hypertension (usually in combination with a diuretic); severe, refractory hypertension; and congestive heart failure.
Pharmacokinetics:	Prodrug for active metabolite enalaprilat. Peak plasma levels: 4 hr. Bioavailability: 40%. Protein binding: 50%. Vd: 1.7 L/kg. Clearance: 4.9 ml/min/kg. $T_{1/2}$: β, 35 hr. 60% urinary excretion.
Pharmacodynamics:	ACE inhibitor.
CNS:	Headache, fatigue.
CVS:	↓ BP, ↓ SVR, ↓ ↓ BP if sodium-depleted, angio-edema.
Pulmonary:	Dry cough.
Renal:	Renal impairment.
GI:	Loss of taste, nausea and diarrhea.
Other:	Skin rash.
Dosage/ Concentrations:	2.5–5.0 mg initially, then 5–40 mg/day p.o. in 1 to 2 doses. Reduce dose if sodium-depleted (e.g., diuretics), in renal impairment and in elderly.
Contraindications:	Porphyria, bilateral renovascular disease, and pregnancy.
Drug Interactions/ Allergy:	Enhanced hypotensive effects of anesthetic agents.

GUANABENZ

Trade Name:	Wytensin
Indications:	Moderate to severe hypertension.
Pharmacokinetics:	Peak plasma levels: 2–5 hr. Protein binding: 90%. 75% absorbed from GI tract, first-pass metabolism ↓ bioavailability. Vd: 100 L/kg. Clearance: 1.3 ml/min/kg. $T_{1/2}$: β, 14 hr. Extensive metabolism. 80% urinary excretion.
Pharmacodynamics:	Centrally acting α_2-adrenergic receptor agonist.

GUANABENZ   *(continued)*

CNS:	Sedation, dizziness.
CVS:	↓ BP, ↓ SVR, ↓ HR.
GI:	Dry mouth.

Dosage/
Concentrations: 8–32 mg/day p.o. in 2 doses. Reduce dose in elderly.

Drug Interactions/   Withdrawal syndrome and rebound increased BP. En-
Allergies: hanced action of other antihypertensive agents, particu-
larly β blockers.

GUANADREL

Trade Name:	Hylorel
Indications:	Moderate to severe hypertension.
Pharmacokinetics:	Peak plasma levels: 1.5–2.0 hr. Protein binding: 20%. Vd: 11.5 L/kg. Clearance: 38 ml/min/kg. $T_{1/2}$: β, 5–45 hr. 85% urinary excretion.
Pharmacodynamics:	Adrenergic-neuron blocking agent.
CVS:	↓ BP, ↓ SVR, orthostatic hypotension, fluid retention.
GI:	Diarrhea.
Other:	Retrograde ejaculation.
Dosage/ **Concentrations:**	20–75 mg/day in 2 to 4 doses.
Drug Interactions/ **Allergy:**	Increased sensitivity to catecholamines. Action antagonized by TCAs and phenothiazines. MAOIs increase BP.

GUANETHIDINE MONOSULFATE

Trade Name:	Ismelin
Indications:	Severe drug-resistant hypertension (combined with a diuretic).
Pharmacokinetics:	Incomplete and variable absorption. Bioavailability: 20%. Protein binding: <10%. Clearance: high. $T_{1/2}$: β, 43 hr. 25%–50% urinary excretion.
Pharmacodynamics:	Adrenergic-neuron blocking agent.
CVS:	↓ BP, ↓ SVR, ↓ cardiac output, fluid retention, orthostatic hypotension, transient ↑ BP after IV dose.
Pulmonary:	Nasal congestion.

GI:	Diarrhea.
Other:	Delayed ejaculation.

Dosage/ Concentrations:	10–50 mg/day p.o. once daily. Reduce dose in elderly.
Contraindications:	Pheochromocytoma.
Drug Interactions/ Allergy:	Action antagonized by TCAs, phenothiazines, and indirect-sympathomimetic agents. MAOIs increase BP. Hypotensive effects of general anesthesia enhanced. Potentiates oral hypoglycemic agents.

GUANFACINE

Trade Name:	Tenex
Indications:	Mild to moderate hypertension (usually combined with a diuretic).
Pharmacokinetics:	Peak plasma levels: 1–4 hr. Bioavailability: 100%. Protein binding: 64%. Vd: 6.5 L/kg. Clearance: 2.6–5.2 ml/min/kg. $T_{1/2}$: β, 12–22 hr. 30%–40% urinary excretion.
Pharmacodynamics:	Centrally acting α_2-adrenergic receptor agonist.
CNS:	Sedation, confusion.
CVS:	↓ BP, ↓ SVR, orthostatic hypotension.
GI:	Dry mouth, constipation.
Other:	Impotence.
Dosage/ Concentrations:	0.5–3.0 mg/day p.o. once daily (at night).
Drug Interactions/ Allergy:	Withdrawal syndrome (minor rebound increased BP).

LISINOPRIL

Trade Name:	Zestril
Indications:	Hypertension (usually in combination with a diuretic); severe, refractory hypertension; and congestive heart failure.
Pharmacokinetics:	Peak plasma levels: 6–8 hr. Bioavailability: 30%. Protein binding: minimal. Vd: 1.8 L/kg. Clearance: 1.5 ml/min/kg. $T_{1/2}$: β, 12 hr. 100% urinary excretion.
Pharmacodynamics:	ACE inhibitor.

LISINOPRIL   *(continued)*

CNS:	Headache, fatigue.
CVS:	↓ BP, ↓ SVR, ↓ ↓ BP if sodium-depleted, angio-edema.
Pulmonary:	Dry cough.
Renal:	Renal impairment.
GI:	Nausea, diarrhea.

Dosage/ Concentrations: 2.5–5.0 mg initially, then 5–40 mg/day p.o. once daily. Reduce dose if sodium-depleted (e.g., diuretics), in renal impairment and in elderly.

Contraindications: Porphyria, bilateral renovascular disease, and pregnancy.

Drug Interactions/ Allergy: Enhanced hypotensive effects of anesthetic agents.

MECAMYLAMINE

Trade Name:	Inversine

Indications: Moderate to severe hypertension and malignant hypertension.

Pharmacokinetics: Well absorbed from GI tract.
Onset: 0.5–2 hr. 50% urinary elimination.

Pharmacodynamics:	Ganglion-blocking agent.
CNS:	Drowsiness, hallucinations, tremor.
CVS:	↓ BP, ↓ SVR, ↓ cardiac output, orthostatic hypotension.
Renal:	Urinary retention.
GI:	Dry mouth, constipation.
Other:	Impotence, glaucoma.

Dosage/ Concentrations: 5–25 mg/day p.o. in 2 to 3 doses.

Drug Interactions/ Allergy: Subarachnoid anesthesia. Decreased action of neostigmine and pyridostigmine in myasthenia gravis.

METHYLDOPA

Trade Name:	Aldomet

Indications: Hypertension.

Pharmacokinetics: Incomplete and variable absorption. Bioavailability: 25%. Protein binding: 15%. Vd: 0.60 L/kg. Clearance:

	3.1 ml/min/kg. $T_{1/2}$: β, 1.38 hr. Hepatic metabolism. Urinary excretion.
Pharmacodynamics:	Centrally acting $α_2$-adrenergic receptor agonist via $α_2$-methylnorepinephrine and $α_2$-methylepinephrine.
CNS:	Sedation, dizziness.
CVS:	↓ BP, ↓ SVR, orthostatic hypotension, fluid retention.
Hepatic:	Abnormal LFTs, necrosis.
GI:	Dry mouth, colitis.
Other:	Positive Coombs' test, hemolytic anemia, drug fever.
Dosage/ Concentrations:	250–2000 mg/day p.o. in 2 to 4 doses. Reduce dose in elderly.
Contraindications:	Acute liver disease and porphyria.
Drug Interactions/ Allergy:	Hypotensive effects of general anesthesia enhanced. Use with MAOIs can cause hyperexcitability and increased BP.

METYROSINE (α-METHYLTYROSINE)

Trade Name:	Demser
Indications:	Preoperative treatment of pheochromocytoma and inoperable pheochromocytoma.
Pharmacokinetics:	Well absorbed from GI tract. Onset: delayed (2–3 days). $T_{1/2}$: β, 3.4–7.2 hr. 69% urinary excretion.
Pharmacodynamics:	Inhibits tyrosine hydroxylase (↓ catecholamine synthesis).
CNS:	Drowsiness, extrapyramidal movements.
CVS:	↓ BP.
Renal:	Crystalluria.
GI:	Dry mouth, nausea and vomiting, diarrhea.
Other:	Impotence.
Dosage/ Concentrations:	1–4 g/day p.o. in 4 doses for 5–7 days prior to surgery.
Drug Interactions/ Allergy:	Arrhythmias during general anesthesia. ↑ action of phenothiazines.

RESERPINE

Trade Name:	Serpasil
Indications:	Hypertension and Raynaud's phenomenon (intra-arterial).

RESERPINE *(continued)*

Pharmacokinetics:	Bioavailability: 30%. Onset: delayed (2–6 wk). $T_{1/2}$: β, 1–2 wk. Extensive metabolism. Slow excretion in urine and feces.
Pharmacodynamics:	Adrenergic-neuron blocking agent.
CNS:	Sedation, nightmares and suicidal depression.
CVS:	↓ BP, ↓ SVR, ↓ cardiac output, ↓ HR.
Pulmonary:	Nasal congestion.
GI:	Abdominal cramps and diarrhea.
Dosage/ Concentrations:	0.1–1.0 mg/day p.o. in 2 doses.
Contraindications:	Depression, colitis.
Drug Interactions/ Allergy:	Hypersensitivity to direct-acting sympathomimetics.

TRIMETHAPHAN

Trade Name:	Arfonad
Indications:	Intraoperative control of hypertension and induced hypotension.
Pharmacokinetics:	Onset: 1–3 min. Duration of action: 5–15 min. 30% urinary excretion.
Pharmacodynamics:	Ganglion-blocking agent.
CVS:	↓ BP, ↓ SVR, ↓ cardiac output, ↑ HR, orthostatic hypotension.
Renal:	Urinary retention.
GI:	Dry mouth, constipation, paralytic ileus.
Other:	Cycloplegia.
Dosage/ Concentrations:	IV: 0.5–6.0 mg/min.
Contraindications:	Severe arteriosclerotic disease.
Drug Interactions/ Allergy:	Inhibits pseudocholinesterase.

10

Antimicrobial Agents

Carl E. Noe, M.D.

ACYCLOVIR*

Trade Name:	Zovirax
Indications:	Herpes simplex encephalitis and other viral infections.
Pharmacokinetics:	Vd: 0.69 ± 0.19 L/kg. Clearance: 0.37 (creatinine); 0.41 ml/min/kg. $T_{1/2}$: 2.4 ± 0.7 hr. Urinary excretion: 75% ± 10%.
Pharmacodynamics:	Viricidal action by inhibition of DNA synthesis.
Dosage/ Concentrations:	IV: up to 10 mg/kg q 8 hr; infusion over 1 hr.
Contraindications:	Allergic reaction.
Drug Interactions/ Allergy:	Encephalopathy with interferon or methotrexate.

AMPHOTERICIN B

Trade Name:	Fungizone
Indications:	Fungal sepsis, pneumonia, and meningitis.
Pharmacokinetics:	Vd: 0.076 ± 0.52 L/kg. Clearance: 0.46 ± 0.20 ml/min/kg. $T_{1/2}$: 18 ± 7 hr. Urinary excretion: 2%–5%.
Pharmacodynamics: Renal: Other:	Disruption of fungal cell membrane impermeability. Renal toxicity, potassium wasting. Fever, rigors.
Dosage/ Concentrations:	IV: After a test dose of 1 mg, dissolved in 20 ml of 5% dextrose, is infused over 20–30 min, escalate dose up to 0.5 to 1.0 mg/kg/day in 3–4 divided doses. If a severe reaction occurs, 0.1 mg/kg per dose; then dose may be increased by 5–10 mg/day as tolerated.
Contraindications:	Life-threatening allergy.
Drug Interactions/ Allergy:	Renal toxicity, potentiated by aminoglycosides.

---

*The information in this chapter has been adapted from USP DI. Copyright 1994. The USP Convention, Inc. with permission.

AMPICILLIN

Trade Names:	Omnipen, Polycillin, Amicill, Unasyn

Indications: Extended-spectrum penicillin (with aminoglycoside), for endocarditis prophylaxis with high-risk patients in pharyngeal or GU procedures; first-line empirical therapy for (with or without aminoglycoside) *Streptococcus agalactiae* (group B) in bacteremia and meningitis; (with aminoglycoside) *Listeria monocytogenes* in meningitis and bacteremia; *Enterococcus* in UTI; (with aminoglycoside) *Enterococcus* in endocarditis or other serious infection (bacteremia); (with beta-lactamase inhibitor); *Branhamella catarrhalis* in otitis, sinusitis, and pneumonia; *Actinomyces israelii* in cervicofacial, abdominal, thoracic, and other lesions; (with aminoglycoside) *Escherichia coli* in UTI and bacteremia; *Proteus mirabilis* in UTI; second-line empirical therapy for (with sulbactam) *Corynebacterium* sp. aerobic and anaerobic (diphtheroids) in endocarditis, infected foreign bodies, and bacteremia; (with sulbactam) *Bacteroides fragilis* in abscesses; (with a penicillinase inhibitor) *E. coli* in UTI and bacteremia; (with a penicillinase inhibitor) *Proteus* sp. in UTI; *Haemophilus influenzae* in otitis media, sinusitis, bronchitis, epiglottitis, pneumonia, and meningitis; third-line empirical therapy for *Salmonella* in typhoid fever, paratyphoid fever, and bacteremia; *Shigella* in acute gastroenteritis; (with a penicillinase inhibitor) *Klebsiella pneumoniae* in pneumonia.

Pharmacokinetics: Vd: 0.28 ± 0.07 L/kg. Clearance: 1.7 (creatinine) + 0.21 ml/min/kg. $T_{1/2}$: 1.3 ± 0.2 hr. Urinary excretion: 82% ± 10%. Fetal/maternal serum concentration: 0.5–1.0. Maternal milk/plasma concentration: 0.5–1.0.

Pharmacodynamics: Bactericidal inhibition of cell wall synthesis.
CNS: Toxicity, myoclonic twitching, seizures.
Renal: Interstitial nephritis.
Other: Eosinophilia, bone marrow suppression.

Dosage/Concentrations: For high-risk endocarditis prophylaxis: Preoperative IV: ampicillin, 2 g, plus gentamicin, 1.5 mg/kg up to 80 mg, followed by oral regimen.

For low-risk endocarditis prophylaxis: Oral: amoxicillin, 50 ml/kg up to 3 g 1 hr before surgery and 25 ml/kg up to 1.5 g q 6 hr after initial dose.

Adult and Adolescent: IM or IV: 250 to 500 mg (base) q 6 hr.

For bacterial meningitis, septicemia: IM or IV: 1 to 2 g (base) q 3–4, 18.75 to 25 mg/kg q 3 hr or 25 to 33.3 mg/kg q 4 hr. Limit: up to 300 mg (base)/kg, or 16 g daily.

AMPICILLIN   *(continued)*

Pediatric:

- Infant up to 20 kg (body weight): IM or IV: 6.25 to 25 mg (base)/kg q 6 hr or 8.3 to 33.3 mg/kg q 8 hr.
- Infant and child ≥ 20 kg. Same as adult and pediatric dose.

  For bacterial meningitis, or septicemia: IM or IV: 18.75 to 25 mg (base)/kg q 3 hr, or 25 to 33.3 mg/kg q 4 hr. Some infants and children may require up to 400 mg (base)/kg daily in divided doses, depending on severity of infection.

Contraindications: β-lactam allergy (penicillins, cephalosporins, imipenem).

Drug Interaction/   Synergism with aminoglycosides against enterococcus.
Allergy: With sulbactam, ampicillin (Unasyn) is a penicillinase inhibitor.

AZTREONAM

Trade Name: Azactam

Indications: Gram-negative coverage; a substitute for aminoglycoside in infections if nephrotoxicity and ototoxicity is a concern; second-line empirical therapy for *Klebsiella pneumoniae* in pneumonia; *Serratia* in nosocomial and opportunistic infections; *Escherichia coli* in bacteremia and other infections, *Enterobacter* sp. in UTI; third-line empirical therapy for *Pseudomonas aeruginosa* in UTI; *Proteus* sp. in UTI.

Pharmacokinetics: Vd: 0.11–0.21 L/kg. $T_{1/2}$: 1.7 hr.

Pharmacodynamics: Interaction with penicillin-binding proteins.

Dosage/
Concentrations:
Adult and Adolescent: IV, > 20–60 min, 2 g q 6–8 hr. Limit: up to maximum of 8 g daily. For severe infection, 2 g q 6–8 hr.

  Adults with impaired renal clearance require a reduced dose as follows:

Creatinine Clearance	Loading Dose	Maintenance Dose
(ml/min)		
>30		Usual adult and adolescent dose
10–30	1–2 g	½ of loading dose
<10	500 mg–2 g	¼ of loading dose. In serious or life-threatening infections, additional ⅛ of loading dose after each hemodialysis period

Pediatric:	2 g q 6–8 hr.
Contraindications:	Allergy.
Drug Interactions/ Allergy:	Rare.

CHLORAMPHENICOL

Trade Name:	Chloromycetin
Indications:	First-line empirical therapy for *Salmonella* in typhoid fever, paratyphoid fever, and bacteremia; *Haemophilus influenzae* in epiglottitis, pneumonia, and meningitis; *Yersinia pestis* in sepsis; *Rickettsia* in typhus fever, murine fever, Brill's disease, and Rocky Mountain spotted fever, Q fever, and rickettsial pox; second-line empirical therapy for (with streptomycin) *Pseudomonas mallei* in glanders; *Pseudomonas pseudomallei* in melioidosis; *Chlamydia psittaci* in psittacosis (ornithosis); third-line empirical therapy for *Streptococcus agalactiae* in meningitis; *Streptococcus* (anaerobic sp.) in bacteremia, endocarditis, brain and other abscesses, and sinusitis; *Streptococcus pneumoniae* (pneumococcus) in meningitis, pneumonia, arthritis, sinusitis, and otitis; *Neisseria meningitidis* (meningococcus) in meningitis and bacteremia; *Listeria monocytogenes* in bacteremia; *Bacillus anthracis* in malignant pustule; *Erysipelothrix rhusiopathiae* in erysipeloid; *Clostridium perfringens* in gas gangrene; *Brucella* in brucellosis; *Yersinia pestis* in plague; *Francisella tularensis* in tularemia; *Vibrio cholerae* in cholera; *Bacteroides fragilis* in brain abscess, lung abscess, intra-abdominal abscess, empyema, bacteremia, and endocarditis; *Fusobacterium nucleatum* in ulcerative pharyngitis, lung abscess, empyema, genital infections, and gingivitis; *Bacteroides* sp. (oral, pharyngeal) in oral disease, sinusitis, brain abscess, and lung abscess; *Streptobacillus moniliformis* in bacteremia, arthritis, endocarditis, and abscesses.
Pharmacokinetics:	Vd: 0.95 $\pm$ 0.06 L/kg. Clearance: 2.4 $\pm$ 0.2 ml/min/kg. $T_{1/2}$: 4.0 $\pm$ 2.0 hr. Urinary excretion: 25% $\pm$ 15%.
Pharmacodynamics: *Hematologic:*	Inhibition of protein synthesis. Bone marrow suppression.

CHLORAMPHENICOL   *(continued)*

Dosage/ Concentrations:	
Adult:	50–100 mg/day in 4 divided doses.
Pediatric:	• Neonate: <2 kg or <1 wk: IV, 25 mg/kg/day.
	• Neonate: >2 kg or >1 wk: IV, 25 mg/kg q 12 hr.
	• Infant: 50–100 mg/day in 4 divided doses.
Contraindications:	Pregnancy, leukopenia, severe anemia, thrombocytopenia, and allergy.
Drug Interactions/ Allergy:	Bone marrow suppression warrants serum level monitoring.

CIPROFLOXACIN

Trade Name:	Cipro
Indications:	First-line empirical therapy for *Pseudomonas aeruginosa* in UTI; *Salmonella* in acute gastroenteritis; *Shigella* in acute gastroenteritis; *Campylobacter jejuni* in enteritis; second-line empirical therapy for *Escherichia coli* in UTI; *Legionella pneumophila* in legionnaires' disease; and third-line empirical therapy for (with rifampin) *Staphylococcus aureus* in abscesses, bacteremia, endocarditis, pneumonia, meningitis, osteomyelitis, and cellulitis; enterococcus in UTI; *Neisseria gonorrhoeae* (gonococcus) in penicillinase-producing and penicillin-sensitive strains; *Neisseria meningitidis* (gonococcus) in post-treatment carrier state; *Branhamella catarrhalis* in otitis, sinusitis, and pneumonia; *Haemophilus influenzae* in otitis media, sinusitis, and bronchitis; *Francisella tularensis* in tularemia; and *Vibrio cholerae* in cholera.
Pharmacokinetics:	Vd: 1.8 ± 0.4 L/kg. Clearance: 6.0 ± 1.2 ml/min/kg. $T_{1/2}$: 4.1 ± 0.9 hr. Urinary excretion: $65\% \pm 12\%$.
Pharmacodynamics:	Interference with DNA synthesis.
Dosage/ Concentrations:	
Adult:	IV, 400 mg q 12 hr over at least 60 min, up to 750 mg b.i.d. If creatinine clearance is 5–30 ml/min, reduce to 200–400 mg q 18–24 hr.
Pediatric:	Not recommended in infants, children, or adolescents.
Contraindications:	Allergy; prepubertal children and pregnant or breast-feeding women.

Drug Interactions/ Allergy:	↑ Bleeding in patients taking warfarin. Inhibition of theophylline metabolism. Synergism against *P. aeruginosa* with imipenem or anti-*Pseudomonas* penicillin (but not with aminoglycoside).

CLINDAMYCIN

Trade Name:	Cleocin
Indications:	First-line empirical therapy for anaerobic coverage; *Fusobacterium nucleatum* in ulcerative pharyngitis, lung abscess, empyema, genital infections, and gingivitis; *Bacteroides fragilis* (and other spp.) in brain abscess, lung abscess, intra-abdominal abscess, empyema, bacteremia, and endocarditis; second-line empirical therapy for *Streptococcus* (anaerobic sp.) in bacteremia, endocarditis, abscesses, and sinusitis; *Clostridium perfringens* and other spp. in gas gangrene; third-line empirical therapy for *Streptococcus pneumoniae* (pneumococcus) in pneumonia, arthritis, sinusitis, and otitis; penicillin-resistant *Staphylococcus; Corynebacterium diphtheriae* in pharyngitis, laryngotracheitis, pneumonia, and other local lesions; *Campylobacter jejuni* in enteritis.
Pharmacokinetics:	Vd: 1.1 ± 0.3 L/kg. Clearance: 4.7 ± 1.3 ml/min/kg. $T_{1/2}$: 2.9 ± 0.7 hr. Urinary excretion: ~87%.
Pharmacodynamics: *GI:* *Musculoskeletal:*	Bacteriostatic inhibition of protein synthesis. Pseudomembranous colitis. Neuromuscular blocking effects.
Dosage/ Concentrations: Adult and Adolescent:	Antibacterial, IM or IV: 300–600 mg (base) q 6–8 hr; or 900 mg q 8 hr.
Pediatric:	• Infants ≤ 1 month: antibacterial, IM or IV: 3.75 to 5 mg (base)/kg q 6 hr or 5 to 6.7 mg/kg q 8 hr.
	• Infants ≥ 1 month: IM or IV: 3.75 to 10 mg (base)/kg or 87.5 to 112.5 mg/m^2 q 6 hr or 5–13.3 mg/kg or 116.7–150 mg/m^2 q 8 hr.
	• Children: Regardless of body weight, minimum recommended dose is 300 mg (base) daily for severe infections. For bone infections: IM or IV, 7.5 mg/kg q 6 hr. Infants: 3.75–10 mg/kg q 6 hr.
Contraindications:	Allergy; infants younger than 1 month of age.
Drug Interactions/ Allergy:	Rare.

ERYTHROMYCIN, ERYTHROMYCIN GLUCEPTATE

Trade Name: Ilotycin Gluceptate

Indications: First-line empirical therapy for *Corynebacterium diphtheriae* in carrier state; *Legionella pneumophila* in legionnaires' disease; *Mycoplasma pneumoniae* in "atypical pneumonia"; second-line empirical therapy for *Streptococcus pneumoniae* (pneumococcus) in pneumonia, arthritis, sinusitis, and otitis; *Streptococcus pyogenes* in pharyngitis, scarlet fever, otitis media, sinusitis, cellulitis, erysipelas, pneumonia, bacteremia, and other systemic infections; *Bacillus anthracis* in malignant pustule and pneumonia; *C. diphtheriae* in pharyngitis, laryngotracheitis, pneumonia, and other local lesions; *Erysipelothrix rhusiopathiae* in erysipeloid; *Borrelia recurrentis* in relapsing fever; *Ureaplasma urealyticum* in nonspecific urethritis; *Chlamydia trachomatis* in lymphogranuloma venereum, trachoma, inclusion conjunctivitis (blennorrhea), and nonspecific urethritis; *Chlamydia pneumoniae* in pneumonia; third-line empirical therapy for *Staphylococcus aureus* in abscesses, bacteremia, endocarditis, pneumonia, meningitis, osteomyelitis, and cellulitis; *Streptococcus agalactiae* in bacteremia; penicillin-sensitive *Neisseria gonorrhoeae*; *Streptococcus* (anaerobic species) in bacteremia, endocarditis, brain abscess, and sinusitis; *Listeria monocytogenes* in bacteremia; *Clostridium tetani* in tetanus; *Streptobacillus moniliformis* in bacteremia, arthritis, endocarditis, and abscesses; *Actinomyces israelii* in cervicofacial, abdominal, thoracic, and other lesions; *Branhamella catarrhalis* in otitis, sinusitis, and pneumonia; *Bacteroides* sp. (oral, pharyngeal) in oral disease, sinusitis, brain abscess, and lung abscess; *Fusobacterium nucleatum* in ulcerative pharyngitis, lung abscess, empyema, genital infections, and gingivitis.

Pharmacokinetics: Vd: 0.78 ± 0.44 L/kg. Clearance: 9.1 ± 4.1 ml/min/kg. $T_{1/2}$: 1.6 ± 0.7 hr. Urinary excretion: $12 \pm 7\%$. Fetal/maternal serum concentration: < 0.3. Maternal milk/plasma concentration: 0.5–1.0.

Pharmacodynamics: Inhibition of protein synthesis.
CNS: Transient auditory impairment.
Hepatic: Cholestatic hepatitis.
GI: Upper gastric distress.
Other: Eosinophilia, fever, skin eruptions.

**Dosage/
Concentrations:**

Adult and Adolescent: Antibacterial (systemic), IV: 250 to 500 mg (base) q 6 hr, or 3.75 to 5 mg/kg q 6 hr. Limit: Up to 4 g (base) daily; doses up to 6 g (base) daily have been used.

Pediatric: Antibacterial (systemic) IV: 3.75 to 5 mg (base)/kg q 6 hr.

Contraindications: Allergy and pregnancy.

**Drug Interactions/
Allergy:** Potentiated effects of carbamazepine, corticosteroids, cyclosporine, digoxin, and warfarin. $\uparrow$ Theophylline concentration.

GENTAMICIN

Trade Name: Garamycin

Indications: First-line empirical therapy for *Enterobacter* sp. in UTI; *Proteus* sp. (other than *mirabilis*) in UTI; *Acinetobacter* in nosocomial infections; *Yersinia enterocolitica* in sepsis; (with ampicillin) *Enterococcus* in endocarditis and bacteremia; (with ampicillin) *Escherichia coli* in UTI and bacteremia; (with penicillin G) *Streptococcus* (viridans group) in endocarditis (bacteremia); (with ampicillin or penicillin) *Listeria monocytogenes* in meningitis and bacteremia; (with broad-spectrum penicillin) *Pseudomonas aeruginosa* in pneumonia and bacteremia; (with cephalosporin) *Klebsiella pneumoniae* in pneumonia; second-line empirical therapy for (with vancomycin) *Enterococcus* in endocarditis and bacteremia; *E. coli* in UTI and bacteremia; *Proteus mirabilis* in UTI; *P. aeruginosa* in UTI; *K. pneumoniae* in UTI.

Pharmacokinetics: Vd: 0.31 ± 0.10 L/kg. Clearance: 0.82 (creatinine) + 0.11 ml/min/kg. $T_{1/2}$: 2–3 hr. Terminal $T_{1/2}$: 53 ± 25 hr (necessitating drug level monitoring). Urinary excretion: > 90%. Fetal/maternal serum concentration: 0.3–0.5 trough drug levels to remain below 2 μg/ml, peak <10 μg/ml. Drug levels: 30 min, 1, 3, 8 hr after loading; then periodically with trough levels; can be used for pharmacokinetic monitoring.

Pharmacodynamics: Inhibition of ribosomal protein synthesis.
CVS: Ototoxicity.
Renal: Renal toxicity, $\downarrow$ sensitivity of collecting duct to ADH.
Musculoskeletal: Neuromuscular blocking effects.

GENTAMICIN   *(continued)*

**Dosage/
Concentrations:**

Adult and Adolescent: Monitor serum levels. Antibacterial (systemic), IV: 1
to 1.7 mg (base)/kg q 8 hr for 7–10 days or more.
   After hemodialysis: supplemental dose of 1–1.7 mg
(base)/kg, depending on severity of infection.
   For severe, life-threatening infections: up to 8 mg
(base)/kg daily.

Pediatric: Dosing intervals may vary from q 4 hr to q 24 hr.
Monitor serum levels. Antibacterial (systemic); IV:
- Premature or full-term neonates ≤ 1 wk of age: 2.5
  mg (base)/kg q 12–24 hr for 7–10 days or more.

- Older Neonates and Infants: 2.5 mg (base)/kg q
  8–16 hr for 7–10 days or more.

- Children: 2–2.5 mg (base)/kg q 8 hr for 7–10 days
  or more.

After hemodialysis: supplemental dose of 2–2.5 mg
(base)/kg, depending on severity of infection.

Contraindications: Allergy and myasthenia gravis.

**Drug Interactions/
Allergy:**   Synergism with bactericidal drugs with a different
mechanism of action (with penicillin or ampicillin
against enterococcus, nafcillin against *Staphylococcus*,
and ticarcillin against *Pseudomonas*). Antagonism with
bacteriostatic drugs (tetracycline, erthromycin, sulfon-
amide).

IMIPENEM-CILASTATIN

Trade Name: Primaxin

Indications: Anaerobic and broad-spectrum coverage, including
Pseudomonas; third-line empirical therapy for *Enterobacter* and *Proteus* spp. in UTI and other infections;
Pseudomonas aeruginosa in pneumonia and bacteremia; *Klebsiella pneumoniae* in pneumonia;
Bacteroides fragilis in brain abscess, lung abscess, intra-abdominal abscess, empyema, bacteremia, and endocarditis.

Pharmacokinetics: Imipenem: Vd: 0.23 ± 0.05 L/kg. Clearance: 2.9 ± 0.3 ml/min/kg. $T_{1/2}$: 0.9 ± 0.1 hr. Urinary excretion:
$69\% \pm 15\%$. Cilastatin: Vd: 0.20 ± 0.03 L/kg. Clear-
ance: 3.0 ± 0.3 ml/min/kg. $T_{1/2}$: 0.8 ± 0.1 hr. Urinary
excretion: $70\% \pm 3\%$.

Pharmacodynamics:	Imipenem: inhibited bacterial cell wall synthesis. Cilastatin: Inhibited renal metabolism.
CNS:	Seizures.
GI:	Nausea, vomiting.

**Dosage/
Concentrations:**

Adult and Adolescent: 500 mg q 6 hr to 1 g q 6–8 hr.

Adults with impaired renal function may require a reduced dose as follows:

Creatinine Clearance (ml/min/1.73 m²)	**Dose**
>70	Adult and Adolescent dose
30–70	500 mg q 6–8 hr
20–30	500 mg q 8–12 hr
0–20	250–500 mg q 12 hr

After hemodialysis: supplemental dose unless next dose is scheduled within 4 hr.

Limit: Up to maximum of 50 mg (imipenem)/kg or 4 g daily, whichever is lower.

Pediatric:	Not established.
Contraindications:	Allergy to either drug.
Drug Interactions/ Allergy:	Antagonism with other β-lactams. Synergism with aminoglycoside against *Pseudomonas*.

METRONIDAZOLE

Trade Name:	Flagyl
Indications:	First-line empirical therapy for *Bacteroides fragilis* in brain, lung, and intra-abdominal abscesses; (oral) for *Clostridium difficile* in antibiotic-associated colitis; second-line empirical therapy for *Bacteroides* (oral) sp. in oral infections, sinus infections, and brain and lung abscesses; *Fusobacterium nucleatum* in ulcerative pharyngitis, lung abscess, empyema, genital infection, gingivitis, trichomonal infection, amebiasis, and giardiasis.
Pharmacokinetics:	Vd: 0.74 ± 0.10 L/kg. Clearance: 0.3 ± 0.3 ml/min/kg. $T_{1/2}$: 8.5 ± 2.9 hr. Urinary excretion: 10% ± 2%. Maternal milk/plasma concentration: 0.5–1.0.
Pharmacodynamics:	Acceptance of electrons from electron transport chain of normal metabolism.
CNS:	Neurotoxicity with numbness or paresthesia.
Other:	Neurotropenia, cancer (in animals).

METRONIDAZOLE   *(continued)*

Dosage/ Concentrations:	IV: loading dose, 15 mg/kg, followed by 7.5 mg/kg q 6 hr.
Contraindications:	Pregnancy and breast-feeding.
Drug Interactions/ Allergy:	Disulfiram-like reaction to alcohol.

NAFCILLIN

Trade Name:	Unipen
Indications:	Penicillinase-resistant penicillin; first-line empirical therapy for *Staphylococcus* in abscesses, bacteremia, endocarditis, pneumonia, meningitis, osteomyelitis, and cellulitis.
Pharmacokinetics:	Penicillinase-resistant penicillin. Vd: 0.35 ± 0.09 L/kg. Clearance: 7.5 ± 1.9 ml/min/kg. $T_{1/2}$: 1.0 ± 0.21 hr. Renal excretion: 27% ± 5%. Fetal/maternal serum concentration: < 0.3.
Pharmacodynamics: *CNS:* *Other:*	Inhibition of cell wall synthesis. Toxicity, myoclonic twitching, seizures. Eosinophilia, bone marrow suppression.
Dosage/ Concentrations: Pediatric:	Adult and Adolescent: IM 500 mg (base) q 4–6 hr. IV: 500 mg–1.5 g (base) q 4 hr. Limit: IM: up to 12 g (base) daily. IV: up to 20 g (base) daily. • Neonates: IM: 10–20 mg (base)/kg q 12 hr. IV: 10–20 mg (base)/kg q 4 hr, or 20–40 mg/kg q 8 hr. • Older Infants and Children: IM: 25 mg (base)/kg q 12 hr. IV: 10 to 20 mg (base)/kg q 4 hr, or 20–40 mg/kg q 8 hr. Some pediatric patients may require up to 200 mg (base)/kg daily in divided doses. For renal dysfunction and dialysis: no need to modify dose.
Contraindications:	β-lactam allergy (penicillin, cephalosporin, imipenem) and jaundice in premature neonates.
Drug Interactions/ Allergy:	Synergism with aminoglycosides against *Staphylococcus*.

PENICILLIN G

Trade Name:	Wycillin

Indications: First-line empirical therapy for *Streptococcus pyogenes* in pharyngitis, scarlet fever, otitis media, sinusitis, cellulitis, erysipelas, pneumonia, bacteremia, and other systemic infections; *Streptococcus* (viridans group) in endocarditis (bacteremia); *Streptococcus agalactiae* (group b) in bacteremia and meningitis; *Streptococcus bovis* in endocarditis, bacteremia; *Streptococcus* (anaerobic sp.) in bacteremia, endocarditis, brain abscess, and sinusitis; *Streptococcus pneumoniae* (pneumococcus) in pneumonia, arthritis, sinusitis, otitis; meningitis and other serious infections; *Enterococcus* in UTI; (with aminoglycoside) *Enterococcus* in endocarditis and other serious infections; penicillin-sensitive *Neisseria gonorrhoeae*, *Neisseria meningitidis* (meningococcus) in meningitis; *Bacillus anthracis* in "malignant pustule" and pneumonia; *Corynebacterium diphtheriae* in pharyngitis, laryngotracheitis, pneumonia, and other lesions; (with aminoglycoside) *Corynebacterium* sp., aerobic and anaerobic (diphtheroids) in endocarditis, infected foreign bodies, and bacteremia; (with or without aminoglycoside) *Listeria monocytogenes* in meningitis; *Erysipelothrix rhusiopathiae* in bacteremia; *Clostridium perfringens* and other spp. in gas gangrene; *Clostridium tetani* in tetanus; *Pasteurella multocida* in wound infection (animal bites), abscesses, bacteremia, and meningitis; *Bacteroides* sp. (oral, pharyngeal) in oral disease, sinusitis, brain abscess, and lung abscess; *Fusobacterium nucleatum* in ulcerative pharyngitis, lung abscess, empyema, genital infections, and gingivitis; *Streptobacillus moniliformis* in bacteremia, arthritis, endocarditis, and abscesses; *Treponema pallidum* in syphilis; *Treponema pertenue* in yaws; *Borrelia burgdorferi* in stage 2 Lyme disease (neurologic and cardiac symptoms, arthritis); *Leptospira* in Weil's disease and meningitis; *Actinomyces israelii* in cervicofacial, abdominal, thoracic, and other lesions; second-line empirical therapy for *C. diphtheriae* in carrier state; (with rifampin) *Corynebacterium* sp. aerobic and anaerobic diphtheroids in carrier state; *B. burgdorferi* in stage 1 Lyme disease (erythema chronica migrans, skin); third-line empirical therapy for *Borrelia recurrentis* in relapsing fever.

Pharmacokinetics: Vd: 0.35 L/kg. Clearance: 3 million U (1.8 g)/hr in adults with normal renal function. $T_{1/2}$: adult, 0.5 hr; neonate, 3 hr. Anuria: 10 hr. Renal excretion: 60%–

PENICILLIN G   *(continued)*

90%. Fetal/maternal serum concentration: 0.5–1.0. Maternal milk/plasma concentration: <0.3.

Pharmacodynamics:	Bactericidal inhibition of bacterial cell wall synthesis.
CNS:	Myoclonic twitching, seizures, dizziness, tinnitus, headache, hallucinations.
Hepatic:	Hepatitis.
Renal:	Interstitial nephritis, hyperkalemia (in renal failure).
Other:	Bone marrow depression, eosinophilia, granulocytopenia, platelet inhibition, fever.

**Dosage/
Concentrations:**

Adult and Adolescent: IM or IV: 1 million to 5 million U (base) q 4–6 hr.

For meningococcal meningitis: 1 million to 2 million U (base) q 2 hr or IV infusion, 20 million to 30 million U (base) daily.

Limit: Up to 100 million U (base) daily.

Pediatric:
- Premature and Full-Term Neonates: IM or IV: 30,000 U (base)/kg body weight q 12 hr.

- Older Infants and Children: IM or IV: 4167 to 16,667 U (base)/kg q 4 hr; or 6250 to 25,000 U (base)/kg q 6 hr.

Some infants and children may require up to 400,000 U (base)/kg daily in divided doses, depending on severity of infection.

Contraindications: β-lactam allergy (penicillin, cephalosporin, imipenem).

**Drug Interactions/
Allergy:**   Synergism with aminoglycosides. ↑ Drug levels with probenecid.

TETRACYCLINE

Trade Name: Terramycin

Indications: First-line empirical therapy *Pseudomonas mallei* in glanders; *Yersinia pestis* in plague; *Vibro cholerae* in cholera; *Borrelia burgdorferi* in Lyme disease; *Borrelia recurrentis* in relapsing fever; *Calymmatobacterium granulomatis* in granuloma inguinale; *Ureaplasma urealyticum* in nonspecific urethritis; *Rickettsia* in typhus fever, murine typhus, Brill's disease, Rocky Mountain spotted fever, Q fever, and rickettsial pox; *Chlamydia psittaci* (ornithosis) in psittacosis; *Chlamydia trachomatis* in lymphogranuloma venereum and nonspecific urethritis; second-line empirical therapy for *Neisseria* *gonorrhoeae* (gonococcus) in penicillin-sensitive; *Bacillus anthracis* in malignant pustule and pneumonia; *Erysipelothrix rhusiopathiae* in erysipeloid; *Clostridium tetani* in tetanus; *Yersinia pestis* in plague; *Francisella tularensis* in tularemia; *Pasteurella multocida* in wound infection (animal bites), abscesses, bacteremia, and meningitis; *Streptobacillus moniliformis* in bacteremia, arthritis, endocarditis, and abscesses; *Treponema pertenue* in yaws; *Leptospira* in Weil's disease and meningitis; *Actinomyces israelii* in cervicofacial, abdominal, and thoracic and other lesions; third-line empirical therapy for *Branhamella catarrhalis* in otitis, sinusitis, and pneumonia; *Listeria monocytogenes* in bacteremia; *Clostridium perfringens* and other spp. in gas gangrene; *Escherichia coli* in UTI; *Haemophilus ducreyi* in chancroid; *Campylobacter jejuni* in enteritis; *Bacteroides* sp. (oral, pharyngeal) in oral disease and sinusitis, brain abscess, and lung abscess; *Fusobacterium nucleatum* in ulcerative pharyngitis, lung abscess, empyema, genital infections, and gingivitis; *Treponema pallidum* in syphilis; *B. burgdorferi* in stage 2 Lyme disease (neurologic and cardiac symptoms, arthritis).

Pharmacokinetics: Vd: 1.5 ± 0.08 L/kg. Clearance: 1.67 ± 0.24 mg/min/kg. $T_{1/2}$: 10.6 ± 1.5 hr. Urinary excretion: 58% ± 8%.

Pharmacodynamics: Inhibition of bacterial protein synthesis.
CNS: Phototoxicity.
Renal: Toxicity.
Hepatic: Toxicity.
GI: Bowel mucosa irritation, diarrhea (versus pseudomembranous colitis from overgrowth of *C. difficile*).
Musculoskeletal: Dental discoloration, ↓ linear bone growth in premature infants.

Dosage/ Concentrations:
Adult: 10–20 mg/kg daily in divided doses up to 2 g/day for severe infection.
Pediatric:
- Child <45 kg: 4.4 mg/kg on first day as loading dose; reduce to 2 mg/kg or less q 12 hr.

- Child >8 yr: 10–20 mg/kg daily in divided doses up to 2 g/day for severe infection.

Contraindications: Children < 8 yr.

Drug Interactions/ Allergy: Phototoxicity.

TICARCILLIN

Trade Names:	Ticar, Timentin
Indications:	Broad-spectrum coverage and first-line empirical therapy for (with aminoglycoside) *Pseudomonas aeruginosa* in pneumonia and bacteremia; *P. aeruginosa* in UTI; second-line empirical therapy for *Enterobacter* sp. in UTI; *Proteus* sp. (other than *mirabilis*) in UTI.
Pharmacokinetics:	Vd: $0.21 + 0.03$ L/kg. Clearance: 2.0 ± 0.2 ml/min/kg. $T_{1/2}$: 1.3 ± 0.1 hr. Urinary excretion: 92% $\pm$ 2%.
Pharmacodynamics:	Bactericidal inhibition of cell wall synthesis.
CNS:	Toxicity, myoclonic twitching, seizures.
CVS:	Congestive heart failure.
Renal:	Fluid retention, compensatory hypokalemia, interstitial nephritis.
Other:	Platelet dysfunction.

**Dosage/
Concentrations:**

Adult and Adolescent:

For septicemia, pneumonia, skin and soft tissue, intra-abdominal, and GU tract infections: IV infusion: 3 g (base) q 3–6 hr; 25–37.5 mg/kg q 3 hr; 33.3–50 mg/kg q 4 hr; or 50–75 mg/kg q 6 hr.

After an initial loading dose of 3 g, adults with impaired renal function may require a reduced dose as follows:

Creatinine Clearance (ml/min)/(ml/sec)	Dose (Base)
>60	3 g q 4 hr
30–60	2 g q 4 hr
10–30	2 g q 8 hr
<10	2 g q 8 hr
<10 with impaired hepatic function	2 g q 24 hr

Limit: Up to 500 mg (base)/kg daily.

Pediatric:
- Neonates up to 2 kg: IM or IV: 100 mg (base)/kg initially, then 75 mg/kg q 8 hr during first week of life; followed by 100 mg/kg q 4 hr thereafter.
- Neonates ≥2 kg: IM or IV: 100 mg (base)/kg initially, then 75 mg/kg q 4–6 hr during first 2 weeks of life, followed by 100 mg/kg q 4 hr thereafter.
- Older children up to 40 kg: IV: 33.3 to 50 mg (base)/kg q 4 hr, or 50 to 75 mg/kg q 6 hr.

Contraindications:	β-Lactam allergy (penicillin, cephalosporin, imipenem).
Drug Interactions/ Allergy:	Synergism with aminoglycoside against *Pseudomonas*.

TRIMETHOPRIM-SULFAMETHOXAZOLE

Trade Names:	Bactrim, Septra
Indications:	First-line empirical therapy for pneumonia in patients with AIDS or at high risk for AIDS; *Escherichia coli* in UTI; *Haemophilus influenzae* in otitis, sinusitis, and bronchitis; *Salmonella* in typhoid fever, paratyphoid fever, and bacteremia; *Haemophilus ducreyi* in chancroid; *Yersinia enterocolitica* in yersiniosis; *Pseudomonas pseudomallei* in melioidosis; *Pneumocystis carinii* in pneumonia in impaired host; *Nocardia asteroides* in abscess and lesions; second-line empirical therapy for *Branhamella catarrhalis* in otitis, sinusitis, and pneumonia; *Listeria monocytogenes* in meningitis; *Salmonella* in acute gastroenteritis; *Shigella* in gastroenteritis; *Brucella* in brucellosis; *Vibrio cholerae* in cholera; *Flavobacterium meningosepticum* in meningitis; *Calymmatobacterium granulomatis* in granuloma inguinale; *Legionella pneumophila* in legionnaires' disease; third-line empirical therapy for *Staphylococcus aureus* in abscesses, bacteremia, endocarditis, pneumonia, and meningitis, osteomyelitis, and cellulitis; *Streptococcus pneumoniae* (pneumococcus) in pneumonia, arthritis, sinusitis, and otitis; *E. coli* in bacteremia; *Klebsiella pneumoniae* in UTI; *Enterobacter* sp. in UTI and other infections; and *H. influenzae* in epiglottitis, pneumonia, and meningitis.
Pharmacokinetics:	Sulfamethoxazole: Vd: 0.21 ± 0.02 L/kg. Clearance: 0.32 ± 0.04 ml/min/kg. $T_{1/2}$: 10.1 ± 4.6 hr. Urinary excretion: $14\% \pm 2\%$. Trimethoprim: Vd: 1.8 ± 0.2 L/kg. Clearance: 2.2 ± 0.6 ml/min/kg. $T_{1/2}$: 11 ± 1.4 hr. Urinary excretion: $69\% \pm 17\%$.
Pharmacodynamics:	Inhibition of folic acid synthesis.
Hepatic:	Jaundice.
GI:	Glossitis, stomatitis.
Other:	Megaloblastosis, leukopenia or thrombocytopenia, exfoliative dermatitis, toxic epidermal necrolysis, Stevens-Johnson syndrome.
Dosage/ Concentrations:	
Adult:	For pneumocystis: 20 mg/kg/day trimethoprim, 100 mg/kg; sulfamethoxazole in equally divided doses q 6 hr for 21 days if AIDS is present.
Pediatric:	IV: 8 mg/kg trimethoprim; 40 mg/kg sulfamethoxazole in 2 divided doses.
Contraindications:	Folate deficiency.

TRIMETHOPRIM-SULFAMETHOXAZOLE   *(continued)*

Drug Interactions/ Allergy:	Rare.

VANCOMYCIN

Trade Name:	Vancocin
Indications:	First-line empirical therapy for methicillin-resistant *Staphylococcus aureus* in abscesses, bacteremia, endocarditis, pneumonia, meningitis, osteomyelitis, cellulitis, and other serious infections; *Clostridium difficile* in antibiotic-associated colitis; *Flavobacterium meningosepticum* in meningitis; second-line empirical therapy for *Enterococcus* in endocarditis or other serious infection (bacteremia) and UTI.
Pharmacokinetics:	Vd: 0.39 ± 0.06 L/kg. Clearance: 0.79 (creatinine) + 0.22 ml/min/kg. $T_{1/2}$: 5.6 ± 1.8 hr. Urinary excretion: 79% ± 11%. Peak effect: 1–2 hr after infusion; 20–50 μg/ml; trough levels, 5–10 μg/ml.
Pharmacodynamics: *CNS:* *CVS:* *Renal:*	Inhibition of cell wall synthesis. ↑ ICP, ototoxicity. Hypotension, histamine release. Nephrotoxicity.
Dosage/ Concentrations: Adult: Pediatric:	IV doses should be monitored. 1 g q 12 hr (if renal function normal). • Neonates: <1 wk: IV, 15 mg/kg q 12 hr. • Infants: 1 wk–1 month: 15 mg/kg q 8 hr. • Older infants and children: 10 mg/kg q 6 hr. For dialysis patients: 1 g q week with monitoring.
Contraindications:	Rapid IV administration in volume-depletion or hypotension.
Drug Interaction/ Allergy:	Additive toxicity and aminoglycosides. Hypotension with or without sign of histamine release (red man syndrome) can be avoided by infusing less than 500 mg/ hr.

First-Generation Cephalosporins

CEFAZOLIN

Trade Names:	Ancef, Kefzol
Indications:	Gram-positive coverage.
Pharmacokinetics:	Vd: 0.12 ± 0.03 L/kg. Clearance: 0.95 ± 0.17 ml/min/kg. $T_{1/2}$: 1.8 ± 0.4 hr. Urinary excretion: 80% ± 16%. Fetal/maternal serum and milk concentration: <0.3.
Pharmacodynamics:	Inhibition of bacterial cell wall synthesis.

**Dosage/
Concentrations:**

Adult and Adolescent: IV: 250 mg–1.5 g (base) q 6–8 hr.

For perioperative prophylaxis: IV infusion, 1 g (base) ½–1 hr before surgery.

After surgery: 500 mg–1 g q hr for up to 24 hr.

After initial loading dose of 500 mg, adults with impaired renal function may require a reduced dose as follows:

Creatinine Clearance (ml/min)	Dose
>55	Usual adult dose
35–54	Full dose q 8 hr or less frequently
11–34	½ usual dose q 12 hr
<10	½ usual dose q 18–24 hr

Pediatric:

- Premature infants and neonates up to 1 month: Not appropriate
- Infants and children 1 month of age and over: IV: 6.25 to 25 mg (base)/kg q 6 hr; or 8.3 to 33.3 mg/kg q 8 hr.

After an initial loading dose, children with impaired renal function may require a reduced dose as follows:

Creatinine Clearance (ml/min)	Dose
>70	Usual pediatric dose
40–70	7.5–30 mg/kg q 12 hr
20–40	3.125–12.5 mg/kg q 12 hr
5–20	2.5–10 mg/kg q 24 hr

Contraindications:	β-Lactam allergy.
Drug Interactions/ Allergy:	Rare.

Second-Generation Cephalosporins

CEFOXITIN

Trade Name:	Mefoxin
Indications:	Surgical prophylaxis and anaerobic coverage.
Pharmacokinetics:	Vd: 0.31 ± 0.12 L/kg. Clearance: 3.3 (creatinine) + 0.19 ml/min/kg. $T_{1/2}$: 0.65 ± 0.09 hr. Urinary excretion: 78%.
Pharmacodynamics:	Inhibition of bacterial cell wall synthesis.
Renal:	Nephrotoxicity.
Other:	Bone marrow suppression with pancytopenia.

Dosage/
Concentrations:

Adult:

For mild or uncomplicated infection: IV: 1 g (base) q 6–8 hr.

For moderately severe or severe infection: IV: 1 g (base) q 4 hr or 2 g q 6–8 hr.

For life-threatening infection: IV: 2 g (base) q 4 hr; or 3 g q 6 hr.

For perioperative prophylaxis, cesarean section: IV: 2 g (base) as soon as umbilical cord is clamped; followed by 2 g 4 hr and 8 hr after first dose.

For perioperative prophylaxis: IV: 2 g (base) ½–1 hr before start of surgery and 2 g q 6 hr after surgery for up to 24 hr.

After initial loading dose of 1 to 2 g (base), adults with impaired renal function may require a reduced dose as follows:

Creatinine Clearance (ml/min)	Dose (Base)
30–50	1–2 g q 8–12 hr
10–29	1–2 g q 12–24 hr
5–9	500 mg–1 g q 12–24 hr
<5	500 mg–1 g q 24–48 hr

Limit: up to 12 g (base) daily.

Pediatric:

- Infants up to 3 months of age: Not established.

- Infants and children up to 3 months of age and over: IV: 13.3 to 26.7 mg (base)/kg q 4 hr or 20 to 40 mg/kg q 6 hr.

For perioperative prophylaxis (>3 months of age): IV: 30–40 mg (base)/kg ½–1 hr before start of surgery and 30–40 mg/kg q 6 hr after surgery for up to 24 hr.

Limit: total daily dose not to exceed 12 g (base). Up to 2 g q 4 hr.

| Contraindications: | Allergy to beta-lactams. |
| Drug Interactions/ Allergy: | Disulfiram-like intolerance of alcohol. |

CEFUROXIME, CEFUROXIME AXETIL

Trade Names:	Zinacef, Kefurox, Ceftin
Indications:	First-line empirical therapy for epiglottitis; second-line empirical therapy for *Streptococcus pneumoniae* (pneumococcus) in meningitis and other serious infections; penicillinase-producing *Neisseria gonorrhoeae* (gonococcus); *Neisseria meningitidis* (meningococcus) in meningitis and bacteremia; *Branhamella catarrhalis* in otitis, sinusitis, and pneumonia; *Haemophilus influenzae* in otitis media, sinusitis, and bronchitis.
Pharmacokinetics:	Cefuroxime sodium: Vd: 0.19 ± 0.04 L/kg. Clearance: 0.94 (creatinine) $\pm$ 0.28 ml/min/kg. $T_{1/2}$: 1.7 ± 0.6 hr. Urinary excretion: $96\% \pm 10\%$.
Pharmacodynamics: *Renal:* *Other:*	Inhibition of bacterial cell wall synthesis. Toxicity. Bone marrow suppression with pancytopenia.
Dosage/ Concentrations: Pediatric:	• Neonates: 10–33.3 mg/kg q 8 hr. • Infants >3 months: 16.7–33.3 mg/kg q 8 hr. Cefuroxime sodium: up to 3 g q 8 hr. Cefuroxime axetil (Ceftin): up to 500 mg q 12 hr.
Contraindications:	β-Lactam allergy.
Drug Interactions/ Allergy:	Rare.

Third-Generation Cephalosporins

CEFOPERAZONE

Trade Name:	Cefobid
Indications:	Broad-spectrum, gram-negative coverage in biliary tree.
Pharmacokinetics:	Vd: 0.09 ± 0.01 L/kg. Clearance: 1.2 ± 0.1 ml/min/kg. $T_{1/2}$: 2.1 ± 0.3 hr.

CEFOPERAZONE   *(continued)*

Pharmacodynamics:	Bactericidal inhibition of cell wall synthesis.
Renal:	Toxicity.
Other:	Bleeding, bone marrow suppression with pancytopenia.

**Dosage/
Concentrations:**

Adult:

    For mild to moderate infection: 1 to 2 g (base) q 12 hr.

    For severe infection: 2 to 4 g (base) q 8 hr or 3 to 6 g q 12 hr.

    For impaired hepatic function or biliary obstruction: not more than 4 g (base) daily.

    For combined hepatic and renal function impairment: not more than 1–2 g (base) daily.

    For patients receiving hemodialysis: dose should follow session.

    Limit: up to 12 g (base) daily (although up to 16 g daily has been given by continuous infusion in severely immunocompromised patients without adverse effect).

Pediatric: Not established.

Contraindications:	None.
**Drug Interactions/
Allergy:**	Disulfiram-like intolerance of alcohol (as noted with cefamandole, cefotetan, moxalactam).

CEFTAZIDIME

Trade Name:	Fortaz
Indications:	In conjunction with aminoglycoside, coverage against *Pseudomonas* and other gram-negative organisms.
Pharmacokinetics:	Vd: 0.23 ± 0.02 L/kg. Clearance: 1.05 (creatinine) + 0.12 ml/min/kg. $T_{1/2}$: 1.6 ± 0.1 hr. Urinary excretion: 84% ± 4%.
Pharmacodynamics:	Bactericidal inhibition of cell wall synthesis.
Renal:	Toxicity.
Other:	Bone marrow suppression with pancytopenia.

**Dosage/
Concentrations:**

Adult and Adolescent: IV: 500 mg–2 g q 8–12 hr.

    For severe infection: 2 g q 8 hr.

    After initial loading dose of 1 g, adults (including dialysis patients) with impaired renal function may require a reduced dose as follows:

Creatinine Clearance (ml/min)	Dose
>50	Usual adult and adolescent dose
31–50	1 g q 12 hr
16–30	1 g q 24 hr
6–15	500 mg q 24 hr
<5	500 mg q 48 hr

Hemodialysis patients:	1 g after each hemodialysis period
Peritoneal dialysis patients:	500 mg q 24 hr

Pediatric:
- Neonates up to 4 wk: IV: 30 mg/kg q 12 hr.
- Infants 1 month–12 yr: IV: 30–50 mg/kg q 8 hr.

Limit: maximum total daily dose not to exceed 6 g.

Contraindications: Allergy.

Drug Interactions/ Allergy: Disulfiram-like intolerance of alcohol.

CEFTRIAXONE

Trade Name: Rocephin

Indications: Coverage against susceptible organisms when a relatively long $T_{1/2}$ is clinically useful; first-line empirical therapy for *Neisseria gonorrhoeae* (gonococcus) in penicillinase-producing strains; second-line empirical therapy for *N. gonorrhoeae* (gonococcus) in penicillin-sensitive strains; *Neisseria meningitidis* (meningococcus) in carrier state (post-treatment); *Haemophilus ducreyi* in chancroid; *Treponema pallidum* in syphilis; third-line empirical therapy for *Borrelia burgdorferi* in Lyme disease (erythema chronica migrans, skin).

Pharmacokinetics: Vd: 0.16 ± 0.03 L/kg. Clearance: 0.24 ± 0.06 ml/min/kg. $T_{1/2}$: 7.3 ± 1.6 hr. Urinary excretion: 46 ± 7%.

Pharmacodynamics: Bactericidal inhibition of bacterial cell wall synthesis.
Renal: Toxicity.
GI: Biliary sludge.
Other: Bone marrow suppression with pancytopenia.

Dosage/ Concentrations:
Adult and Adolescent: IV: 1–2 g (base) q 24 hr or 500 mg–1 g q 12 hr.
Limit: Up to 4 g (base) daily.

CEFTRIAXONE   *(continued)*

Pediatric: IV: 25–37.5 mg (base)/kg q 12 hr, with or without a
                              loading dose of 75 mg/kg or 80 mg/kg q 12 hr for 3
                              doses, then every 24 hr.
                                  Limit: maximum total daily dose not to exceed 4 g
                              (base) for meningitis or 2 g for other infections.

Contraindications: β-Lactam allergy.

Drug Interactions/   Disulfiram-like intolerance of alcohol.
Allergy:

11

Antineoplastics and Immunosuppressants

Yifeng Ding, M.D.

Antineoplastics

AMINOGLUTETHIMIDE

Trade Name:	Cytadren
Indications:	Breast and prostatic carcinoma, Cushing syndrome.
Pharmacokinetics:	Absorption: Rapidly and completely absorbed after oral administration. Vd: 76 L. Clearance: 3.49 L/hr. $T_{1/2}$: α, 15.5 hr.
Pharmacodynamics:	Inhibition of enzymatic conversion of cholesterol to pregnenolone and inhibition of estrogen production from androgens.
CNS:	Lethargy, somnolence, vertigo, nystagmus, ataxia.
CVS:	Orthostatic hypotension, tachycardia.
Hepatic:	↑ SGPT, ↑ SGOT.
GI:	Vomiting.
Musculoskeletal:	Myalgia.
Other:	Leukopenia, agranulocytosis.
Dosage/ Concentrations:	Tablets: 100 per bottle. Each tablet contains 250 mg of aminoglutethimide. Dose: 250 mg p.o. q.i.d.
Contraindications:	None known.
Drug Interactions/ Allergy:	↑ Clearance rates of warfarin, antipyrine, theophylline, and digitoxin.

ASPARAGINASE

Trade Name:	Elspar
Indications:	Induction of remission of acute lymphocytic leukemia in children.
Pharmacokinetics:	Vd: minimal distribution out of the vascular compartment. Clearance: rapid binding of enzyme to perivascular and intravascular binding sites slowly and unpredictably cleared from the plasma; poor extravascular tissue penetration. $T_{1/2}$: α, 4–9 hr; β, 1.4–1.8 days.
Pharmacodynamics:	Breakdown of asparagine, to aspartic acid and ammonia and interference with protein, DNA, and RNA synthesis.
CNS:	Confusion, drowsiness, hallucination, mental depression, nervousness, and unusual tiredness (mostly in adults).

CVS:	Hypotension.
Pulmonary:	Laryngeal constriction, asthma.
Hepatic:	Liver function abnormalities, fatty hepatocellular meta-morphosis, hypoalbuminemia.
Renal:	Hyperuricemia or uric acid nephropathy, renal failure.
GI:	Nausea, vomiting, weight loss, acute pancreatitis.
Other:	Slight anemia, leukopenia, or thrombocytopenia, ↓ blood clotting factors.

Dosage/Concentrations: Sterile 10-ml vial containing 10,000 IU of asparaginase and 80 mg mannitol. Asparaginase, 1000 IU/kg/day IV, for 10 successive days beginning on day 22 of treatment period in combination with other chemotherapeutic agents.

Contraindications: Pancreatitis or a history of pancreatitis.

Drug Interactions/Allergy: Anaphylactic or hypersensitivity reaction (laryngeal constriction, hypotension, diaphoresis, edema, asthma, loss of consciousness).

BUSULFAN

Trade Name: Myleran

Indications: Chronic myelogenous leukemia.

Pharmacokinetics: Adults: Vd: 0.60 L/kg. Clearance: 95 ml/min/m². $T_{1/2}$: α, 2.3 hr. Children: Vd: 1.42 L/kg. Clearance: 197 ml/min/m². $T_{1/2}$: α, 1.5 hr.

Pharmacodynamics: Alkylation, cross-linking of DNA strands, and myelosuppression.

CNS:	Generalized seizure.
CVS:	Endocardial fibrosis.
Pulmonary:	Interstitial pulmonary fibrosis.
Hepatic:	Transient ↑ hepatic enzymes; fatal hepatoveno-occlusive disease; hyperbilirubinemia.
Renal:	Cytologic dysplasia of renal tubule cells.
GI:	Nausea and vomiting, cheilosis, glossitis, anhidrosis.
Other:	Transient autoimmune disorders (rash, arthritis), pancytopenia.

Dosage/Concentrations: Tablet: 2 mg. Dose: 4–8 mg/day for several weeks.

Contraindications: Prior resistance to the drug.

Drug Interactions/Allergy: None known.

CARMUSTINE

Trade Name:	BiCNU
Indications:	Brain tumor, multiple myeloma, Hodgkin's disease, and non-Hodgkin's lymphomas.
Pharmacokinetics:	Vd: 3.25 L/kg. Clearance: 56 ml/min/m^2. T$_{1/2}$: α, 6.1 min; β, 21.5 min.
Pharmacodynamics:	Alkylation and interference with DNA and RNA function.
CNS:	Encephalopathy, seizures, hyperprolactinemia, dementia.
CVS:	Thrombophlebitis.
Pulmonary:	Pulmonary fibrosis, severe interstitial pneumonitis, frequent opportunistic infections.
Hepatic:	↑ Transaminase, ↑ alkaline phosphatase, ↑ bilirubin levels.
Renal:	Azotemia, ↓ kidney size, renal failure.
GI:	Transient nausea and vomiting.
Other:	Delayed myelosuppression, acute leukemia, bone marrow dysplasias, hypothyroidism, and optic neuroretinitis.
Dosage/ Concentrations:	Lyophilized powder, 100 mg, in 30-ml amber vials along with a separate 3.5-ml vial of absolute alcohol diluent. Dose: 75–100 mg/m^2 for 2 consecutive days or 200 mg/m^2 in a single injection.
Contraindications:	None known.
Drug Interactions/ Allergy:	In combination with amphotericin B, may increase therapeutic ratio; H2 antihistamine may potentiate toxicity of carmustine in experimental settings.

CISPLATIN

Trade Name:	Platinol
Indications:	Metastatic testicular and ovarian tumors and advanced bladder cancers.
Pharmacokinetics:	Clearance: In first two phases, free drug is cleared from plasma; in third phase, cisplatin is probably removed from plasma proteins. T$_{1/2}$: α, 20 min; β, 48–70 min; γ, 24 hr.
Pharmacodynamics:	Cross-linking and interference with DNA and RNA functions and stimulation of the host immune system.
CNS:	"Glove-and-stocking" type neuropathy; numbness,

	tingling, and a sensory loss distally in arms and legs; focal encephalopathy with cortical blindness, seizures, and aphasia.
CVS:	ST-T wave abnormalities, bundle branch block; atrial fibrillation, supraventricular tachycardia, vascular toxicities (MI, CVA, thrombotic microangiopathy, cerebral arteritis, Raynaud's phenomenon).
Hepatic:	↑ Serum bilirubin, ↑ alkaline phosphatase, ↑ SGOT, steatosis, cholestasis, periportal edema.
Renal:	Hyperuricemia or uric acid nephropathy; ↑ BUN, ↑ creatinine, acute renal failure.
GI:	Nausea, vomiting.
Other:	Myelosuppression (Coombs-positive hemolytic anemia, leukopenia, and thrombocytopenia).
Dosage/ Concentrations:	A single-dose vial contains either 50 mg or 100 mg of ciplastin. For metastatic testicular tumors: 20 mg/m², in combination with bleomycin and vinblastine. For metastatic ovarian tumors: 50 mg/m² and doxorubicin. For advanced bladder cancers: 50–70 mg/m² as a single agent.
Contraindications:	Preexisting renal impairment, myelosuppression, hearing impairment, and allergic reactions.
Drug Interactions/ Allergy:	Renal tubular damage, affects other drugs eliminated renally.

DACARBAZINE

Trade Name:	DTIC-Dome
Indications:	Malignant melanoma, Hodgkin's lymphomas, and soft tissue sarcomas.
Pharmacokinetics:	Vd: 0.2 L/kg. Clearance: 15.4 ml/kg/min. $T_{1/2}$: α, 2.9 min; β, 41 min.
Pharmacodynamics:	Inhibition of DNA and RNA synthesis.
CVS:	Fatal thrombosis, allergic vasculitis, hypotension.
Hepatic:	Hepatic vein thrombosis, hepatocellular necrosis, delayed hepatic failure.
GI:	Severe nausea and vomiting.
Musculoskeletal:	Myalgias.
Other:	Myelosuppression, nadir of leukopenia and thrombocytopenia, anemia, flu-like syndrome.
Dosage/ Concentrations:	10-ml or 20-ml vials containing 100 mg or 200 mg.

DACARBAZINE *(continued)*

	For malignant melanoma: 2–4.5 mg/kg for 10 days. For Hodgkin's lymphomas: 150 mg/m² for 5 days.
Contraindications:	None known.
Drug Interactions/ Allergy:	May cause additive hypouricemic effects when used with allopurinol and potentially increased toxicity if given concomitantly with azathioprine or 6-mercapto-purine.

ETOPOSIDE

Trade Name:	VePesid
Indications:	Refractory testicular tumors and small cell lung cancer.
Pharmacokinetics:	Adults: Vd: 15.7 L/m². Clearance: 27 ml/min/m². $T_{1/2}$: α, 70 min. β, 7 hr. Children: Vd: 10 L/m². Clearance: 39 ml/min/m². $T_{1/2}$: α, 35 min; β, 3.4 hr.
Pharmacodynamics:	Inhibition of DNA synthesis.
CNS:	Ataxia, numbness or tingling in fingers and toes, weakness.
CVS:	Hypotension.
Pulmonary:	Bronchospasm and dyspnea.
Hepatic:	Hepatotoxicity, metabolic acidosis.
GI:	Nausea, vomiting.
Other:	Dose-response anemia, leukopenia, thrombocytopenia.
Dosage/ Concentrations:	20–100 mg/5 ml sterile multiple dose vial for injection. Oral dose: 40- to 50-mg capsules. Injection: 5–100 mg/m²/day.
Contraindications:	None known.
Drug Interactions/ Allergy:	Anaphylactic reaction or symptoms of hypersensitivity: tachycardia, bronchospasm, dyspnea, hypertension, flushing.

FLUOROURACIL

Trade Name:	Adrucil
Indications:	Carcinoma of the colon, rectum, breast, stomach, pancreas, bladder, prostate, ovary, cervix, endometrium, and lung, and liver and head and neck tumors.
Pharmacokinetics:	May be eliminated by a two- or three-compartment model.

Pharmacodynamics:	Conversion to active metabolite, inhibition of DNA and RNA synthesis.
CNS:	Acute cerebellar syndrome, nystagmus, headache.
CVS:	Myocardial ischemia, angina, dysrhythmias.
Pulmonary:	Cough, shortness of breath.
GI:	Ulcerative stomatitis, esophagopharyngitis, ulceration and bleeding, nausea and vomiting (intractable), diarrhea.
Musculoskeletal:	Palmar-plantar dysesthesia.
Other:	Leukopenia (primarily granulocytopenia), thrombocytopenia.
Dosage/ Concentrations:	Single-use vials (10 ml) containing 500 mg FU. Conventional bolus: 12 mg/kg. Maintenance: 6 mg/kg.
Contraindications:	Poor nutritional state, depressed bone marrow function, and potentially serious infections.
Drug Interactions/ Allergy:	Leucovorin increases therapeutic and toxic effects of FU. Anaphylaxis and generalized allergic reactions may occur.

FLUTAMIDE

Trade Name:	Eulexin
Indications:	Metastatic prostatic carcinoma.
Pharmacokinetics:	Metabolism: extensively metabolized. Major species identified is an α-hydroxylated active metabolite, hydroxyflutamide. $T_{1/2}$: α, 0.8 hr; β, 7.8 hr.
Pharmacodynamics:	Inhibition of androgen activity and interference with testosterone.
CNS:	Drowsiness, confusion, depression, anxiety, nervousness.
CVS:	Hypertension.
Hepatic:	↑ SGPT, ↑ SGOT.
GI:	Nausea, vomiting, diarrhea.
Other:	Anemia, leukopenia, thrombocytopenia.
Dosage/ Concentrations:	Capsules: 100 and 500 per bottle. Each capsule contains 125 mg flutamide. Dose: 2 capsules t.i.d.
Contraindications:	None known.
Drug Interactions/ Allergy:	None known.

LEVAMISOLE

Trade Name:	Ergamisol
Indications:	Colorectal carcinoma and malignant melanoma.
Pharmacokinetics:	Metabolism: liver; less than 5% of the unmetabolized drug is detected in urine and feces. $T_{1/2}$: α, 4 hr.
Pharmacodynamics:	Augmentation of T-cell, monocyte, macrophage, and neutrophil activity.
CNS:	Ataxia, blurred vision, confusion, paranoia, paresthesias, seizures, tardive dyskinesia, CSF pleiocytosis, psychiatric symptoms.
Hepatic:	Hyperbilirubinemia.
GI:	Nausea, vomiting, diarrhea, stomatitis, anorexia.
Other:	Agranulocytosis, leukopenia, flu-like syndrome (due to agranulocytosis).
Dosage/ Concentrations:	White, coated tablets containing the equivalent of 50 mg of levamisole. Dose: 50 mg p.o. q 8 hr administered alone or in combination with fluorouracil (FU) in a different regimen for postoperative treatment.
Contraindications:	None.
Drug Interactions/ Allergy:	Levamisole enhances coumarin's effect on prolongation of PT. When given with alcohol, a disulfiram-like syndrome develops. Levamisole plus 5-FU increases plasma levels of phenytoin.

MECHLORETHAMINE

Trade Name:	Mustargen
Indications:	Hodgkin's and non-Hodgkin's lymphomas.
Pharmacokinetics:	Rapid chemical transformation in water or body fluids and combines with water or reactive compounds of cells.
Pharmacodynamics:	Cytotoxic action and inhibition of protein synthesis.
CNS:	Weakness, drowsiness, fever, headache, tinnitus, deafness, temporary aphasia and paresis.
CVS:	Thrombophlebitis, hemorrhagic diathesis.
Hepatic:	Jaundice, $\downarrow$ hepatic function.
Renal:	Hyperuricemia, $\downarrow$ renal function.
GI:	Nausea, vomiting.
Other:	Leukopenia and thrombocytopenia, maculopapular skin eruption.

Dosage/ Concentrations:	10-mg vials. IV, 0.4 mg/kg as a single dose or four separate (0.1 mg/kg) on successive days. In MOPP regimen, 6.0 mg/m² on days 1 and 8 of a 14-day combination drug program. Limited use in children.
Contraindications:	Infectious diseases.
Drug Interactions/ Allergy:	Glutathione-depleting agents increase the alkylating activity of nitrogen mustard in experimental settings.

MERCAPTOPURINE

Trade Name:	Purinethol
Indications:	Remission induction and maintenance therapy of acute lymphatic leukemia.
Pharmacokinetics:	Children: Vd: 0.9 ± 0.8 L/kg. Clearance: 719 ± 610 ml/min/m². $T_{1/2}$: α, 0.9 ± 0.3 hr.
Pharmacodynamics: Hepatic:	Inhibition of DNA and RNA synthesis. Jaundice, hepatitis, biliary stasis, hyperbilirubinemia, intrahepatic cholestasis, centrolobular necrosis.
Renal:	Hematuria, crystalluria, renal tubule defect.
GI:	Anorexia, nausea, vomiting, mucositis, stomatitis, profound diarrhea, sprue-like condition.
Other:	Leukopenia, thrombocytopenia, anemia, immunosuppression.
Dosage/ Concentrations: Adult and Pediatric:	Off-white, scored tablets containing 50 mg of 6-MP. Initial dose, 2.5 mg/kg/day; may be increased up to 5 mg/kg/day.
Contraindications:	Prior resistance to MP.
Drug Interactions/ Allergy:	Allopurinol creates a metabolic blockade in 6-MP metabolism. 6-MP antagonizes anticoagulant effects of warfarin. In combination with doxorubicin in adult acute leukemia, the incidence of hepatotoxicity was greater than 50%. There is usually complete cross-resistance between MP and Tabloid brand thioguanine.

METHOTREXATE

Trade Name:	Folex, Mexate
Indications:	Neoplastic diseases, psoriasis, and rheumatoid arthritis.
Pharmacokinetics:	Vd: initial, 0.18 L/kg; steady state, 0.4–0.8 L/kg. Clear-

METHOTREXATE *(continued)*

ance: renal, 70–100 ml/min; urinary, 60%–100% of a dose; fecal, 1%–9% of a dose; biliary, <20% of a dose. $T_{1/2}$: α, <1 hr; β, 3–4 hr.

Pharmacodynamics:	Inhibition of DNA, RNA, thymidylate, and protein synthesis.
CNS:	↑ CSF pressure, leukoencephalopathy, demyelination, or chemical arachnoiditis (back pain, blurred vision, confusion, convulsion, dizziness, drowsiness, headache, unusual tiredness or weakness).
CVS:	Cutaneous vasculitis.
Pulmonary:	Pulmonary fibrosis, pneumonitis.
Hepatic:	Liver atrophy, necrosis, cirrhosis, fatty changes, periportal fibrosis.
Renal:	Renal failure, azotemia, hyperuricemia, severe nephropathy.
Metabolic:	Fever, osteoporosis.
GI:	Ulceration and bleeding, enteritis, intestinal perforation, loss of appetite, nausea, vomiting.
Other:	Marked bone marrow depression, with resultant anemia, leukopenia, or thrombocytopenia.
Dosage/ Concentrations:	20-, 50-, and 500-mg and 1-g vials and sterile water MTX given by numerous dosing schedules.
Contraindications:	Pregnancy; breast-feeding; severe, chronic liver diseases; bone marrow depression.
Drug Interactions/ Allergy:	Salicylates, sulfonamides, phenytoin, and *p*-aminobenzoic acid cause small increase in levels of free drug. Antibiotics used in gut sterilization eliminate slow phase of excretion. Ethyl alcohol increases MTX-induced hepatoxicity. Warfarin levels may be greatly potentiated by MTX.

TAMOXIFEN

Trade Name:	Nolvadex
Indications:	Breast carcinoma, metastatic breast cancer, and alternative treatment to oophorectomy or ovarian irradiation.
Pharmacokinetics:	$T_{1/2}$: α, 7–14 hr; β, 4 or more days.
Pharmacodynamics:	Alteration of estrogen receptors, inhibition of DNA and RNA activity.
CNS:	Depression, dizziness, lightheadedness, headache.

CVS:	↓ Low-density lipid cholesterol levels, thromboembolic events.
Hepatic:	Cholestatic liver damage, ↑ SGPT, ↑ SGOT.
GI:	Nausea, vomiting.
Musculoskeletal:	Bone pain along with hypercalcemia in patients with bony disease.
Other:	Myelosuppression, slight and transient thrombocytopenia and leukopenia.
Dosage/ Concentrations:	Tablets: 60 and 250 per bottle. Each tablet contains 10 mg of tamoxifen. Dose: 1 or 2 10-mg tablets b.i.d.
Contraindications:	None known.
Drug Interactions/ Allergy:	May potentiate the mild hepatotoxicity induced by chronic allopurinol therapy.

THIOTEPA

Trade Name:	Thioplex
Indications:	Adenocarcinoma of breast and ovary, intracavitary effusions due to diffuse or localized neoplastic disease of various serosal cavities, and superficial papillary carcinoma of the urinary bladder.
Pharmacokinetics:	Vd: 0.25 L/kg. Clearance: 186 ml/min/m^2. T$_{1/2}$: α, 7.7 min; β, 125 min.
Pharmacodynamics:	Cytotoxic action and inhibition of protein synthesis.
CNS:	Inappropriate behavior, confusion, somnolence, headache, dizziness, paresthesias.
CVS:	Septicemia, hemorrhage.
Pulmonary:	Bronchoconstriction in patients with hypersensitivity.
Hepatic:	"Bronzing" or hyperpigmentation of skin, ↑ transaminase, ↑ bilirubin.
Renal:	Chemical or hemorrhagic cystitis.
GI:	Nausea, vomiting, anorexia.
Other:	Leukopenia, thrombocytopenia, anemia.
Dosage/ Concentrations:	15-mg vials. IV: is 0.3–0.4 mg/kg at 1- to 4-wk intervals.
Contraindications:	Hepatic, renal, or bone marrow damage.
Drug Interactions/ Allergy:	↓ Pseudocholinesterase levels. Severe and cumulative platelet toxicity when combined with sargramostim. Prolonged apnea after succinylcholine administered prior to surgery.

VINBLASTINE

Trade Names:	Velban, Velsar
Indications:	Generalized Hodgkin's disease, lymphocytic lymphoma, mycosis fungoides, advanced carcinoma of the testis, Kaposi's sarcoma, Letterer-Siwe disease (histiocytosis X), resistant choriocarcinoma, unresponsive carcinoma.
Pharmacokinetics:	Vd: 27.3 ± 14.9 L/kg. Clearance: 0.74 ± 0.319 L/kg/hr. $T_{1/2}$: α, 0.062 ± 0.04 hr; β, 1.64 ± 0.34 hr; γ, 24.8 ± 7.5 hr.
Pharmacodynamics:	Blocking of mitosis and interference with amino acid metabolism.
CNS:	Paresthesias, peripheral neuropathy, depression, headache, malaise, urinary retention, convulsions, vocal cord paralysis, cranial nerve paralysis.
CVS:	Hypertension, tachycardia, orthostatic hypotension, Raynaud's phenomenon.
Pulmonary:	Acute shortness of breath, severe bronchospasm.
Hepatic:	Transient hepatitis.
Renal:	Hyperuricemia or uric acid nephropathy.
GI:	Nausea, vomiting, constipation, adynamic ileus, abdominal pain, rectal bleeding, hemorrhagic colitis, bleeding from a previously existing peptic ulcer.
Musculoskeletal:	Muscle pain.
Other:	Leukopenia, thrombocytopenia, ↓ platelets, ↓ erythrocytes, myelosuppression.
Dosage/ Concentrations:	10-ml vials containing 10 mg. Dose: 0.1–0.5 mg/kg/wk.
Contraindications:	Pregnancy, significant granulocytopenia, bacterial infection.
Drug Interactions/ Allergy:	↑ Cellular uptake of methotrexate by some malignant cells, enhances cell kill with bleomycin, and decreases plasma phenytoin levels.

Immunosuppressants

AZATHIOPRINE

Trade Name:	Imuran
Indications:	Renal homotransplantation, rheumatoid arthritis.
Pharmacokinetics:	Metabolism and Elimination: Cleaved in vivo to mer-

captopurine; both compounds rapidly eliminated from blood and are oxidized or methylated in erythrocytes and liver; no azathioprine or mercaptopurine detectable in urine after 8 hr. $T_{1/2}$: α, 5 hr.

Pharmacodynamics:	Inhibition of mitosis; inhibited synthesis of DNA, RNA, and protein; and interference with cellular metabolism.
Pulmonary:	Pneumonitis.
Hepatic:	Hepatitis or biliary stasis, hepatic veno-occlusive disease (stomach pain, swelling of feet or lower legs).
GI:	Loss of appetite, nausea, vomiting, hypersensitivity pancreatitis (severe abdominal pain with nausea and vomiting).
Musculoskeletal:	Arthralgias.
Other:	Severe leukopenia or thrombocytopenia, macrocytic anemia, severe bone marrow depression, unusual bleeding or bruising, serious infections, skin rash.
Dosage/ Concentrations:	100 tablets per bottle or 20-ml vial containing either 50 or equivalent of 100 mg. Initial dose: 3–5 mg/kg daily. Maintenance dose: 1–2 mg/kg.
Contraindications:	Pregnancy.
Drug Interactions/ Allergy:	Reduced to ¼ to ⅓ of usual dose if allopurinol is given concomitantly. Azathioprine inhibits cAMP phosphodiesterase and thus alters effects of adrenergic or other agents on neuromuscular transmission. Nondepolarizing blockers are inhibited by azathioprine; in contrast, succinylcholine may be enhanced. Hypersensitivity reactions: fast heart beat, sudden fever, muscle or joint pain, redness, or skin blisters.

CYCLOSPORINE

Trade Name:	Sandimmune
Indications:	Organ transplant rejection.
Pharmacokinetics:	Vd: Distributed largely outside the blood volume. Metabolism: extensively metabolized but no major metabolic pathway. Adults: $T_{1/2}$: α, 19 hr. Children: $T_{1/2}$: α, 7 hr.
Pharmacodynamics:	Inhibition of interleukin-2.
CNS:	Convulsions.
CVS:	Hypertension.
Hepatic:	↑ SGPT, ↑ SGOT, ↑ bilirubin.

CYCLOSPORINE   *(continued)*

Renal:	Hemolytic-uremic syndrome (microangiopathic hemolytic anemia, renal failure, and thrombocytopenia).
GI:	Anorexia, gastritis, peptic ulcer.
Musculoskeletal:	Muscle pain.

Dosage/ Concentrations:	Soft gelatin capsules, oral solution, and IV ampule. Single dose: 15 mg/kg 4–12 hr prior to transplantation. Daily single dose: 14–18 mg/kg after transplantation.
Contraindications:	None.
Drug Interactions/ Allergy:	The following drugs, in combination with cyclosporine, may increase risk of renal failure: cimetidine, erythromycin, ketoconazole, miconazole, NSAIDs, blood from blood bank, diuretics, and other immunosuppressants. Anaphylactic reactions: flushing of face and upper thorax, acute respiratory distress with dyspnea and wheezing, BP changes, and tachycardia.

FILGRASTIM

Trade Name:	Neupogen
Indications:	Patients with nonmyeloid malignancies receiving myelosuppressive anticancer drugs, general and AIDS-associated neutropenia.
Pharmacokinetics:	Follows first-order pharmacokinetic modeling without apparent concentration dependence. Vd: 150 ml/kg. Clearance: 0.5–0.7 ml/min/kg. $T_{1/2}$: α, 3.5 hr.
Pharmacodynamics:	Alteration of progenitor cells and receptors.
CVS:	Transient supraventricular arrhythmia, vasculitis.
Musculoskeletal:	Mild to moderate medullary bone pain.
Other:	Excessive leukocytosis, splenomegaly.
Dosage/ Concentrations:	Single-dose vial containing 300 μg (1 ml) or 480 μg (1.6 ml). Starting dose: 5 μg/kg/day.
Contraindications:	Known hypersensitivity to *Escherichia coli*–derived protein.
Drug Interactions/ Allergy:	May potentiate the release of neutrophils. Allergic reactions: rare.

LYMPHOCYTE IMMUNE GLOBULIN

Trade Name:	Atgam
Indications:	Renal transplantation; aplastic anemia.
Pharmacokinetics:	Administered with other immunosuppressive agents and measured as horse serum IgG. $T_{1/2}$: α, 5.7 ± 3 days.
Pharmacodynamics:	Antilymphocytic effect.
CNS:	Headache, dizziness, seizures, paresthesias.
CVS:	Hypertension, hypotension, tachycardia, clotted arteriovenous fistula, peripheral thrombophlebitis, iliac vein obstruction, renal artery thrombosis, hemolysis.
Pulmonary:	Dyspnea, pulmonary edema.
GI:	Nausea, vomiting, hiccoughs, epigastric pain.
Musculoskeletal:	Myalgia.
Other:	Leukopenia, thrombocytopenia.
Dosage/ Concentrations:	Ampules: 5 ml; contain 50 mg of horse gamma globulin/ml.
Adult:	10–30 mg/kg daily.
Pediatric:	5–25 mg/kg daily.
Contraindications:	Severe systemic reaction to equine gamma globulin preparations.
Drug Interactions/ Allergy:	Diluted in dextrose injection, USP, because low salt concentrations may cause precipitation. The use of highly acidic infusion solutions is not recommended because of possible physical instability over time. Respiratory distress, pain in chest, flank or back, and hypotension indicate an anaphylactoid reaction.

12

Benzodiazepines and Antagonists

Ronald H. Wender, M.D.
Paul E. Wender, M.D.

CHLORDIAZEPOXIDE

Trade Name:	Librium
Indications:	Anxiety and anxiety disorders, alcohol withdrawal, and premedication.
Pharmacokinetics:	Vd: 0.3 L/kg. Clearance: 0.5 ml/kg/min. Metabolism: conjugated in liver. Elimination: metabolites excreted in urine.
Pharmacodynamics:	
CNS:	Sedation, anxiolysis, drowsiness, ataxia, confusion.
CVS:	Hypotension (overdose).
Pulmonary:	Upper airway obstruction, $\downarrow$ ventilation.
Hepatic:	Hepatic dysfunction.
Other:	Agranulocytosis.
Dosage/ Concentrations:	Tablets: 5, 10, and 25 mg. Powder: 100 mg in 5-ml ampule with 2 ml of special IM dilutent; do not use IM dilutent for IV administration.
Adults:	Oral, 5–25 mg 3–4 times daily. IV/IM, 50–100 mg, then 25–50 mg q 6–8 hr.
Pediatric:	Oral, 5 mg 2–4 times daily.
Geriatric:	Oral, 5 mg 2–4 times daily. IV/IM, 25–50 mg.
Contraindications:	Hepatic failure. Limit dose in elderly patients, critically ill patients, and patients with impaired hepatic reserve.
Drug Interactions/ Allergy:	Clearance impaired by liver disease, cimetidine, and advanced age.

DIAZEPAM

Trade Name:	Valium
Indications:	Anxiety disorders, ethanol withdrawal, conscious sedation, relief of muscle spasms, seizure therapy, preoperative medication, and induction and maintenance of anesthesia.
Pharmacokinetics:	Vd: 0.7–1.7 L/kg. Clearance: 0.2–0.5 ml/kg/min. $T_{1/2}$: β, 20–50 hr. Metabolism: biotransformation by oxidative reduction in liver.
Pharmacodynamics:	
CNS:	Sedation, anxiolysis. $\downarrow$ $CMRO_2$, $\downarrow$ CBF.

DIAZEPAM   *(continued)*

CVS:	↓ SVR, ↓ MAP, venous irritation, phlebitis.
Pulmonary:	↓ Tidal volume, ↓ minute volume, ↑ Pa_{CO_2}.
Musculoskeletal:	Central muscle relaxant properties.

**Dosage/
Concentrations:**　　5 mg/ml in 2- and 10-ml containers.

Adult: Premedication, oral 0.1–0.2 mg/kg. Induction, 0.3–0.5 mg/kg. Maintenance, 0.1 mg/kg q 1–2 hr p.r.n. Sedation, 2–5 mg p.r.n.

Pediatric: Premedication, oral 0.1–0.2 mg/kg. Anticonvulsant, 0.1–0.3 mg/kg IV.

Geriatric: Reduce dose, and titrate slowly.

Contraindications:　　Acute glaucoma.

**Drug Interactions/
Allergy:**　　Clearance impaired by cimetidine, alcohol, and advanced age.

FLUMAZENIL

Trade Name: Romazicon

Indications: Reversal of residual benzodiazepine sedation and amnesia and therapy for benzodiazepine overdose.

Pharmacokinetics: Short-acting, rapid onset. Vd: 0.6–1.6 L/kg. Clearance: 5–20 ml/kg/min. $T_{1/2}$: β, 0.7–1.3 hr. Metabolism: hepatic (rapid).

Pharmacodynamics:

CNS: Benzodiazepine receptor antagonist.
Headaches; dizziness.

Pulmonary Partial reversal of respiratory effects of agonists.

GI: Nausea and vomiting.

**Dosage/
Concentrations:**　　5-ml and 10-ml multidose vials at a concentration of 0.1 mg/ml.

Adult: Infusion 30–60 μg/min (0.5 to 1.0 μg/kg/min).

For overdose: bolus of 0.2 mg (2ml), wait 30 seconds, then 0.3 mg (3ml), then 0.5 mg (5 ml) up to cumulative dose of 3 mg. May need additional doses as resedation occurs in 60–90 min.

For reversal of conscious sedation: bolus of 0.2 mg (2 ml). May repeat up to 1 mg. Observe for resedation.

Pediatric:	12 μg/kg IV.
Geriatric:	Same as adult dosage.

Contraindications: Chronic benzodiazepine use or abuse, TCA overdose, and patients receiving benzodiazepines for seizure.

Drug Interactions/ Allergy: May precipitate seizures in patients chronically using or abusing benzodiazepines or in TCA overdose.

LORAZEPAM

Trade Name: Ativan

Indications: Preoperative medication, ICU sedation, convulsions, alcohol withdrawal.

Pharmacokinetics: Intermediate-acting. Metabolism: rapidly conjugated to lorazepam glucuronide. Metabolite excreted in urine. Vd: 0.8–1.3 L/kg. Clearance: 0.8–1.8 ml/kg/min. $T_{1/2}$: β, 11–22 hr.

Pharmacodynamics:
CNS: Sedation, anxiolysis, amnesia, ↓ $CMRO_2$, ↓ CBF.
CVS: ↓ BP, ↓ SVR.
Pulmonary: ↑ RR at low-dose, ↓ RR at high-dose; ↓ minute ventilation, upper airway obstruction.
Musculoskeletal: Spinally mediated central muscle relaxant properties.

Dosage/ Concentrations: Tablets: 0.5, 1, and 2 mg.
Tubex: 2 and 4 mg/ml.
Vials: 2 and 4 mg/ml as 1 ml vials.

Adult: IM: 0.05 mg/kg to a maximum of 4 mg, 1–2 hr prior to procedure.
 IV: initially 0.044 mg/kg up to 2 mg: for further effect, 0.05 mg/kg up to 4 mg.
 Induction of general anesthesia: 0.1 mg/kg.
 Maintenance: 0.02 mg/kg p.r.n.

Pediatric: For sedation; IV: 0.03–0.05 mg/kg q 6 hr p.r.n.; oral: 0.05 mg/kg for 6-yr-olds and up.

Geriatric: Reduce doses, titrate in small increments.

Contraindications: Acute narrow-angle glaucoma and renal or hepatic failure. Use with caution in elderly and ICU patients.

Drug Interactions/ Allergy: Additive with other CNS depressants. Clearance impaired by cimetidine, alcohol, and advanced age.

MIDAZOLAM

Trade Name:	Versed
Indications:	Preoperative medication, conscious sedation; ICU sedation, induction and maintenance of general anesthesia.
Pharmacokinetics:	Short-acting. Oxidized rapidly in liver. Elimination: inactive metabolites renally excreted. Vd: 1.1–1.7 L/kg. Clearance: 7.5 ml/kg/min. $T_{1/2}$: β, 2–4 hr.

Pharmacodynamics:

CNS:	Sedation, anxiolysis, amnesia, hypnosis, ↓ CBF, ↓ $CMRO_2$.
CVS:	↓ MAP, ↓ SV, ↓ SVR, ↓ cardiac output, hypotension in critically ill patients.
Pulmonary:	↑ RR at low-dose, ↓ RR at high-dose; ↓ tidal volume, ↓ minute volume, apnea.
Musculoskeletal:	Spinally mediated muscle relaxant properties.
Dosage/ Concentrations:	1 mg/ml in 2-ml vials; 5 mg/ml in 2-ml vials.
Adult:	Premedication: IV/IM: 1–5 mg. Induction: IV, 0.1–0.2 mg/kg. ICU sedation: 0.25–1.5 μg/kg/min infusion.
Pediatric:	Premedication: Oral, 0.5–1.0 mg/kg p.o. in syrup elixir. Intranasal, 0.2–0.3 mg/kg. IV, 0.03 mg/kg p.r.n. Induction: IV, 0.1–0.2 mg/kg
Geriatric:	Premedication: 1–2.5 mg IV; divided doses of 0.5 mg.
Contraindications:	Acute narrow-angle glaucoma.
Drug Interactions/ Allergy:	With opioids, ethanol, and CNS depressants, ↑ respiratory depression. With inhalational agents, 10%–25% ↓ MAC requirement. Clearance impaired by cimetidine, alcohol, and advanced age.

13

Beta Blockers

Michael Guertin, M.D.

ACEBUTOLOL

Trade Name:	Sectral
Indications:	Hypertension, ventricular and supraventricular cardiac arrhythmias, angina, and reduction of cardiovascular mortality after acute phase of MI.
Pharmacokinetics:	Vd: 1.6–3 L/kg. Oral absorption: 70%. Bioavailability: 35%–50%. Distribution: placenta and milk; minimal into CSF. Clearance: 7–11 ml/min/kg ($\downarrow$ in elderly). $T_{1/2}$: α, 3 hr; β, 6–12 hr (average, 11 hr). Elimination: extensive hepatic metabolism (active metabolite = diacetolol); excreted in feces and urine ($\downarrow$ in renal or hepatic disease).
Pharmacodynamics:	Selective β_1 antagonist.
CNS:	Fatigue, dizziness, headaches, mental depression.
CVS:	Negative chronotropic and inotropic effects. $\downarrow$ Systolic and diastolic BP and HR, membrane-stabilizing effect on heart, antiarrhythmic activity (class II).
Pulmonary:	$\uparrow$ Airway resistance in asthma or COPD and at high doses.
Renal:	Slight $\downarrow$ RBF.
GI:	Constipation, dyspepsia, nausea, diarrhea.
Dosages/ Concentrations:	Capsules = 200 and 400 mg. For hypertension: 200–400 mg daily (single daily dose). For ventricular arrhythmias: 200 mg b.i.d. For angina: 200–400 mg b.i.d.
Contraindications:	Impaired myocardial function, second- or third-degree AV block, severe bradycardia, and bronchospastic disease (use with caution).
Drug Interactions/ Allergy:	Use with other antihypertensive agents may exaggerate hypotensive effect. Acute withdrawal may cause rebound $\uparrow$ HR and $\uparrow$ BP. May mask signs of hyperthyroidism and hypoglycemia. May antagonize bronchodilation produced by β agonists. May $\downarrow$ hypoglycemic action of glyburide.

ATENOLOL

Trade Name:	Tenormin
Indications:	Hypertension, angina, reduction of cardiovascular mortality after acute phase of MI, and acute alcohol withdrawal.

Pharmacokinetics:	Vd: 1.1 L/kg. Oral absorption: 50%–60%. Bioavailability: 50%–60%. Distribution: placenta and milk; minimal into CSF and brain. $T_{1/2}$: β, 6–7 hr. Elimination: excreted in urine unchanged (no hepatic metabolism); ↓ as creatinine clearance ↓.
Pharmacodynamics:	Selective $β_1$ antagonist.
CNS:	Dizziness, fatigue, mental depression, headaches.
CVS:	Negative chronotropic and inotropic effects, ↓ systolic and diastolic BP and HR at rest and during exercise.
Pulmonary:	↑ Airway resistance in asthma or COPD and at high doses.
Renal:	↓ Plasma renin/aldosterone activity, ↓ RBF, ↓ GFR.
GI:	Nausea, diarrhea.
Dosages/ Concentrations:	Tablets: 25 mg, 50 mg, and 100 mg. IV: 0.5 mg/ml. For hypertension: 25–100 mg p.o. daily (single daily dose). For angina: 50–100 mg p.o. daily. For MI: 5 mg IV over 5 min; may repeat after 10 min, then 50 mg p.o. b.i.d. Reduce doses in renal disease.
Contraindications:	Impaired myocardial function, second- or third-degree AV block, severe bradycardia, and bronchospastic disease (use with caution).
Drug Interactions/ Allergy:	Use with other antihypertensive agents may exaggerate hypotensive effect. Acute withdrawal may cause rebound ↑ HR and ↑ BP. May mask signs of hyperthyroidism and hypoglycemia. May antagonize bronchodilation produced by β agonists.

BETAXOLOL

Trade Names:	Kerlone, Betoptic (ophthalmic solution)
Indications:	Hypertension and chronic open-angle glaucoma and ocular hypertension.
Pharmacokinetics:	Vd: 4.9–9.8 L/kg. Oral absorption: 80%–90%. Bioavailability: 90%. Minimal systemic absorption after topical eye application. $T_{1/2}$: β, 14–22 hr (↑ in hypertension and renal or hepatic disease). Elimination: hepatic metabolism (minimally active metabolite); renal and biliary excretion.
Pharmacodynamics:	Selective $β_1$ antagonist.
CNS:	Dizziness, fatigue, mental depression, headaches, ↓ IOP.

BETAXOLOL   *(continued)*

CVS:	Negative chronotropic and inotropic effects, ↓ systolic and diastolic BP and HR at rest and during exercise.
Pulmonary:	↑ Bronchial airway resistance in asthma or COPD.
Dosages/ Concentrations:	Eye solution (Betoptic): 0.5%. Tablets (Kerlone): 10 and 20 mg.
	For hypertension: 5–20 mg p.o. daily (single daily dose).
	For open-angle glaucoma or ocular hypertension: 1–2 drops b.i.d. Dose may need to be adjusted if renal disease is present.
Contraindications:	Impaired myocardial function, second- or third-degree AV block, severe bradycardia, cardiogenic shock, and bronchospastic disease or COPD (use with caution).
Drug Interactions/ Allergy:	Acute withdrawal may cause rebound ↑ HR and ↑ BP. May mask signs of hyperthyroidism and hypoglycemia.

BISOPROLOL

Trade Name:	Zebeta
Indications:	Hypertension.
Pharmacokinetics:	Oral absorption: 80%–90%. Bioavailability: 90%. $T_{1/2}$: β, 9–12 hr. Elimination: renal (↓ as creatinine clearance ↓).
Pharmacodynamics:	Selective β_1 antagonist.
CNS:	Dizziness, fatigue, mental depression, headaches.
CVS:	Negative chronotropic and inotropic effect, ↓ systolic and diastolic BP and HR at rest and during exercise.
Pulmonary:	↑ Airway resistance in asthma or COPD and at high doses.
Renal:	↓ RBF.
Dosages/ Concentrations:	Tablets: 5 and 10 mg.
	For hypertension: 25–100 mg p.o. daily (single daily dose).
Contraindications:	Impaired myocardial function, second- or third-degree AV block, severe bradycardia, bronchospastic disease.
Drug Interactions/ Allergy:	Use with other antihypertensive agents may exaggerate hypotensive effect. Acute withdrawal may cause rebound ↑ HR and ↑ BP. May mask signs of hyperthy-

roidism and hypoglycemia. May antagonize bronchodilation produced by β agonists.

CARTEOLOL

Trade Name:	Cartrol Filmtabs
Indications:	Hypertension.
Pharmacokinetics:	Oral absorption: 80%. Bioavailability: 85%. $T_{1/2}$: β, 6 hr. Elimination: minimal hepatic metabolism (active metabolite); 50%–70% excreted in urine unchanged (removed by hemodialysis).
Pharmacodynamics: *CVS:*	Nonselective β antagonist. Negative chronotropic and inotropic effects, ↓ systolic and diastolic BP and HR during exercise, ↓ effect on resting HR.
Pulmonary:	↑ Airway resistance (bronchospasm).
Dosages/ Concentrations:	Tablets: 2.5 and 5 mg. For hypertension: initial dose, 2.5 mg p.o. daily (single daily dose); usual maintenance dose, 10 mg daily. Reduce dose in patients with renal impairment.
Contraindications:	Impaired myocardial function, second- or third-degree AV block, severe bradycardia, and bronchospastic disease (asthma).
Drug Interactions/ Allergy:	Use with other antihypertensive agents may exaggerate hypotensive effect. Acute withdrawal may cause rebound ↑ HR and ↑ BP. May mask signs of hyperthyroidism and hypoglycemia. May antagonize bronchodilation produced by β agonists.

ESMOLOL

Trade Name:	Brevibloc
Indications:	Hypertension, SVT, and acute MI.
Pharmacokinetics:	Vd: 3 L/kg. Distribution: placenta and milk not known; minimal into CSF. $T_{1/2}$: α, 2 min; β, 9 min (5–23 min). Clearance: 300 ml/min/kg. Metabolism: red blood cell esterases. Elimination: Renal.
Pharmacodynamics: *CNS:*	Selective β₁ antagonist. Dizziness, somnolence, headaches, confusion.
CVS:	Negative chronotropic and inotropic effects,

ESMOLOL *(continued)*

	↓ systolic and diastolic BP and HR at rest and during exercise.
GI:	Nausea.
Dosages/ Concentrations:	IV infusion: 250 mg/ml. IV injection: 10 mg/ml. 　For intraoperative and postoperative hypertension or tachycardia: 1 mg/kg IV bolus, then 150 μg/kg/min. 　For SVT: 500 μg/kg/min for 1 min, then 50 μg/kg/ min for 4 min. 　Reduce doses in renal disease.
Contraindications:	Impaired myocardial function, second- or third-degree AV block, severe bradycardia, and bronchospastic disease.
Drug Interactions/ Allergy:	Use with other antihypertensive agents may exaggerate hypotensive effect. May mask signs of hyperthyroidism and hypoglycemia. May antagonize bronchodilation produced by β agonists.

LABETALOL

Trade Names:	Normodyne, Trandate
Indications:	Hypertension, controlled hypotension during anesthesia.
Pharmacokinetics:	Oral absorption: 90%–100%. Bioavailability: 30%–40% (extensive first-pass metabolism). Vd: 3.2–16 L/kg. Distribution: placenta and milk; minimally across blood-brain barrier. $T_{1/2}$: α, 6–44 min; β, 5–8 hr. Elimination: extensive hepatic metabolism; 55%–60% excreted in urine; remainder excreted in bile.
Pharmacodynamics:	Nonselective $β_1$ and $β_2$ antagonist and $α_1$ antagonist.
CNS:	Dizziness, fatigue.
CVS:	Negative chronotropic and inotropic effects, ↓ SVR, ↓ systolic and diastolic BP and HR during rest and exercise.
Pulmonary:	↑ Airway resistance (bronchospasm).
GI:	Nausea, dyspepsia, vomiting, ↑ LFTs.
Other:	↑ Plasma glucose (no change in serum insulin level).
Dosages/ Concentrations:	Tablets: 100, 200, 300 mg. IV: 5 mg/ml. 　For hypertension: oral: initial dose, 100 mg b.i.d.; usual maintenance dose, 200–400 mg b.i.d. 　For severe hypertension (IV):

- Initial dose: 5–20 mg by slow IV push.

- Additional doses: 20–80 mg q 10 min, titrated to desired effect.

- Continuous IV infusion: 2 mg/min (alternative to IV push).

- Usual effective cumulative dose: 50–300 mg.
Reduce doses in patients with hepatic impairment and severe renal impairment.

Contraindications: Impaired myocardial function, second- or third-degree AV block, severe bradycardia, and bronchospastic disease (asthma).

Drug Interactions/   Use with other antihypertensive agents may exagerate
Allergy: hypotensive effect. Concomitant use with cimetidine significantly ↑ bioavailability of labetalol. May antagonize bronchodilation produced by β agonists. May cause symptomatic orthostatic hypotension. Acute withdrawal may cause rebound ↑ HR and BP. May mask signs of hyperthyroidism and hypoglycemia. May exacerbate Raynaud's phenomenon.

LEVOBUNOLOL

Trade Name: Betagan Liquifilm ophthalmic solution

Indications: Reduction of IOP.

Pharmacokinetics: Systemic absorption with topical eye application.

Pharmacodynamics: Nonselective $β_1$ and $β_2$ antagonist.
CNS: ↓ IOP.
CVS: *   Negative chronotropic and inotropic effects,
                            ↓ systolic and diastolic BP at rest and during exercise.
Pulmonary: ↑ Airway resistance (bronchospasm).

Dosages/   Ophthalmic solution = 0.25%, 0.5%. Initial dose:
Concentrations: 0.5% solution, 1 or 2 drops once daily.

Contraindications: Angle-closure glaucoma unless used in combination with a miotic agent.

Drug Interactions/   Use with systemic antihypertensive agents may exag-
Allergy: gerate hypotensive effect.

*If absorbed systemically.

METOPROLOL

Trade Names:	Lopressor, Toprol XL (extended release)
Indications:	Hypertension, cardiac arrhythmias, angina, and reduction of cardiovascular mortality after acute phase of MI.
Pharmacokinetics:	Oral absorption: 95%. Bioavailability: 50% of oral dose (large first-pass metabolism). Distribution: placenta and milk; crosses blood-brain barrier. $T_{1/2}$: β, 3–7 hr. Elimination: hepatic (little activity in metabolites); metabolites excreted in urine (not removable by hemodialysis).

Pharmacodynamics:	Selective β_1 antagonist.
CNS:	Fatigue, dizziness, headaches, mental depression.
CVS:	Negative chronotropic and inotropic effects, ↓ systolic and diastolic BP and HR at rest and during exercise.
Renal:	↓ Plasma renin activity.
GI:	Constipation, dyspepsia, nausea, diarrhea.

Dosages/ Concentrations:	Tablets: 50 and 100 mg. Extended-release tabs: 47.5, 95, and 190 mg. Parenteral: 1 mg/ml. For hypertension: initial dose: 50–100 mg p.o. daily (increase at weekly intervals). Usual effective dose: 100–450 mg p.o. daily. For acute MI: 5 mg IV 3 doses q 2–5 min, then 100 mg p.o. b.i.d. For angina: 100–400 mg p.o. daily.
Contraindications:	Impaired myocardial function, second- or third-degree AV block, severe bradycardia, and bronchospastic disease (asthma).
Drug Interactions/ Allergy:	Use with other antihypertensive agents may exaggerate hypotensive effect. Acute withdrawal may cause rebound ↑ HR and ↑ BP. May mask signs of hyperthyroidism and hypoglycemia

NADOLOL

Trade Name:	Corgard
Indications:	Hypertension and angina.
Pharmacokinetics:	Oral absorption: 30%–40%. Bioavailability: 30%–50%. Distribution: placenta and milk; crosses blood-brain

barrier. $T_{1/2}$: β, 20–24 hr. Elimination: excreted in urine unchanged (removed by hemodialysis).

Pharmacodynamics:	Nonselective β antagonist.
CNS:	Dizziness, fatigue.
CVS:	Negative chronotropic and inotropic effects, ↓ systolic and diastolic BP and HR during rest and exercise.
Pulmonary:	↑ Airway resistance (bronchospasm).
GI:	Nausea, diarrhea, abdominal discomfort, constipation.
Other:	Inhibited release of free fatty acids and insulin.

Dosages/ Concentrations:
Tablets: 20, 40, 80, 120, and 160 mg.
For hypertension: initial dose: 20–40 mg daily (single daily dose). Usual maintenance: 40–80 mg daily.
For angina: 40–80 mg daily.
Reduce dose in patients with renal impairment.

Contraindications:
Impaired myocardial function, second- or third-degree AV block, severe bradycardia, and bronchospastic disease (asthma).

Drug Interactions/ Allergy:
Use with other antihypertensive agents may exaggerate hypotensive effect. Acute withdrawal may cause rebound ↑ HR and ↑ BP. May mask signs of hyperthyroidism and hypoglycemia. May antagonize bronchodilation produced by β agonists. May antagonize hypoglycemic effects of oral hypoglycemic agents.

PENBUTOLOL

Trade Name:	Levatol
Indications:	Hypertension.
Pharmacokinetics:	Oral absorption: 100%. Bioavailability: 100% (little first-pass metabolism). $T_{1/2}$: β, 5 hr. Elimination: hepatic metabolism (conjugation and oxidation); renal excretion of metabolites (not removable with hemodialysis).
Pharmacodynamics:	Nonselective β antagonist.
CVS:	Negative chronotropic and inotropic effects, ↓ systolic and diastolic BP and HR during exercise, and less effect on resting HR.
Pulmonary:	↑ Airway resistance (bronchospasm).

Dosages/ Concentrations:
Tablets: 20 mg.
For hypertension: Initial dose: 20 mg daily. Usual maintenance dose: 20–40 mg daily. Reduce doses if hepatic impairment but not renal disease.

PENBUTOLOL   *(continued)*

Contraindications:	Impaired myocardial function, second- or third-degree AV block, severe bradycardia, and bronchospastic disease (asthma).
Drug Interactions/ Allergy:	Use with other antihypertensive agents may exaggerate hypotensive effect. Acute withdrawal may cause rebound ↑ HR and ↑ BP. May mask signs of hyperthyroidism and hypoglycemia.

PINDOLOL

Trade Name:	Visken
Indications:	Hypertension and angina.
Pharmacokinetics:	Vd: 1.2–2 L/kg. Oral absorption: 95%. Bioavailability: 50%–95%. $T_{1/2}$: β, 3–4 hr (3–11 hr. with renal failure, 7–15 hr. in elderly). Elimination: 60%–65% hepatic metabolism; 35%–50% excreted in urine unchanged (removed by hemodialysis).
Pharmacodynamics:	Nonselective β antagonist.
CNS:	Fatigue, dizziness, insomnia, anxiety, hallucinations.
CVS:	Negative chronotropic and inotropic effects, ↓ systolic and diastolic BP and HR during exercise, membrane-stabilizing effect on heart.
Pulmonary:	↑ Airway resistance (bronchospasm).
GI:	Nausea, abdominal discomfort. ↑ Serum AST and ALT.
Other:	Inhibited release of free fatty acids and insulin.

Dosages/ Concentrations:	Tablets: 5 and 10 mg.
	    For hypertension: initial dose: 5 mg b.i.d.; usual maintenance dose: 10–30 mg daily.
	    For angina: 15–40 mg daily.
	    Reduce doses in patients with renal or hepatic impairment.

Contraindications:	Impaired myocardial function, second- or third-degree AV block, severe bradycardia, and bronchospastic disease (asthma).
Drug Interactions/ Allergy:	Use with other antihypertensive agents may exaggerate hypotensive effect. Acute withdrawal may cause rebound ↑ HR and ↑ BP. May mask signs of hyperthyroidism and hypoglycemia. May precipitate severe, acute hyperglycemia.

PROPRANOLOL

Trade Name:	Inderal
Indications:	Hypertension, angina, cardiac arrhythmias, hypertrophic subaortic stenosis, pheochromocytoma, thyrotoxicosis, migraine, reduction of cardiovascular mortality after acute phase of MI, and essential tremor.
Pharmacokinetics:	Oral absorption: 90%. Bioavailability: 30%. Distribution: placenta and milk; crosses blood-brain barrier. $T_{1/2}$: α, 10 min; β, 3–5 hr (long-acting capsules, 8–11 hr). Elimination: hepatic metabolism (active metabolites).

Pharmacodynamics: Nonselective β_1 and β_2 antagonist.
CNS: Fatigue, dizziness, depression.
CVS: Negative chronotropic and inotropic effects, ↓ systolic and diastolic BP and HR at rest and during exercise, membrane-stabilizing effect on heart.
Pulmonary: ↑ Airway resistance (bronchospasm).
Hepatic: ↓ Hepatic blood flow.
Renal: ↓ Plasma renin activity.
GI: Constipation, nausea, diarrhea.
Other: Inhibited glycogenolysis, release of free fatty acids and insulin.

Dosages/Concentrations: Extended-release capsules: 60, 80, 120, and 160 mg.
Tablets: 10, 20, 40, 60, 80, and 90 mg.
Oral solution: 20 mg/5 ml, 40 mg/5 ml, and 80 mg/ml.
IV: 1 mg/ml.
  For hypertension: initial dose: 20–40 mg b.i.d. (tablets) or 60–80 mg daily (extended-release capsules). Usual maintenance: 160–480 mg daily (tablets); 120–160 mg daily (extended-release capsules).
  For angina: 160–240 mg daily (start 10–20 mg t.i.d. or q.i.d.).
  For arrhythmias (life-threatening): 0.5–3 mg IV; may repeat after 2 min.
  For MI: 180–240 mg daily.
  For migraine: 80–240 mg daily.

Contraindications: Impaired myocardial function, second- or third-degree AV block, severe bradycardia, bronchospastic disease (asthma), and hepatic or renal impairment (use with caution).

Drug Interactions/Allergy: Use with other antihypertensive agents may exaggerate hypotensive effect. Acute withdrawal may cause rebound ↑ HR and ↑ BP. May potentiate effects of neuromuscular blocking agents (tubocurarine). May reduce clearance of theophylline. May mask signs of hy-

PROPRANOLOL   *(continued)*

perthyroidism and hypoglycemia. May antagonize bronchodilation produced by β agonists. May decrease hypoglycemic action of glyburide.

SOTALOL

Trade Name:	Betapace
Indications:	Ventricular arrhythmias.
Pharmacokinetics:	Bioavailability: 90%–100%. $T_{1/2}$: β, 12 hr. Elimination: excreted in urine unchanged (removed by hemodialysis).
Pharmacodynamics:	Nonselective β antagonist.
CNS:	Fatigue, dizziness.
CVS:	Prolonged repolarization and refractoriness (conduction unchanged), torsades de pointes, negative chronotropic and inotropic effects.
Pulmonary:	↑ Airway resistance (bronchospasm).
GI:	Nausea, vomiting.
Other:	Inhibited release of free fatty acids and insulin.
Dosages/ Concentrations:	Tablets: 80, 160, and 240 mg. Initial dose: 80 mg b.i.d. (adjust individually). May increase up to 320 mg daily. Reduce dose in patients with renal impairment.
Contraindications:	Impaired myocardial function, second- or third-degree AV block, severe bradycardia, and bronchospastic disease (asthma).
Drug Interactions/ Allergy:	Can precipitate torsades de pointes. Acute withdrawal may cause rebound ↑ HR and ↑ BP. May mask signs of hyperthyroidism and hypoglycemia. May antagonize bronchodilation produced by β agonists.

TIMOLOL

Trade Names:	Blocadren, Timoptic (ophthalmic solution)
Indications:	Hypertension, angina, reduction of cardiovascular mortality after acute phase of MI, prophylactic treatment of common and classic migraine headache, and reduction of IOP.
Pharmacokinetics:	Oral absorption: 90%. Systemic absorption with topical eye application. Bioavailability: 50%–75% (exten-

sive first-pass metabolism). $T_{1/2}$: β, 3–4 hr.
Distribution: milk. Elimination: 80% hepatic metabolism (inactive metabolites); 20% unchanged drug and metabolites excreted in urine (not removed by hemodialysis).

Pharmacodynamics: Nonselective β antagonist.

CNS: Fatigue, dizziness, asthenia, ↓ IOP.

CVS: Negative chronotropic and inotropic effects,
↓ systolic and diastolic BP and HR at rest and during exercise.

Pulmonary: ↑ Airway resistance (bronchospasm).

GI: Constipation, nausea, abdominal discomfort.

Renal: ↓ Plasma renin activity, ↓ GFR, ↓ RBF.

**Dosages/
Concentrations:** Tablets: 5, 10, and 20 mg. Ophthalmic solution: 0.25% and 0.5%.

For hypertension: initial dose: 10 mg b.i.d. Usual maintenance dose: 20–40 mg daily.

For angina: 15–45 mg daily.

For MI: 10 mg b.i.d.

For migraine headache: 10 mg b.i.d.

For ophthalmic use: Initial dose: 0.25% solution,
1 drop b.i.d.

Reduce doses in patients with renal or hepatic impairment.

Contraindications: Impaired myocardial function, second- or third-degree AV block, severe bradycardia, bronchospastic disease (asthma), angle-closure glaucoma unless used in combination with a miotic agent.

**Drug Interactions/
Allergy:** Use with other antihypertensive agents may exaggerate hypotensive effect. Acute withdrawal may cause rebound ↑ HR and ↑ BP. May mask signs of hyperthyroidism and hypoglycemia. May antagonize bronchodilation produced by β agonists. May increase muscle weakness in patients with myasthenia.

14

Blood Substitutes

Harbhej Singh, M.D.

ALBUMIN

Trade Names:	Albutein 5%; Albutein 25%; Albuminar-5; Albuminar-25; Buminate 5%; Buminate 25%; Plasbumin-5; Plasbumin-25; Albumin Human 5%; and Albumin Human 25%.
Indications:	Hypovolemia, isovolemic hemodilution, adjunct to crystalloid pump prime, ARDS, hemodialysis, red blood cell suspension, hypoproteinemia, severe burns, neonatal hyperbilirubinemia, ascites, nephrosis, pancreatitis, and liver failure.
Pharmacokinetics:	Onset: 15 min for blood volume expansion. Duration: longer duration of volume expansion in patients with reduced initial blood volume. Distribution: extracellular compartment. $T_{1/2}$: intravascular: 24 hr; elimination: 15–20 days.
Pharmacodynamics:	
CVS:	Blood volume support. 5% Albumin iso-oncotic with human plasma and ↑ blood volume equivalent to volume of albumin infused; 25% albumin oncotically equivalent to ~ 5 times the volume of human plasma and draws into circulation an amount of fluid ~ 3.5 times the volume of the albumin infused.
Hematologic:	↓ Hematocrit and blood viscosity due to ↑ blood volume
Other:	Binds reversibly to endogenous and exogenous substances, including bilirubin, fatty acids, hormones, enzymes, drugs, dyes, and trace metals.
Dosages/ Concentrations:	2 g/kg/24 hr. 5% solution in 50, 250, 500, and 1000 ml; 25% solution in 20, 50, and 100 ml.
Contraindications:	Severe anemia, cardiac failure, hypervolemia, and pulmonary edema.
Drug Interactions/ Allergy:	Incompatible with verapamil hydrochloride, alcohol-containing solutions, amino acid solutions, fat emulsions, and protein hydrolysates.

F-DECALIN (FDC); F-TRIPROPYLAMINE (FTPA); F-N-METHYL-DECAHYDROISOQUINOLINE (FMIQ); PERFLUBRON (PFOB)

Trade Names:	Fluosol-DA (FDC + FTPA), Oxygent (PFOB), Oxyfluor
Indications:	Protection of the myocardium from ischemia during

F-DECALIN (FDC); F-TRIPROPYLAMINE (FTPA); F-N-METHYL-DECAHYDROISOQUINOLINE (FMIQ); PERFLUBRON (PFOB) *(continued)*

	PTCA, possible acute isovolemic hemodilution and clinical blood replacement therapy (Oxygent, Oxyflor), increase of tumor cells' susceptibility to radiation and chemotherapy, ARDS, and organ preservation.
Pharmacokinetics:	Exhalation (low MW) and phagocytosis (high MW); excretion rate dependent on MW of fluorocarbon: $T_{1/2}$: β, 4–65 days (PFOB—4 days, FDC—7 days, FTPA—65 days).
Pharmacodynamics:	Fluorocarbon-based oxygen carrier.
CVS:	Myocardial protection.
Hematologic:	Straight oxyhemoglobin-dissociation curve (ODC); oxygen-carrying capacity dependent upon concentration of fluorocarbon.
Other:	Phagocytosis of high-molecular-weight fluorocarbons by reticuloendothelial system results in "foamy macrophages" in liver and spleen.

Dosage/ Concentrations:	Water-insoluble emulsions (0.1–0.3 μm diameter). Fluosol (20% intravascular perfluorochemical emulsion) consists of three components that must be mixed before administration:
	   1. Fluosol emulsion—400 ml in plastic bag
	   2. Solution 1—30 ml in glass vial
	   3. Solution 2—70 ml in glass vial
	Only Fluosol approved for use during PTCA.

Contraindications:	None known.
Drug Interactions/ Allergy:	Anaphylaxis to Pluronic F-68 in Fluosol-DA.

HEMOGLOBIN-BASED OXYGEN CARRIER

Trade Name:	N/A
Indications:	Possible clinical blood replacement therapy and acute isovolemic hemodilution.
Pharmacokinetics:	Unmodified hemoglobin tetramers ($\alpha_2\beta_2$) rapidly dissociate into dimers ($\alpha\beta$) outside red blood cells. $T_{1/2}$: β, 1–2 hr. Intravascular retention times up to 36 hr can be achieved by intramolecular cross-linking, binding of large molecules to α or β chains, and polymerization by intermolecular cross-linking.

Pharmacodynamics:

CNS:	Altered histology and enzymatic changes in retina.
CVS:	Interference with EDRF/nitric oxide system; coronary vasoconstriction; maintenance of constant cardiac output during hemodilution; altered histology and enzymatic changes in heart.
Pulmonary:	Altered histology and enzymatic changes in lungs.
Hepatic:	Altered histology and enzymatic changes in liver.
Renal:	Renal vasoconstriction, ↓ GFR, renal toxicity.
Other:	Altered histology and enzymatic changes in spleen.

Dosage/ Concentrations: N/A.

Contraindications: Coronary artery disease.

Drug Interactions/ Allergy: ↑ Immunogenicity of enlarged hemoglobin molecules. Complement activation.

HETASTARCH

Trade Name: Hespan Injection

Indications: Acute isovolemic hemodilution and plasma volume expansion (non-oxygen-carrying blood replacement therapy).

Pharmacokinetics: Onset: immediate. $T_{1/2}$: β, 25.5 hr. Elimination: renal; molecules < 50,000 daltons excreted rapidly. <10% detected intravascularly after 2 wk. Tissue $T_{1/2}$: 10–15 days; larger molecules degraded enzymatically in liver and spleen by amylase.

Pharmacodynamics:

CNS:	Headache.
CVS:	↑ Arterial and venous pressures, ↑ cardiac index, ↑ LV stroke work index, ↑ PCWP.
Pulmonary:	Pulmonary edema, volume overload.
Hepatic:	↑ Serum bilirubin level.
GI:	↑ Serum amylase level (temporary), vomiting.
Musculoskeletal:	Muscle pain.
Other:	↑ Plasma volume in excess of volume infused, ↑ temperature, impaired reticuloendothelial system, ↑ PT, ↑ PTT, interference with platelet function.

Dosages/ Concentrations: Maximum dose: 20 ml/kg/day (1500 ml); 500-ml bags of 6% hetastarch in 0.9% NaCl.

HETASTARCH   *(continued)*

Contraindications: Bleeding disorders, congestive heart failure, and renal failure.

Drug Interactions/   Urticaria, anaphylactoid reactions.
Allergy:

15

Bronchodilators and Antiasthmatics

Eugene Y. Lai, M.D.
Ahmed F. Ghouri, M.D.

ALBUTEROL

Trade Names:	Proventil, Ventolin
Indications:	Bronchodilation in asthma and COPD exacerbation, symptoms of hyperkalemic familial periodic paralysis.
Pharmacokinetics:	Onset: 5–15 min (oral inhaler). Peak effect: 1–2 hr. Duration: 3–4 hr. Elimination: hepatic ($T_{1/2}$: 3.8 hr).
Pharmacodynamics:	β_2-Selective bronchodilation.
CNS:	Tremor, nervousness, headache, vertigo, hyperactivity insomnia, pupillary dilation, irritability.
CVS:	β_1 effects: tachycardia, hypertension.
Pulmonary:	Cough, drying of secretions, paradoxical bronchospasm.
Hepatic:	Transient hyperglycemia.
Renal:	Transient hypokalemia, difficult micturition.
GI:	Nausea, vomiting, oropharyngeal edema.
Dosage/ Concentrations:	Each actuation of inhaler delivers 90 μg.
Adult and Pediatric (>4 yr):	1–2 puffs q 4–6 hr. Safety and efficacy not established in children < 4 yr of age.
Contraindications:	Discontinue if tachyphylaxis occurs. Use with caution or avoid if other sympathomimetics are administered, especially in patients with congestive heart failure, dysrhythmias, coronary artery disease, hypertension, hyperthyroidism, and seizure disorders.
Drug Interactions/ Allergy:	Effects antagonized by β-adrenergic blockers. ↑ Dysrhythmias or side effects when used with other sympathomimetics (especially theophylline). Use with extreme caution in patients taking MAOIs and TCAs.

AMINOPHYLLINE

Trade Name:	N/A
Indications:	Prevention and treatment of acute bronchospasm.
Pharmacokinetics:	Aminophylline is converted to theophylline, a methylxanthine bronchodilator; inhibiting phosphodiesterase increases levels of cAMP in bronchial smooth muscle. Onset: 3–4 min (IV); 30 min (p.o.). Peak effect: 60 min (IV); 2 hr (p.o.). Duration: 2–4 hr (IV); 4–8 hr (p.o.). Elimination: hepatic. Toxic level: >20 μg/ml; therapeutic level: 10–20 μg/ml.
Pharmacodynamics:	Bronchodilation.

CNS:	Headaches, seizures, excitement, irritability, SIADH.
CVS:	↑ Cardiac output, angina, congestive heart failure, tachycardia, ventricular and supraventricular dysrhythmias, ↓ PVR.
Pulmonary:	↑ Diaphragmatic contractility, tachypnea, bronchodilation.
Hepatic:	Hyperglycemia.
GI:	Dyspepsia, nausea, vomiting, abdominal pain.
Musculoskeletal:	↑ Muscle contractility.

Dosage/ Concentrations: Loading dose: 5 mg/kg IV over 20 min; 6 mg/kg p.o. Maintenance dose: 0.5–1.0 mg/kg/hr IV; 2–4 mg/kg q 6–12 hr p.o. Use lower end of dosing in infants and elderly, with congestive heart failure, and in those already taking theophylline. Use higher end of dosing range in smokers and children.

Contraindications: Use with caution in patients with cardiac dysfunction.

Drug Interactions/ Allergy: Effects antagonized by β-adrenergic blockers. ↑ Effects of sympathomimetics. ↑ Toxicity in patients taking cimetidine, quinolones, allopurinol, contraceptives, β blockers, corticosteroids, and erythromycins. ↑ Toxicity in patients with liver insufficiency. ↑ Dose in patients taking rifampin, phenobarbital, phenytoin, other hepatic enzyme-inducing agents and in smokers. Concomitant use of volaatile anesthetics, especially halothane, ↑ dysrhythmogenicity.

BECLOMETHASONE

Trade Names: Beclovent, Vanceril

Indications: Bronchospasm.

Pharmacokinetics: Onset (inhaler): undetermined. Duration (inhaler): ~ 4–6 hr. Topical effect only. Rapid hepatic inactivation of systemically absorbed dose. Partial metabolism by lung esterases. Continuous use for 1–4 wk may be required for maximal benefit.

Pharmacodynamics:	
CNS:	Hypothalamic-pituitary-adrenal suppression, Cushing syndrome.
Pulmonary:	↓ Airway inflammation, paradoxical bronchospasm, ↑ colonization, localized infections of larynx or bronchi with opportunistic organisms, dysphonia due to steroid myopathy of laryngeal muscles.
GI:	↑ Colonization; localized infections of mouth, phar-

BECLOMETHASONE   *(continued)*

ynx, and esophagus with opportunistic organisms (e.g., *Candida*).

Dosage/ **Concentrations:**	Each actuation of inhaler delivers 42 μg. Dose may be doubled in severe asthma; subsequently taper.
Adult:	Initial dose: 2 puffs t.i.d.
Pediatric:	1 puff t.i.d. (6–12 yr). Safety and efficacy not established in children <6 yr.

Contraindications: Not efficacious in acute bronchospasm. When switching from systemic steroids to inhaler, use a taper.

Drug Interactions/ **Allergy:**   Used safely with β agonists. Hypothalamic-pituitary-adrenal suppression and Cushing syndrome with concomitant systemic steroids.

CROMOLYN SODIUM

Trade Name: Intal

Indications: Prevention of bronchospasm.

Pharmacokinetics: Absorption: 5%–10% of inhaled dose is absorbed systemically (depends on proficiency of patient, degree of bronchoconstriction, and presence of mucous plugging). Absorption $T_{1/2}$ from lungs: 1 hr. Elimination $T_{1/2}$: 81 min. with equal excretion in urine and bile.

Pharmacodynamics:	↓ Release of histamine and SRS-A from mast cells.
CNS:	Dizziness, headache.
CVS:	Angina (from propellant), dysrhythmias.
Pulmonary:	Bronchospasm, eosinophilic pneumonia.
Renal:	Nephrosis.
GI:	GI distress in lactase-deficient patients, throat dryness and irritation.
Musculoskeletal:	Myalgias, joint pain, swelling.

Dosage/ **Concentrations:**	Each actuation of inhaler delivers 800 μg.
Adult and Pediatric (>5 yr):	1.6 mg (2 puffs) q.i.d. Not recommended <2 yr of age. Administer 10–15 min prior to known precipitant of bronchospasm (e.g., exercise, allergen).

Contraindications: Not to be used as a bronchodilator (for asthma prophylaxis only). Use with caution in patients with coronary artery disease or dysrhythmias.

Drug Interactions/ **Allergy:**   Use lactose-free preparations in lactase-deficient patients.

IPRATROPIUM BROMIDE

Trade Name:	Atrovent
Indications:	To augment bronchodilation produced by β_2 agonists.
Pharmacokinetics:	Onset: 30–60 min (oral inhaler). Peak effect: 2 hr. Duration: 3–4 hr. Elimination: hepatic. Absorption: Very little systemically when inhaled.
Pharmacodynamics:	Bronchodilation.
CNS:	Mydriasis, dizziness, insomnia, tremor, anxiety.
CVS:	Vagolysis, tachycardia, dysrhythmias, hypertension.
Pulmonary:	↓ Airway secretions, paradoxical bronchospasm, bronchitis, coughing.
Renal:	Urine retention.
GI:	Drying of secretions, nausea, constipation.
Musculoskeletal:	Arthritis.
Dosage/ Concentrations:	Each actuation of inhaler delivers 80 μg.
Adult and Pediatric (>12 yr):	2–4 puffs q 3–4 hr. Maximum daily dose: 2000 μg. Safety and efficacy not established in children <12 yr.
Contraindications:	Narrow-angle glaucoma, bladder neck obstruction, prostatic hypertrophy.
Drug Interactions/ Allergy:	Used safely with methylxanthines, corticosteroids, and β-adrenergic agonists. Antagonizes miotics. May increase efficacy without lowering safety profile when used concurrently with β agonists.

ISOPROTERENOL

Trade Name:	Isuprel
Indications:	Refractory bronchospasm.
Pharmacokinetics:	Onset: immediate (IV); 2–5 min (inhalation). Duration: 1–5 min (IV); 30–120 min (inhalation). Elimination: hepatic and renal.
Pharmacodynamics:	β_1- and β_2-Adrenergic agonist (no α effects); bronchodilation.
CNS:	Tremors, vertigo, headache.
CVS:	Tachycardia, ↑ contractility, ↑ cardiac output, angina, ↑ automaticity, ↓ SVR. ↓ or ↑ BP (depending on baseline vascular tone), Cheyne-Stokes attacks.
Pulmonary:	Paradoxical bronchospasm, pulmonary edema, tachyphylaxis.

ISOPROTERENOL   *(continued)*

Hepatic:	↑ Glycogenolysis and insulin secretion.
Renal:	Prolonged effects in renal failure.
GI:	Irritability, nausea, vomiting.

**Dosage/
Concentrations:**
Each actuation of inhaler delivers 120 μg.

Adult and Pediatric: 1–2 puffs q 3–4 hr (maximum 6 puffs/hr). IV infusion: start at 0.02 μg/kg/min, titrate to lowest effective dose.

Contraindications: Heart block caused by digitalis intoxication and tachyarrhythmias.

**Drug Interactions/
Allergy:**
Effects antagonized by β-adrenergic blockers.
↑ Dysrhythmias when used with volatile anesthetics and other sympathomimetics. Sulfites in drug may cause anaphylaxis or paradoxical bronchospasm.

METAPROTERENOL

Trade Names: Alupent, Metaprel

Indications: Bronchodilation in asthma and COPD exacerbation.

Pharmacokinetics: Onset: 1 min (oral inhaler), 5–30 min (nebulizer).
Peak effect: 1 hr (both). Duration: 60–150 min (both).
Elimination: hepatic and renal.

Pharmacodynamics: β_2-Mediated bronchodilation.
CNS: Tremor, nervousness, headache, fatigue, vertigo.
CVS: β_1 effects: tachycardia, palpitations, hypertension, cardiac dysrhythmias, ischemia.
Pulmonary: Paradoxical bronchospasm, cough, tachyphylaxis.
GI: Throat irritation, bad taste, nausea, vomiting.
Musculoskeletal: Muscular cramping.

**Dosage/
Concentrations:**
Each actuation of inhaler delivers 0.65 mg.

Adult and Pediatric
(>6 yr):   2–3 puffs q 3–4 hr. Safety and efficacy not established in children <6 yr.

Contraindications: Discontinue if tachyphylaxis occurs. Use with caution or avoid if other sympathomimetics are administered, especially in congestive heart failure, dysrhythmias, coronary artery disease, hypertension, hyperthyroidism, and seizure disorders.

**Drug Interactions/
Allergy:**
Effects antagonized by β-adrenergic blockers.
↑ Dysrhythmias or side effects when used with other sympathomimetics (especially theophylline).

TERBUTALINE

Trade Names:	Brethine, Brethaire, Bricanyl
Indications:	Bronchodilation in acute bronchospasm.
Pharmacokinetics:	Onset: 5–30 min (oral inhaler), 15 min (SC). Peak effect: 1–2 hr (inhaled), 30–60 min (SC). Duration: 3–6 hr (inhaled), 90 min–4 hr (SC). Elimination: hepatic; complete in 72–96 hr.
Pharmacodynamics:	β_2-Selective bronchodilation and β_1 effects.
CNS:	Tremor, nervousness, vertigo, headache, anxiety, drowsiness, tinnitus, seizures, unusual taste.
CVS:	β_1 effects: tachycardia, palpitations, hypertension, cardiac dysrhythmias, ischemia, peripheral vasodilation, diaphoresis.
Pulmonary:	Cough, drying of secretions, paradoxical bronchospasm.
Renal:	Transient hypokalemia.
GI:	Drying of secretions, nausea, dyspepsia.
Musculoskeletal:	Potent uterine tocolytic effects.
Dosage/ Concentrations:	Each actuation of inhaler delivers 200 μg.
Adult and Pediatric (>12 yr):	2 puffs q 4–6 hr. 0.25 mg SC q 30 min; maximum dose: 0.5 mg/4 hr. Not recommended for children <12 yr.
Contraindications:	Tachyphylaxis. Use with caution or avoid in patients with dysrhythmias, angina, congestive heart failure, diabetes mellitus, seizures, hypokalemia, and hyperthyroidism.
Drug Interactions/ Allergy:	Effects antagonized by β-adrenergic blockers. ↑ Dysrhythmias and side effects when used with volatile anesthetics and other sympathomimetics (especially theophylline). Use with extreme caution in patients taking MAOIs, TCAs. Risk of hypokalemia in patients taking potassium-depleting diuretics. Paradoxical bronchoconstriction with repeated excessive use of inhalational preparations.

16

Calcium Channel Blockers

William B. Kelly, M.D.

AMLODIPINE BESYLATE

Trade Name:	Norvasc
Indications:	Angina and essential hypertension.
Pharmacokinetics:	MW: 567.1. pKa: 8.6. Slightly water-soluble, sparingly soluble in ethanol. Absolute bioavailability: 64%–90%. Time to peak plasma concentration: 6–12 hr. Protein binding: 93%. Metabolism: 90% converted to inactive metabolites. Extensively metabolized by hepatic P-450 system. $T_{1/2}$: 30–50 hr. Elimination: breast milk; 10% excreted unchanged in urine.

Pharmacodynamics:	
CNS:	Headache, fatigue, lethargy.
CVS:	Myocardial contractility, ↑ cardiac output, ↓ PVR, palpitations.

Dosage/ Concentrations:	Tablets: 2.5, 5.0, and 10.0 mg. For hypertension: usual dose: 5 mg p.o. q.d.; may be taken without regard to meals; maximum dose: 10 mg p.o. q.d.; for elderly or patients with hepatic insufficiency: begin at 2.5 mg p.o. q.d.; titrate over 7–14 days. For angina: 5–10 mg p.o. q.d.; for elderly or patients with hepatic insufficiency: lower dose.

Contraindications:	Sick sinus syndrome, second- or third-degree AV block (with pacemaker), hypotension, and impaired hepatic function (use with caution).

Drug Interactions/ Allergy:	Drugs that affect hepatic enzyme system affect blood levels and clearance. Hypotension or ↑ fluid requirements with opioids. General anesthetics ↓ lithium serum levels.

BEPRIDIL

Trade Name:	Vascor
Indications:	Chronic stable angina.
Pharmacokinetics:	MW: 421.02. Slightly water-soluble; very soluble in ethanol, methanol, and chloroform. Absorption: ~ 100%. Absolute bioavailability: 59%. Onset: 60 min (oral). Time of protein plasma levels: 2–3 hr. Protein binding: >99%. Therapeutic serum level: 1–2 mg/ml. $T_{1/2}$: 24 hr. Elimination: excreted in breast milk.

BEPRIDIL *(continued)*

Pharmacodynamics:

CNS:	Dizziness, lightheadedness, nervousness, headache, asthenia.
CVS:	↓ PVR, prolonged atrial effective refractory period, AV nodal conduction time, prolonged PR interval, ↓ myocardial contractility, palpitations, prolonged QT interval, ↓ HR, torsades de pointes.
Pulmonary:	Shortness of breath.
Hepatic:	↑ LFT results.
GI:	Nausea, diarrhea.
Other:	Hypokalemia, peripheral edema.

Dosage/Concentrations: Tablets: 200, 300, and 400 mg. Starting dose 200 mg p.o. q.d.; can increase to 300 (max 400 mg) p.o. q.d. with increased dosage at 10-day intervals.

Contraindications: Serious ventricular arrhythmias, sick sinus syndrome; second- or third-degree heart block, uncompensated cardiac failure, hypotension, prolonged QT interval or drugs that prolong QT interval, and recent (<3 months) MI.

Drug Interactions/Allergy: Prolonged QT interval with TCAs, procainamide, quinidine, and cardiac glycosides.

DILTIAZEM

Trade Names: Cardizem, Cardizem CD, Cardizem SR, Dilacor XR

Indications: Angina and essential hypertension. Unlabeled use: Raynaud's phenomenon.

Pharmacokinetics: MW: 450.98. Clearance: ↓ by 40% if hepatic disease present. Absorption: 80%–90%. Absolute bioavailability: 40%–67%. Onset: 30–60 min. Time to peak plasma level: 2–3 hr; SR, 6–11 hr. Protein binding: 70%–80%. Therapeutic serum level: 50–200 ng/ml. $T_{1/2}$: 3.5–6 hr; SR, 5–7 hr. Metabolism: major metabolite, desacetyl diltiazem; has 25%–50% pharmacologic activity of diltiazem. Elimination: excreted in breast milk.

Pharmacodynamics:

CNS:	Dizziness, headache, asthenia.
CVS:	↓ PVR, ↓ (slight) HR, slight ↓ SA node automaticity, ↓ AV nodal conduction, prolonged PR interval, second- or third-degree AV block.

Hepatic:	↑ LFT results, may ↓ P_{450} metabolism.
Other:	Dermatitis, flushing, erythema multiforme.

**Dosage/
Concentrations:**

Trade Name	Dose Available	Starting Dose		Optimal Dose
		Hypertension	*Angina*	
Cardizem	30, 60, 90, 120 mg	30 mg p.o. q.i.d.		180–360 mg q.d.
Cardizem CD	120, 180, 240,	180–240 mg p.o.	120–180 mg	≥480 mg q.d.
(dual release)	300 mg	q.d.	p.o. q.d.	
Cardizem SR		60–120 mg p.o.	60–120 mg p.o.	
(extended release)	60, 90, 120 mg	b.i.d.	b.i.d.	
Dilacor XR		180–240 mg p.o.		
(extended release)	120, 180, 240 mg	q.d.		

Adult:	IV: Infusion: dilute in 0.9% Nacl, 5% dextrose; infuse at 5–10 mg/hr. For antiarrhythmic effect: 0.25 mg/kg over 2 min and ECG monitoring. May repeat at dose to 0.35 mg/kg in 15 min. Can follow with infusion.
Pediatric:	Safety not established.
Contraindications:	Sick sinus syndrome; second- or third-degree AV block; MI (<3 months); elderly; and congestive heart failure, β blockade, digoxin use, AV conduction anomalies, or hepatic or renal dysfunction (use with caution).
**Drug Interactions/
Allergy:**	Digoxin and cyclosporine levels. Drugs that alter hepatic cytochrome P_{450} system will alter diltiazem clearance.

FELODIPINE

Trade Name:	Plendil
Indications:	Essential hypertension.
Pharmacokinetics:	MW: 384.26. Insoluble in water; freely soluble in dichloromethane and ethanol. Absorption (oral): ~100%. Absolute bioavailability: 20%. Onset: 120–300 min. Time of peak plasma level: 2.5–5.0 hr. Protein binding: 99%. Metabolism: six metabolites identified (inactive). Elimination: <0.5% excreted unchanged in urine. $T_{1/2}$: 11–16 hr.
Pharmacodynamics: *CNS:*	Dizziness, headache, asthenia.

FELODIPINE *(continued)*

CVS:	↓ SVR, reflexive ↑ in cardiac output, ↑ myocardial contractility, mild ↑ HR, hypotension.
Hepatic:	↓ Clearance by 40% in patients with hepatic disease.
GI:	Abdominal discomfort.
Other:	Flushing, peripheral edema.

Dosage/ Concentrations: Tablets: 2.5, 5, and 10 mg. Do not crush.
Initial dose: 5 mg p.o. q.d.; increase at 2-wk intervals.
Usual adult dose: ≤20 mg p.o. q.d.
For elderly (>60 yr) and patients with hepatic insufficiency, not to exceed 10 mg p.o. q.d.

Contraindications: Pregnant and pediatric patients.

Drug Interactions/ Allergy: ↓ Clearance of metoprolol. Usually well tolerated when given concomitantly with β blockers, including metoprolol. Hydantoins and barbiturates ↓ bioavailability of felodipine. Erythromycin ↑ effects of felodipine. Felodipine ↑ serum digoxin levels.

ISRADIPINE

Trade Name: DynaCirc

Indications: Essential hypertension.

Pharmacokinetics: MW 371.39. Practically insoluble in water; soluble in ethanol, acetone, chloroform, and methylene chloride. Absorption (oral): 90%–95%. Absolute bioavailability: 15%–24%. Bioavailability: ↑ in elderly (>60 yr) and in patients with hepatic impairment. Onset (oral): 120 min. Time to peak plasma concentration: 1.5 hr. Protein binding: 95%. Elimination: 0% excreted in urine unchanged. $T_{1/2}$: 8 hr.

Pharmacodynamics:
CNS:	Dizziness.
CVS:	↓ SVR, improved cardiac output, palpitations.
Hepatic:	↑ LFT values.
Other:	Peripheral edema, flushing.

Dosage/ Concentrations: Capsules: 2.5 and 5.0 mg. Initial dose: 2.5 mg p.o. b.i.d. alone or in combination with thiazide diuretic. May adjust upward in increments of 5 mg/day at intervals of 2–4 wk to maximum of 20 mg/day. Adverse effects and limited additional response at doses >10 mg/day.

Contraindications:	Ventricular dysfunction, hepatic dysfunction, and in elderly, pregnant, pediatric, and breast-feeding patients (use with caution).
Drug Interactions/ Allergy:	Severe hypotension in patients receiving fentanyl, Ca^{2+} channel blockers, and β blockers.

NICARDIPINE

Trade Names:	Cardene, Cardene SR
Indications:	Angina, essential hypertension, and short-term therapy in NPO patients with hypertension. Unlabeled use: CHF.
Pharmacokinetics:	Oral: absorption: ~100%. Absolute bioavailability: 35%. Onset: 20 min. Time to peak plasma levels: 0.5–2 hr. Protein binding: >95%. Therapeutic serum levels: 28–50 mg/ml. Elimination: $T_{1/2}$: 2–4 hr; <1% excreted unchanged in urine; excreted in breast milk. IV: $T_{1/2}$: α, 2.7 min; β, 44.8 min, γ, 14.4 hr.
Pharmacodynamics:	
CNS:	Dizziness, headache, asthenia.
CVS:	↓ SVR, improved cardiac output, coronary vasodilation, negative inotropic effect, ↑ HR, prolonged QT interval, tachycardia, palpitations, angina.
Renal:	↓ GFR.
Other:	Peripheral edema, flushing.
Dosage/ Concentrations:	Oral: 20–40 mg q 8 hr. Capsules: 20 and 30 mg. IV: 25 mg in 10 cc ampules (2.5 mg/cc). Dilute each ampule with 240 cc fluid (not compatible with NaHCO₃ or lactated Ringer's solution) to give final concentration of 0.1 mg/ml. Infusion rate: 0.5–2.2 mg/hr. Reaches 50% ultimate decrease in ~45 min. If infusion discontinued, will have 50% offset of that BP change within 30 ± 7 min with declining antihypertensive effects for up to 50 hr.
Contraindications:	Recent intracranial hemorrhage and aortic stenosis. Use with caution in pregnant and pediatric patients. Passed in breast milk.
Drug Interactions/ Allergy:	H2 antagonists ↑ serum levels of nicardipine. Monitor digoxin and cyclosporine levels closely.

NIFEDIPINE

Trade Names:	Procardia, Procardia XL, Adalat
Indications:	Angina and essential hypertension. Unlabeled uses: migraine headache, Raynaud's phenomenon, congestive heart failure, and cardiomyopathy.
Pharmacokinetics:	MW: 346.3. Absorption: 90%. Absolute bioavailability: 45%–70%; SR, 86%. Bioavailability: ↑ in hepatic insufficiency; ↑ by ethanol. Onset: (oral): 20 min. Time to peak plasma concentration: 5 hr; SR 6 hr. Protein binding: 92%–98%. Therapeutic serum levels: 25–100 mg/ml. Elimination: 1%–2% excreted unchanged in urine; excreted in breast milk. $T_{1/2}$: 2–5 hr.

Pharmacodynamics:

CNS:	Dizziness, headache.
CVS:	Angina, ↓ SVR, MI, congestive heart failure, ↑ HR, negative effect in myocardial contractility, improved cardiac output.
Pulmonary:	Shortness of breath, wheezing.
Hepatic:	↑ LFT values.
Renal:	↓ Renal function, ↑ plasma concentration.
GI:	Nausea.
Other:	↓ Platelet aggregation; ↑ bleeding time, dermatologic changes, peripheral edema, flushing.

Dosage/ Concentrations:	For acute hypertension: 10–20 mg.

- Adalat (10, 20 mg capsules): 30–60 mg p.o. q.d. on an empty stomach.
- Procardia (10, 20 mg capsules): 10–30 mg p.o. t.i.d.
- Procardia XL: 30–60 p.o. q.d. 24-hr delivery system: don't destroy tablet.

Contraindications:	Congestive heart failure, aortic stenosis, concomitant β blocker use, and pregnant and pediatric patients.
Drug Interactions/ Allergy:	Ethanol increases bioavailability. Monitor cardiac glycosides closely. Agents that inhibit cytochrome P_{450} system can increase bioavailability. Can elevate phenytoin levels, leading to toxicity.

NIMODIPINE

Trade Name:	Nimotop
Indications:	Subarachnoid hemorrhage. Unlabeled use: migraine headache.

Pharmacokinetics:	MW: 418.5. Practically insoluble in water. Absolute bioavailability: 13%. Time to peak plasma level: 1 hr. Protein binding: >95%. Elimination: <1% excreted unchanged in urine. $T_{1/2}$: 1–2 hr.
Pharmacodynamics:	
CNS:	Anticonvulsant activity, headache, psychiatric disturbances.
CVS:	↓ BP.
Hepatic:	↑ Clearance time if hepatic insufficiency present.
GI:	Nausea, abdominal discomfort.
Other:	Peripheral edema, dermatitis, rash.

Dosage/ Concentrations:	Capsule: 30 mg.
	    For subarachnoid hemorrhage: begin within 96 hr of event. Usual dose: 60 mg p.o. on empty stomach q 4 hr for 21 days. If patient cannot swallow, withdraw contents of capsule with needle and syringe, dilute with 30 cc saline, and administer per NG tube. If hepatic insufficiency, reduce dose to 30 mg p.o. q 4 hr.
	    For prevention of migraine: 120 mg/day; prophylactic effect usually apparent within 1–2 months.

Contraindications:	None.
Drug Interactions/ Allergy:	Use caution in pregnant, breast-feeding, and pediatric patients. Can potentiate effects of other Ca^{2+} channel blockers. ↑ Serum phenytoin levels. Exacerbates toxicity; monitor levels.

VERAPAMIL

Trade Names:	Calan, Calan SR, Isoptin, Isoptin SR, Verelan
Indications:	Angina, essential hypertension, arrhythmias, PSVT, and hypertrophic cardiomyopathy. Unlabeled use: migraine headache.
Pharmacokinetics:	MW: 491.08. Absorption: 90%. Onset: 30 min (oral). Time to peak plasma concentration: oral, 1–2.2 hr; IV, 3–5 min. Protein binding: 83%–92%. Therapeutic serum level: 80–300 mg/ml. Metabolites: norverapamil has 20% pharmacologic activity of parent. Excreted in breast milk. $T_{1/2}$: 3–7 hr.
Pharmacodynamics:	
CNS:	Dizziness, headache.
CVS:	↓ ↓ SA node automaticity, ↓ ↓ ↓ AV nodal conduction, ↑ PR interval, ↓ SVR, hypotension, bradycardia.
GI:	Constipation, altered GI transit time, ↓ P_{450} activity.

VERAPAMIL   *(continued)*

Other:	Erythema multiforme, Stevens-Johnson syndrome, peripheral edema.

Dosage/ Concentrations:
Adult:
Pediatric:

IV infusion over 3 min. Continuous ECG monitoring. For SVT:

5–10 mg IV (0.075–0.15 mg/kg), repeat in 15–30 min.

- 1–15 yr: 2–5 mg IV (0.1–0.3 mg/kg); repeat in 30 min.

- <1 yr: 0.75–2 mg (0.1–0.2 mg/kg).

For chronic atrial flutter or fibrillation: 240–320 mg total in 3–4 divided doses.

For prevention of PSVT in adults: 240–480 mg p.o. total in 3–4 divided doses.

For angina: starting dose: 80 mg p.o. q 6–8 hr; usual range: 320–480 mg total q.d.

For hypertension: oral dose: 40–80 mg p.o. b.i.d. Extended-release formulations: 120–240 mg p.o. every morning. If hepatic or renal impairment, hypertension in elderly, 70%.

Contraindications:

Sick sinus syndrome, ventricular tachycardia, atrial flutter or fibrillation with necessary pathway, severe LV dysfunction, second- or third-degree heart block. Use with caution in congestive heart failure and pseudohypertrophic muscular dystrophy and in pregnant and pediatric patients.

Drug Interactions/ Allergy:

↑ Bioavailability of metoprolol, digoxin, carbamazepine, theophylline, and cyclosporine. Potentiates neuromuscular blocking agents. Can result in excessive hypotension if used with quinidine, disopyramide, and dantrolene.

17

Central Stimulants

Steven J. Luke, M.D.

BACLOFEN

Trade Name:	Lioresal
Indications:	Spasticity from multiple sclerosis and spinal cord diseases.
Pharmacokinetics:	Onset: hours to weeks. Duration: 2.5–4 hr. Elimination: renal; 70%–85% excreted unchanged in 24 hr.

Pharmacodynamics:

CNS:	Generalized CNS depressant; ↓ release of excitatory neurotransmitters.
CVS:	Hypotension (rare).
Renal:	Urinary frequency.
GI:	Nausea, constipation.
Musculoskeletal:	Relief of flexor spasm.

Dosage/ Concentrations:

Adult:	Up to 20 mg 4 times a day.
Contraindications:	Spasm from rheumatism, stroke, cerebral palsy, and parkinsonism. Use with caution in elderly with poor renal function.
Drug Interactions/ Allergy:	Augments action of other CNS depressants.

BROMOCRIPTINE

Trade Name:	Parlodel
Indications:	Hyperprolactinemia, prevention of lactation, acromegaly, Parkinson's disese.
Pharmacokinetics:	Onset: slow p.o. Duration: 8–12 wk. Elimination: hepatic.

Pharmacodynamics:

CNS:	Inhibition of prolactin secretion, drowsiness.
CFS:	Hypotension.
GI:	Diarrhea, cramps.
Musculoskeletal:	Cold-sensitive digital vasospasm.
Dosage:	2.5–15 mg/day.
Contraindications:	Pregnancy, uncontrolled hypertension.
Drug Interactions/ Allergy:	↓ Efficacy with phenothiazines and butyrophenones.

DISULFIRAM

Trade Name:	Antabuse
Indications:	Chronic alcoholism.
Pharmacokinetics:	Onset: 1–2 hr. Duration: up to 14 days. Elimination: primarily renal.

Pharmacodynamics:
CNS:	Intense throbbing, pulsating headache.
CVS:	Hypotension, syncope.
Pulmonary:	Difficulty breathing.
Hepatic:	Inhibition of hepatic microsomal enzymes.
Renal:	Renal elimination.
GI:	Nausea, vomiting.
Other:	Heat and flushing felt in face.

**Dosage/
Concentrations:**
Adult:	125–500 mg daily.
Contraindications:	Children and pregnant women. Use with caution in elderly with renal impairment.
Drug Interactions/ Allergy:	With alcohol, accumulation of acetaldehyde. With alfentanil, ↓ clearance. With anticoagulants, ↑ effect.

DOXAPRAM

Trade Name:	Dopram
Indications:	Drug-induced postanesthetic respiratory depression, respiratory and CNS depression from drug overdose, and acute respiratory insufficiency in COPD.
Pharmacokinetics:	Onset: 20–40 sec. Duration: 5–12 min. Elimination: extensively metabolized; less than 5% unchanged in urine.

Pharmacodynamics:	Stimulation of peripheral carotid chemoreceptors.
CNS:	Seizures.
CVS:	Hypertension, tachycardia, dysrhythmias.
Pulmonary:	↑ Minute ventilation (↑ TV, no change in respiratory rate).
Renal:	Transient flushing, warmth, or pain in genital area.
Other:	↓ Postanesthetic shivering.

**Dosage/
Concentrations:**
Adult:	1 mg/kg bolus, 2–3 mg/min as infusion.

DOXAPRAM   *(continued)*

Contraindications:	Seizure disorder, CNS tumor, coronary artery disease, congestive heart failure, pheochromocytoma, and asthma. Use with caution in elderly. Not for use in neonates or premature infants.
Drug Interactions/ Allergy:	With MAOIs, hypertension, tachycardia, seizures. ↑ Action of vasopressors.

ERGOTAMINE, DIHYDROERGOTAMINE, METHYLERGONOVINE, METHYSERGIDE

Trade Names:	Cafergot, D.H.E. 45, Methergine, Sansert
Indications:	Migraine headache, uterine hemorrhage.
Pharmacokinetics:	Onset: slow p.o.; rapid IV. Duration: 2–21 hr. Elimination: hepatic.

Pharmacodynamics:

CNS:	Cerebral vasoconstriction.
CVS:	Vasoconstriction.
Hepatic:	Ergot poisoning with hepatic impairment.
GI:	Severe nausea, vomiting.
Musculoskeletal:	Ischemia and gangrene.
Other:	Uterine contraction.

Dosage/ Concentrations:	Ergotamine: 1 mg with 100 mg caffeine. Dihydroergotamine: 0.5 mg IV. Methylergonovine: 0.2 mg IV/IM 0.2 mg p.o. t.i.d. Methysergide: 4–8 mg/day.
Contraindications:	Hypertension, coronary artery disease, and peripheral vascular disease.
Drug Interactions/ Allergy:	Avoid use with vasoconstrictors.

LEVODOPA, L-DOPA, CARBIDOPA

Trade Names:	Dopar, Larodopa, Sinemet
Indications:	Parkinson's disease.
Pharmacokinetics:	Onset: rapidly absorbed from small bowel. Peak concentration: 30 min–2 hr. Duration: $T_{1/2}$: 1–3 hr. Elimination: renal excretion; 95% decarboxylated in

periphery by L-amino acid decarboxylase. Extensive first-pass metabolism. Less than 1% penetrates CNS.

Pharmacodynamics:

CNS: ↓ Tremor, ↓ rigidity, and ↓ bradykinesia; prolactin secretion.

CVS: Orthostatic hypotension, cardiac stimulation.

Pulmonary: Improved pulmonary function.

Renal: Urine red, then black, on exposure to air or alkali.

GI: Sluggish gastric emptying; ↓ bioavailability if hyperacidity; anorexia, nausea, and vomiting in early treatment.

Musculoskeletal: Improved posture, gait, facial expression, handwriting.

Dosage/ Concentrations:

Adult: Levodopa alone: 2–3 g/day.
Carbidopa: one tablet t.i.d.

Contraindications: Bronchial asthma, severe cardiovascular disease, glaucoma, melanoma, peptic ulcer, psychosis, renal insufficiency, and urinary retention; concomitant use with MAOI.

Drug Interactions/ Allergy: Pyridoxine in diet enhances extracellular metabolism of levodopa. Antipsychotic drugs can cause parkinsonism-like effect, nullifying action of levodopa. MAOIs exaggerate central effect, causing hypertension and hyperpyrexia.

METHYLPHENIDATE, DEXTROAMPHETAMINE, METHAMPHETAMINE

Trade Names: Ritalin, Ritalin-SR, Dexedrine, Desoxyn

Indications: Attention deficit disorder and narcolepsy.

Pharmacokinetics: Methylphenidate: rapid onset: $T_{1/2}$: 2 hr; renal elimination. Dextroamphetamine: rapid onset. Methamphetamine: rapid onset; duration: 4–5 hr; renal elimination.

Pharmacodynamics: Blockade of reuptake at dopaminergic neurons; generalized CNS stimulation.

CNS: Enhanced ability to pay attention.

CVS: ↑ Systolic and diastolic BP.

Pulmonary: Weak bronchodilation.

GI: Diarrhea, nausea, vomiting, cramps, constipation.

Musculoskeletal: ↓ Motor restlessness.

Dosage/ Concentrations:

Adult: Methylphenidate:
20–30 mg/day.

METHYLPHENIDATE, DEXTROAMPHETAMINE, METHAMPHETAMINE *(continued)*

Pediatric:	Begin 5 mg/day, increase to effect.
	Dextroamphetamine:
Adult:	5–60 mg once a day.
Pediatric:	5–15 mg once a day.
	Methamphetamine:
Adult:	20–25 mg/day.
Pediatric:	Begin 5 mg/day, increase to effect.

Contraindications: Marked anxiety, tension, agitation, and Tourette's syndrome. Do not use within 14 days of last dose of MAOI.

Drug Interactions/ Allergy: β Blockers can cause unopposed α stimulation. Meperidine can cause coma, convulsions, hyperpyrexia. MAOIs can cause prolonged, intense cardiac stimulant and vasopressor effects.

METHYLXANTHINES (THEOPHYLLINE, CAFFEINE)

Trade Names: Theo-Dur, Slo-bid, NōDōz, Vivarin

Indications: Asthma, reversible bronchoconstriction, COPD, fatigue, and drowsiness.

Pharmacokinetics: Onset: 1–2 hr orally. Duration: 3–9 hr in children and adults, 50 hr in premature infants; $T_{1/2}$ prolonged in elderly. Elimination: metabolized in liver; more rapid metabolism in smokers. 10% unchanged in urine.

Pharmacodynamics:

CNS:	Clearer, more rapid thought; stimulation of medullary respiratory center.
CVS:	↑ HR, ↓ PVR.
Pulmonary:	Bronchodilation; ↑ vital capacity, ↑ diaphragmatic contraction.
Renal:	Diuresis; bladder and uterine relaxation.
GI:	Suppression of small- and large-bowel motility; relaxation of lower esophageal sphincter.
Musculoskeletal:	↑ Contractility of striated muscle.

Dosage/ Concentrations: Theophylline:

Adult:	IV, 5 mg/kg bolus, 0.5–1.0 mg/kg/hr infusion; p.o., 16 mg/kg/day.
Pediatric:	16 mg/kg/day in 2 divided doses; titrate up or down to effect.
Geriatric:	Lower dose may be needed.

Contraindications:	Active peptic ulcer disease and untreated seizure disorders.
Drug Interactions/ Allergy:	↑ Metabolism of methylxanthines with tobacco, nicotine, phenytoin, and phenobarbital.

NICOTINE

Trade Names:	Nicorette, Habitrol, Nicoderm
Indications:	Smoking cessation.
Pharmacokinetics:	Onset: 15–30 min chewing; 5–6 hr transdermally. Duration: 1–2 hr nicotine, 15–20 hr metabolites. Elimination: hepatic.

Pharmacodynamics:
CNS:	Stimulation, tremor.
CVS:	↑ HR, ↑ BP.
Pulmonary:	↑ Bronchial secretions, ↑ ventilation.
GI:	Injury to dental work, nausea, vomiting.
Musculoskeletal:	Tremor.

Dosage/ Concentrations:
Adult:	Gum, 10 pieces of 2 mg gum/day. Transdermal patch, 15–21 mg/day.
Contraindications:	Angina pectoris, cardiac arrhythmias, post MI, pregnant women, and children.
Drug Interactions/ Allergy:	↑ Absorption of insulin. Smoking cessation reduces metabolism of bronchodilators, propranolol, and propoxyphene.

SELEGILINE (DEPRENYL)

Trade Name:	Eldepryl
Indications:	Parkinson's disease (must be used concurrently with levodopa).
Pharmacokinetics:	Onset: 0.5 to 2 hr. Elimination: 45% appears in urine in 24 hr.
Pharmacodynamics:	Irreversible inhibition of MAO-B (↑ central dopamine levels).
CNS:	Preservation of dopamine in basal ganglia.
CVS:	Hypertensive crisis, angina, dysrhythmias.
Pulmonary:	Asthma.

SELEGILINE (DEPRENYL) *(continued)*

Renal:	Urinary retention.
GI:	Dry mouth.
Musculoskeletal:	Improvement in motor symptoms of parkinsonism.

Dosage/ Concentrations: Adult: — Not to exceed 10 mg/day.

Contraindications: Peptic ulcer disease, concurrent use of meperidine.

Drug Interactions/ Allergy: With fluoxetine (Prozac), serotonin syndrome (confusion, myoclonus, hyperreflexia, fever, convulsions). With meperidine (Demerol), excitation, sweating, rigidity, convulsion, fever, coma. With tyramine, doses of selegiline > 20 mg/day cause hypertensive crisis. Enhances side effects of levodopa and levodopa/carbidopa.

TRIHEXYPHENIDYL, BENZTROPINE, BIPERIDEN, ETHOPROPAZINE, PROCYCLIDINE

Trade Names: Artane, Cogentin, Akineton, Parsidol, Kemadrin

Indications: Drug-induced extrapyramidal reactions, mild cases of parkinsonism.

Pharmacokinetics: Trihexyphenidyl: onset: p.o., 1 hr; duration: p.o. 6–12 hr. Benztropine: onset: p.o., 1 hr; IV, minutes; duration: 24 hr. Biperiden: onset: IM, 10–30 min; IV, minutes; duration: IV, 1–8 hr. Ethopropazine: duration: p.o., 4 hr. Procyclidine: duration: p.o., 4 hr.

Pharmacodynamics:	Blockade of central (striatal) cholinergic receptors.
CNS:	Improved tremor, blurred vision, ↑ IOP; confusion, delirium, hallucinations, somnolence.
CVS:	Tachycardia, dysrhythmia.
Renal:	Urinary retention.
GI:	Dry mouth, constipation.
Musculoskeletal:	Improvement of tremor.

Dosage/ Concentrations: Trihexyphenidyl: 1–15 mg/day.
Benztropine: 0.5–6 mg/day.
Biperiden: 2–8 mg/day.
Ethopropazine: 50–600 mg/day.
Procyclidine: 7.5–20 mg/day.

Contraindications: Glaucoma, tardive dyskinesia, myasthenia gravis, cardiovascular instability, intestinal obstruction, and urinary retention.

**Drug Interactions/
Allergy:**

Alcohol can increase sedation. Use caution with other anticholinergics. Antacids may adsorb drug, reducing bioavailability.

18

Cholinesterase Inhibitors

Ralph A. Farina, M.D.

BETHANECHOL CHLORIDE

Trade Names:	Duvoid, Urecholine
Indications:	Postoperative or postpartum period, nonobstructive urinary retention, and neurogenic atony of bladder with retention.
Pharmacokinetics:	Onset: p.o., 30–90 min; SC, SQ 5–15 min. Peak: p.o., 1 hr; SC, 15–30 min. Duration: p.o., 6 hr; SC, 2 hr.

Pharmacodynamics:
CNS: Dizziness, headache, seizures.
CVS: Hypotension with reflex tachycardia.
Pulmonary: Wheezing, bronchoconstriction.
GI: Abdominal cramping, diarrhea, nausea, vomiting.
Musculoskeletal: Body ache.
Other: Flushing, sweating.

Dosage/ Concentrations:	Oral: 10–15 mg t.i.d., q.i.d. SC: 2–5 mg q 4–6 hr. Tablets: package: 10–50 mg.
Contraindications:	Hyperthyroidism, peptic ulcer disease, asthma, pronounced bradycardia or coronary artery disease, parkinsonism, epilepsy, and GI obstruction (mechanical).
Drug Interactions/ Allergy:	With ganglionic blocking agents, combination may lead to precipitous fall in BP. Procainamide or quinidine may antagonize anticholinergic activity of bethanechol.

CARBACHOLINE (CARBAMOYLCHOLINE CHLORIDE)

Trade Names:	Miostat Intraocular, Isopto Carbachol
Indications:	Reduction of IOP in open-angle glaucoma and emergency treatment of angle-closure glaucoma prior to surgery.
Pharmacokinetics:	After topical administration, miosis occurs within 10–20 min and persists 4–8 hr. Maximum reduction in IOP within 2 hr. After intraocular injection, peak effect for miosis is 2–5 min and lasts 24 hr.

Pharmacodynamics:
CNS: Seizures, headaches.
CVS: Hypotension, bradycardia.
Pulmonary: Bronchoconstriction, excessive secretions.
GI: Nausea, vomiting, cramps.

CARBACHOLINE (CARBAMOYLCHOLINE CHLORIDE)   *(continued)*

Musculoskeletal:	Muscle cramping, weakness.
Other:	Blurred vision, painful ciliary spasm.

Dosage/ Concentrations:	Injection (intraocular): 100 μg/ml–0.5 ml. Solution: 0.75%, 1.5%, 2.25%, and 3%; 1–2 drops q 8 hr.
Contraindications:	Risk of retinal detachment, hypersensitivity to miotics, and acute iritis. Use with caution in asthma, corneal abrasion, hyperthyroidism, urinary tract obstruction, and significant coronary artery disease.
Drug Interactions/ Allergy:	Additive effects in combination with topical epinephrine, timolol, or carbonic anhydrases.

DEMECARIUM BROMIDE

Trade Name:	Humorsol
Indications:	Glaucoma and convergent strabismus.
Pharmacokinetics:	Miosis occurs within 15–60 min. Maximum miosis: 2–4 hr; persists 3–10 days. Maximum reduction in IOP within 24 hr. pH, 5–7.5.
Pharmacodynamics:	
CNS:	Headache, vertigo.
CVS:	Bradycardia, hypotension.
Pulmonary:	Bronchoconstriction, secretions, nasal congestion.
Renal:	Urinary frequency.
GI:	Nausea, diarrhea, cramping.
Dosage/ Concentrations:	0.125%–0.25% per drop. For glaucoma: dosing individualized; range, 2 times a week to 2 times a day.
Adult:	1–2 drops.
Pediatric:	1 drop. For convergent strabismus: 1 drop q.d. for 2–3 wk; follow q.o.d. for 2–4 wk; and follow 2 times/wk for several months.
Contraindications:	Risk of retinal detachment, hypersensitivity to miotics, marked vagotonia, asthma, hyperthyroidism, and cardiac failure.
Drug Interactions/ Allergy:	Additive effects with ocular hypotensive agents and systemic cholinesterase inhibitors; possibly with some general anesthetic agents. Use caution with succinylcholine. Hyperactivity in some Down's syndrome patients.

ECHOTHIOPHATE IODIDE

Trade Name:	Phospholine Iodide
Indications:	Open-angle glaucoma and convergent strabismus.
Pharmacokinetics:	Miosis, 10–30 min; persists several days. ↓ IOP within 4–8 hr. Maximal reduction of IOP within 24 hr. Bound to serum and ocular tissues. Oxidized and hydrolyzed by phosphoryl phosphatases.

Pharmacodynamics:

CNS:	Headache, vertigo, hyperactivity in Down's syndrome.
CVS:	Bradycardia, hypotension.
Pulmonary:	Bronchoconstriction, secretions, nasal congestion.
Renal:	Urinary frequency.
GI:	Nausea, diarrhea, cramping.

Dosage/ Concentrations:	1.5 mg–12.5 mg (0.03%–0.25%). 1 drop q 12–48 hr. For glaucoma: usually 2 doses/day. For convergent strabismus: 1 drop 0.125% solution each eye h.s. for 1–5 yr.
Contraindications:	Risk of retinal detachment, hypersensitivity to miotics, marked vagotonia, asthma, hyperthyroidism, and cardiac failure.
Drug Interactions/ Allergy:	Additive effect with ocular hypotensive agents and systemic cholinesterase inhibitors; possibly with some general anesthetic agents. Use caution with succinylcholine.

EDROPHONIUM CHLORIDE

Trade Names:	Tensilon, Enlon
Indications:	Differential diagnosis of myasthenia gravis, evaluation of emergency treatment of myasthenic crisis, and reversal of neuromuscular blockade of nondepolarizing muscle relaxants.
Pharmacokinetics:	Vd: 1.1 L/kg. Clearance: 9.6 ml/min/kg. $T_{1/2}$: α, 7.2 min; β, 110 min.

Pharmacodynamics:

CNS:	Convulsions, dysarthria, dysphonia, dysphasia.
CVS:	Bradycardia, ↓ cardiac output.
Pulmonary:	↑ Secretions, laryngospasm, bronchiolar constriction.
GI:	↑ Salivary and gastric secretions, nausea, vomiting, ↑ peristalsis, cramping.
Musculoskeletal:	Weakness, fasciculations.

EDROPHONIUM CHLORIDE   *(continued)*

Dosage/ Concentrations:	10 mg/ml concentration. For neuromuscular blockade reversal: 10–40 mg, 10 mg over 45 sec; or 0.5–1.0 mg/kg.
Contraindications:	Asthma, mechanical urinary tract or intestinal obstruction, and cardiac dysrhythmias (AV block, bradycardia).
Drug Interactions/ Allergy:	With digitalis, additive vagomimetic effects on heart. With succinylcholine, prior treatment with edrophonium may cause prolonged phase 1 block of depolarizing muscle relaxants.

ISOFLUROPHATE

Trade Name:	Floropryl
Indications:	Glaucoma and convergent strabismus.
Pharmacokinetics:	Miosis occurs after 5–10 min, maximal miosis after 15–20 min; persists for 1–4 wk. Maximal reduction in IOP within 24 hr. Rapidly decomposes with moisture to hydrogen fluoride.
Pharmacodynamics: *CNS:* *CVS:* *Pulmonary:* *Renal:* *GI:*	 Headache, vertigo. Bradycardia, hypotension. Bronchoconstriction, secretions, nasal congestion. Urinary frequency. Nausea, diarrhea, cramping.

Dosage/
Concentrations:
	0.25% concentration.
	   For glaucoma: 0.5 cm ointment every 8–72 hr.
	   For convergent strabismus: 0.5 cm to each eye q.d. h.s. for 2 wk for up to 5 yr.

Contraindications:	Risk of retinal detachment, hypersensitivity to miotics, marked vagotonia, asthma, hyperthyroidism, and cardiac failure.
Drug Interactions/ Allergy:	Additive effects with ocular hypotensive agents and systemic cholinesterase inhibitors; possibly with some general anesthetic agents. Use caution with succinylcholine.

NEOSTIGMINE BROMIDE (ORAL), NEOSTIGMINE METHYLSULFATE (IV)

Trade Name: Prostigmin

Indications: Myasthenia gravis; reversal of effects of nondepolarizing neuromuscular blocking agents after surgery; and postoperative distention and urinary retention after mechanical obstruction has been excluded.

Pharmacokinetics: Vd: 1.0 L/kg. Clearance: 9.6 ml/min/kg. $T_{1/2}$: β, 104 min.

Pharmacodynamics:
CNS: Dizziness, convulsions, headache, miosis, visual changes.
CVS: Arrhythmias (bradycardia, tachycardia, AV block, nodal rhythm), cardiac arrest, hypotension.
Pulmonary: ↑ Oral secretions, ↑ bronchial secretions, respiratory depression, bronchospasm.
Renal: Urinary frequency.
GI: Nausea, emesis, flatulence, ↑ peristalsis.
Musculoskeletal: Muscle cramps, spasms.
Other: Rash, urticaria.

Dosage/   0.25 mg/ml; 1–10 ml vials; 0.5 mg/ml; 1.0 mg/ml.
Concentrations: For myasthenia gravis:
Adult: Oral, 15 mg q 3–4 hr.
Pediatric: 2 mg/kg/day.
                               For reversal of neuromuscular blockade:
Adult: 50–70 μg/kg.
Pediatric: 0.01–0.04 mg/kg.

Contraindications: Peritonitis or mechanical obstruction of the GI tract.

Drug Interactions/   Prolonged phase 1 block of depolarizing muscle relaxants.
Allergy:

PHYSOSTIGMINE SALICYLATE

Trade Names: Antilirium, Eserine Salicylate

Indications: Glaucoma, atropine intoxication, TCA intoxication, postoperative somnolence, and reversal of nondepolarizing muscle relaxation.

PHYSOSTIGMINE SALICYLATE   *(continued)*

Pharmacokinetics:	$T_{1/2}$: β, 20–30 min. Tertiary amine; crosses blood-brain barrier. Destroyed by hydrolysis at ester linkage.

Pharmacodynamics:

CNS:	Anxiety, delirium, hallucinations, seizures, blurred vision, miosis.
CVS:	Bradycardia, tachycardia.
Pulmonary:	Bronchoconstriction.
Renal:	Urge to urinate.
GI:	Emesis, diarrhea, nausea, hypersalivation.

Dosage/ Concentrations:	Package: 2-ml vials (1 mg/ml).
Adult:	0.5–1 mg IM/IV ≤ 1 mg/min.
Pediatric:	0.02 g/kg IM/slow IV.
Contraindications:	Asthma, gangrene, diabetes, CVS disease, bowel obstruction, corneal injury, and sensitivity to physostigmine.
Drug Interactions/ Allergy:	With echothiophate, duration of action may be shortened by physostigmine. Belladonna alkaloids may antagonize antiglaucoma and miotic action. With succinylcholine, prior dose of physostigmine prolongs phase 1 block of depolarizing muscle relaxants.

PYRIDOSTIGMINE BROMIDE

Trade Names:	Regonol, Mestinon
Indications:	Myasthenia gravis, postoperative urinary retention, and antagonism of nondepolarizing muscle relaxants.
Pharmacokinetics:	Vd: 1.1 L/kg. Clearance: 8.6 ml/min/kg. $T_{1/2}$: α, 6.8 min; β, 112 min. Duration: anticholinesterase activity may be prolonged in elderly.

Pharmacodynamics:

CNS:	Confusion, seizures, nervousness, miosis.
CVS:	Bradycardia.
Pulmonary:	Wheezing, ↑ secretions.
GI:	Cramping, nausea, vomiting, diarrhea.
Musculoskeletal:	Weakness, muscle cramping.

Dosage/ Concentrations:	Package: 5 mg/ml.
Adult:	10–20 mg/70 kg
Pediatric:	Antimyasthenic: IM, 0.05–0.15 mg/kg q 4–6 hr.

Contraindications: Asthma, pneumonia, cardiac dysrhythmia (AV block, bradycardia), and intestinal obstruction.

Drug Interactions/   ↓ Metabolism of local anesthetics (ester types). With
Allergy: succinylcholine, prior treatment with pyridostigmine prolongs phase 1 block. With quinine, enflurane, halothane, and aminoglycosides, the neuromuscular blocking action of these medications may antagonize pyridostigmine's antimyasthenic effect on skeletal muscle.

19

Cutaneous-Topical Drugs

Harbhej Singh, M.D.

BENZOCAINE

Trade Names:	Hurricaine, Cetacaine
Indications:	Topical anesthesia.
Pharmacokinetics:	Onset: 15–30 sec. Duration: 12–15 min. Systemic absorption: minimal. Elimination: hydrolysis by plasma pseudocholinesterase to alcohol and PABA.
Pharmacodynamics:	
CNS:	Stabilization of neuronal membrane; seizures.
CVS:	Dose-dependent depression of myocardial contractility; vasodilation.
Other:	Methemoglobinemia.

**Dosages/
Concentrations:**

- Hurricaine topical anesthetic aerosol spray: 2% benzocaine.

- Cetacaine topical anesthetic: 14% benzocaine, 2% butyl aminobenzoate, 2% tetracaine HCl.

- Average dose: 200–400 mg (over 1–2 sec).

Contraindications:	IV or intraocular use.
Drug Interactions/ Allergy:	Inhibition of action of sulfonamides by PABA. Urticaria, pruritus, and anaphylactoid reactions.

CAPSAICIN

Trade Names:	Zostrix, Zostrix-HP
Indications:	Pain, reflex sympathetic dystrophy syndrome.
Pharmacodynamics:	
CNS:	Blocks conduction of painful impulses by depleting and preventing reaccumulation of substance P in peripheral sensory neurons.

**Dosages/
Concentrations:**
Apply cream locally to affected area t.i.d. or q.i.d.
- Zostrix: 0.025%.

- Zostrix-HP: 0.075%.

Contraindications:	Intraocular use or application on open skin surface.
Drug Interactions/ Allergy:	Initial burning sensation at the site of application.

CLONIDINE TRANSDERMAL

Trade Names:	Catapres-TTS-1, Catapres-TTS-2, Catapres-TTS-3
Indications:	Hypertension, supplementation of regional and general anesthesia, perioperative hemodynamic stability, and postoperative analgesia.
Pharmacokinetics:	Onset: 2–3 days after initial application. $T_{1/2}$: 12.7 ± 7 hr. Elimination: 50% of the absorbed drug metabolized in liver, remainder excreted unchanged in urine.
Pharmacodynamics:	
CNS:	Selective agonist action on postsynaptic α_2 receptors. Reduced sympathetic outflow, sedation, inhibition of spinal substance P release.
CVS:	↓ SVR, ↓ HR, ↓ BP, ↓ cardiac output.
GI:	Dry mouth.
Dosages/ Concentrations:	Apply to a hairless area of skin on upper arm or torso once every 7 days; apply each new application onto a different skin site. The 3.5, 7, and 10.5 cm² systems contain clonidine, 2.5, 5.0, and 7.5 mg (Catapres-TTS-1, -2, and -3), and deliver clonidine, 0.1, 0.2, and 0.3 mg/day, respectively.
Contraindications:	Use with caution in coronary artery disease, recent MI, CVS disease, chronic renal failure and pregnancy.
Drug Interactions/ Allergy:	TCA therapy may exaggerate the rebound hypertension associated with discontinuation of clonidine therapy. Clonidine therapy may enhance the CNS depressant effects of alcohol, barbiturates, and other sedatives. In patients receiving β blockers and clonidine concurrently, β blockers should be discontinued several days before cessation of clonidine administration to prevent rebound hypertension.

COCAINE HYDROCHLORIDE

Trade Name:	Cocaine Viscous topical solution
Pharmacokinetics:	Onset: <1 min. $T_{1/2}$: 60–90 min. Metabolized by liver and plasma pseudocholinesterase.
Indications:	Topical anesthesia of nasal mucosa.
Pharmacodynamics:	
CNS:	Blocks initiation and conduction of nerve impulses. CNS stimulation and/or depression, leading to vom-

	iting, euphoria, tremors, excitement, seizures, mydriasis, pyrexia, and respiratory failure.
CVS:	CVAs, bradycardia, hypertension, tachycardia, tachyarrhythmias, ventricular fibrillation, ↓ uterine blood flow.
Dosages/ Concentrations:	Maximum safe dose: 3 mg/kg. Reduce dosages for children, elderly, debilitated, and acutely ill. 4% and 10% Topical solution: 4-ml unit dose bottle, 10 ml multiple-dose bottle.
Contraindications:	Patients with addiction potential, coronary artery disease, and intraocular or IV use. Use with caution in patients with traumatized mucosa and sepsis in the region of application and in patients taking MAOIs.
Drug Interactions/ Allergy:	Sensitizes myocardium to catecholamines. Use with caution with concomitant MAOI and epinephrine therapy, idiosyncrasy, and decreased tolerance.

FENTANYL TRANSDERMAL

Trade Name:	Duragesic
Indications:	Chronic pain.
Pharmacokinetics:	Vd: 6 L/kg. Clearance: 46 L/hr. Metabolized in liver by *N*-dealkylation to norfentanyl and other inactive metabolites. Peak serum levels: 24–72 hr after single application. Steady-state serum concentration: after several sequential 72-hr applications; serum fentanyl concentrations decline by ≃ 50% 17 hr after system removal. Released slowly into blood from accumulated stores in skeletal muscle and fat.
Pharmacodynamics: *CNS:*	Analgesia, sedation, altered mood, depression of respiratory center and cough reflex, constriction of pupils.
CVS:	Bradycardia, orthostatic hypotension.
Pulmonary:	Hypoventilation.
GI:	Nausea and vomiting, constipation, ↑ biliary tract pressure.
Dosages/ Concentrations:	For patients without opioid tolerance, 25 μg/hr. For patients taking other narcotics for chronic pain, equivalent doses following conversion. Each dose may be worn continuously for 72 hr. A new system is applied to a different skin site on upper torso after removal of the previous system. Delivery systems available in the following four strengths:

FENTANYL TRANSDERMAL   *(continued)*

Dose/Drug Release (µg/hr)	Size (cm²)	Fentanyl content (mg)
25	10	2.5
50	20	5
75	30	7.5
100	40	10

Contraindications:	↑ ICP. Use with caution in chronic pulmonary disease. Head injury.
Drug Interactions/ Allergy:	Concomitant use of other CNS depressants (e.g., sedatives, hypnotics, general anesthetics, phenothiazines, other opioids, tranquilizers, sedating antihistamines, alcoholic beverages) may produce additive depressant effects. Clinically significant histamine release (rare).

LIDOCAINE/PRILOCAINE

Trade Name:	Emla Cream
Indications:	Topical analgesia.
Pharmacokinetics:	Onset: 1 hr after application. Peak: 2–3 hr. Duration: up to 1–2 hr after removal. Systemic blood levels: $1/20$–$1/50$ of toxic levels when used as recommended.
Pharmacodynamics: *CVS:*	Inhibition of ion fluxes during initiation and conduction of impulses.
Other:	Methemoglobinemia.
Dosages/ Concentrations: Adult:	Available as 5- and 30-g tubes; each gram contains lidocaine, 25 mg; prilocaine, 25 mg; fatty acid esters; a thickening agent; sodium hydroxide; and water. For minor procedures (venipuncture), apply 2.5 g over 20–25 cm² of skin surface under occlusive dressing for at least 1 hr. For major procedures (split-thickness skin graft), 2 g over 10 cm² of skin surface under occlusive dressing for at least 2 hr.
Pediatric:	• <10 kg: single application not to be applied to an area > 100 cm².
	• 10–20 kg: single application not to be applied to an area > 600 cm².

Contraindications:	Sensitivity to amide local anesthetics; congenital or idiopathic methemoglobinemia; and G-6-P deficiency. Use with caution in breast-feeding patients.
Drug Interactions/ Allergy:	Patients taking methemoglobin-inducing drugs (e.g., sulfonamides, acetaminophen, nitrates, nitrites, nitrofurantoin, nitroglycerin, nitroprusside, phenacetin, phenobarbital, phenytoin) are at greater risk for methemoglobinemia. Blanching, erythema, edema, itching, and altered skin temperature at site of application.

LIDOCAINE HYDROCHLORIDE

Trade Name:	Xylocaine
Indications:	Topical anesthesia of mucous membranes. Lubrication of endotracheal tubes.
Pharmacokinetics:	Absorption: rapid after intratracheal administration. $T_{1/2}$: 1.5–2 hr (may be prolonged in liver dysfunction). Elimination: metabolized in liver by oxidative N-dealkylation to less potent metabolites, monoethylglycinexylidide and glycinexylidide.
Pharmacodynamics: *CNS:*	Inhibition of sodium flux during initiation and conduction of nerve impulses, lightheadedness, apprehension, euphoria, confusion, dizziness, drowsiness, tinnitus, blurred vision, vomiting, tremor, convulsions, unconsciousness, and respiratory depression and arrest.
CVS:	Bradycardia, hypotension, cardiovascular collapse.
Dosages/ Concentrations:	Maximum dose: 4.5 mg/kg, not to exceed a total of 300 mg. Reduce dosage for children, elderly, and acutely ill.

- Xylocaine 2% jelly: 30-ml collapsible tubes.
- Xylocaine 10% oral spray: 26.8-ml aerosol container (each actuation of the metered dose valve delivers lidocaine, 10 mg).
- Xylocaine 2% viscous solution: 20-, 100-, and 450-ml polyethylene squeeze bottles.
- Xylocaine 4% topical solution: 50-ml screw-cap bottle.

Contraindications:	Sensitivity to amide local anesthetics. Use with caution in patients with potentially full stomach, severe shock, heart block, sepsis, or traumatized mucosa in the area of application.

LIDOCAINE HYDROCHLORIDE   *(continued)*

Drug Interactions/ Allergy:	Additive or antagonistic cardiac interaction with phenytoin, procainamide, propranolol, or quinidine. Potentiates neuromuscular blocking effects of succinylcholine and tubocurarine. ↓ Clearance with concomitant use of β blockers and cimetidine. ↑ Seizure threshold with benzodiazepines. Urticaria, pruritus, cutaneous lesions, angioneurotic edema, and anaphylactoid reactions. Allergic reactions due to sensitivity to either lidocaine or to methylparaben/propylparaben (in formulation).

NITROGLYCERIN

Trade Names:	Deponit, Minitran, Nitrodisc, Transderm-Nitro (transdermal patches), Nitro-Bid, Nitrol (ointments)
Indications:	Angina pectoris.
Pharmacokinetics:	Steady-state level: within 1 to 2 hr of application of ointment and patch, respectively. Duration: ≈ 12 hr. Vd: 3 L/kg. $T_{1/2}$: 3 min. Clearance: greater than hepatic blood flow.
Pharmacodynamics:	
CNS:	Headache.
CVS:	Peripheral vasodilation, hypotension, venous pooling, ↓ venous return to heart, ↓ LVEDP, ↓ PCWP, ↓ SVR, ↓ MAP (afterload), coronary vasodilation.
Dosages/ Concentrations:	Ointment (Nitro-Bid): 20- and 60-g tubes; 2.5 cm (1 inch) of ointment = 15 mg of nitroglycerin; apply 7.5–30 mg (½–2 inches) on 36 square inches of truncal skin; apply twice a day 6 hr apart.
	Transdermal systems (patches) deliver 0.1–0.6 mg/hr. After 24 hr, each patch has delivered 10%–15% of original nitroglycerin content. Initial dose: 0.2–0.4 mg/hr. Dose of 0.4–0.8 mg/hr is effective for 10–12 hr daily for at least 1 month. Apply patch daily for 12 hr on and 12 hr off periods.
Contraindications:	Allergy. Use with caution in volume-depletion, hypotension, hypertrophic cardiomyopathy, and pregnancy.
Drug Interactions/ Allergy:	Vasodilating effects of nitroglycerin may be additive with those of other vasodilators, especially alcohol. Marked orthostatic hypotension when used in

conjunction with calcium channel blockers. Contact dermatitis and fixed drug eruptions.

OXYMETAZOLINE HYDROCHLORIDE

Trade Name:	4-Way Long Lasting (nasal spray)
Indications:	Nasal decongestion.
Pharmacokinetics:	Duration: 12 hr.
Pharmacodynamics:	Directly acting sympathomimetic amine. Nasal mucosal vasoconstriction.
Dosages/ Concentrations:	Supplied as ½ fl. oz. atomizer and metered pump in a concentration of 0.05%; 2–3 metered doses sprayed into each nostril, not to exceed 2 applications over 24 hr.
Contraindications:	Hypertension, coronary artery disease, diabetes mellitus, thyroid disease, and urinary retention due to benign prostatic hypertrophy.
Drug Interactions/ Allergy:	Cross-sensitivity to other nasal decongestants.

PHENYLEPHRINE HYDROCHLORIDE

Trade Name:	4-Way Fast Acting (nasal spray)
Indications:	Nasal decongestion.
Pharmacokinetics:	Duration: 30 min–4 hr.
Pharmacodynamics:	Directly acting sympathomimetic amine. Nasal mucosal vasoconstriction.
CNS:	Sedation if swallowed in children < 12 yr.
Respiratory:	Burning, sneezing, stinging, excessive nasal discharge.
Dosage/ Concentrations:	Drops: available in 0.125%, 0.16%, 0.2%, 0.25%, 0.5%, and 1%. Spray: 0.125%, 0.25%, 0.5%, and 1%.
Adult and Adolescent:	• Drops: 2–3 drops of 0.25%–0.5% solution into each nostril not more often than q 6 hr.
	• Spray: 1–2 drops of 0.25%–0.5% solution into each nostril.
Pediatric:	• Up to 6 yr: Drops: 2–3 drops of 0.125% solution into each nostril.

PHENYLEPHRINE HYDROCHLORIDE   *(continued)*

- 6–12 yr: Drops: 2–3 drops of 0.25% solution into each nostril. Spray: 1–2 sprays of 0.25% solution into each nostril.

Contraindications: Sensitivity to nasal decongestants. Use cautiously in coronary artery disease, hypertension, diabetes mellitus, hyperthyroidism, and urinary retention due to prostate enlargement.

Drug Interactions/ Allergy: Potentiation of the pressor effect in presence of MAOIs (pargyline, furazolidone, procarbazine), guanethidine, and TCAs on significant systemic absorption. Cross-sensitivity with other nasal decongestants.

20

Dermatologic Drugs

Rui Sun, M.D., Ph.D.

ANTHRALIN

Trade Names:	Drithocreme, Dritho-Scalp, Lasan
Indications:	Psoriasis and alopecia areata.
Pharmacokinetics:	Absorption: low; through skin.
Pharmacodynamics:	Antipsoriatic activity.
Dosage/ Concentrations:	Available as cream and ointment.
Adult:	Apply (0.1%–1%) to skin, once or twice/day.
Pediatric:	Not established.
Contraindications:	Acute eruptions or presence of skin inflammation.
Drug Interactions/ Allergy:	Photosensitizing effects, skin rash.

BENZOYL PEROXIDE

Trade Names:	Desquam, Ben-Aqua, Acne-10, Benzac, Panoxyl, Clearasil 10%, Clearasil Maximum Strength, Noxzema
Indications:	Acne vulgaris and decubital or stasis ulcers.
Pharmacokinetics:	Absorption and metabolism: in skin. Elimination: 5% excreted as benzoic acid in urine.
Pharmacodynamics:	Keratolytic activity.
Dosage/ Concentrations:	Available as cream, gel, lotion, cleansing bar, facial mask, and stick.
Adult and Adolescent:	Apply (2.5%–20%) to skin, one to four times/day.
Pediatric:	<12 yr: not established.
Contraindications:	Acute inflammation of skin and denuded skin.
Drug Interactions/ Allergy:	Excessive skin irritation from concurrent use of peeling, desquamating, or abrasive agents.

CHLOROXINE

Trade Name:	Capitrol
Indications:	Seborrheic dermatitis and dandruff.
Pharmacokinetics:	Absorption: through scalp.
Pharmacodynamics:	Antibacterial, antifungal, and antiseborrheic activity.
Dosage/ Concentrations:	Available as shampoo.
Adult:	Apply (2%) to scalp twice/week.
Pediatric:	Not established.
Contraindications:	Acute inflammation and exudative scalp lesions.
Drug Interactions/ Allergy:	None.

COAL TAR

Trade Names:	Alphosyl, AquaTar, DHS Tar
Indications:	Seborrheic dermatitis (dandruff), atopic dermatitis, eczema, and psoriasis.
Pharmacokinetics:	N/A.
Pharmacodynamics: CVS:	Antipsoriatic, antiseborrheic, and vulnerary activity. Vasoconstriction.
Dosage/ Concentrations:	Available as lotion, cream, gel, cleansing bar, ointment solution, suspension and shampoo.
Adult:	Apply (1%–25.5%) to skin one to four times/day.
Pediatric:	Not established.
Contraindications:	Acute inflammation, open wounds, and skin infection.
Drug Interactions/ Allergy:	Photosensitizing effects of other drugs enhanced by coal tar.

ETRETINATE

Trade Name:	Tegison
Indications:	Psoriasis and lichen planus.
Pharmacokinetics:	Absorption: in small intestine; increased by milk or high-fat diet. Highly bound to plasma protein. Metabolism: significant first-pass metabolized to the pharmacologically active acid form. $T_{1/2}$: >4 months, primarily biliary.

Pharmacodynamics: Antiseborrheic activity.
CNS: Mood or mental changes.
Hepatic: Hepatitis, hepatic fibrosis, enorosis, cirrhosis.
GI: Nausea.
Musculoskeletal: Hyperostosis.
Other: Hypertriglyceridemia, hypercholesterolemia, ↓ HDL level.

Dosage/
Concentrations: Supplied as 10- or 25-mg tablets.
Adult: Initial dose: 0.75–1.0 mg/kg/day p.o.
Maintenance dose: 0.5–0.75 mg/kg/day in divided dose p.o.

Contraindications: CVS disease, diabetes mellitus, hepatic disease, hypertriglyceridemia, or sensitivity to vitamin A derivatives. Not for use in children.

Drug Interactions/
Allergy: Alcohol increases incidence of hypertriglyceridemia. Additive toxic effects by isotretinoin, tretinoin, and vitamin A. ↑ Potential for hepatotoxicity by other hepatotoxic medications or for pseudotumor cerebri by tetracyclines.

HYDROXYPROPYL CELLULOSE

Trade Name:	Lacrisert
Indications:	Keratoconjunctivitis sicca, corneal erosions, decreased corneal sensitivity, and exposure keratitis.
Pharmacokinetics:	Not absorbed.
Pharmacodynamics:	Ocular moisturizing effect.

Dosage/
Concentrations:

Adult and Pediatric: Apply 5 mg to conjunctiva once/day.

Contraindications: None.

Drug Interactions/ None.
Allergy:

ISOTRETINOIN

Trade Name: Accutane

Indications: Acne vulgaris, rosacea, gram-negative folliculitis, and suppurative hidradenitis.

Pharmacokinetics: Absorption: rapidly, from GI tract; extremely high protein binding. Peak plasma concentration: 3 hr after oral dose. Metabolism: hepatic. $T_{1/2}$: 10–20 hr. Elimination: liver and kidneys.

Pharmacodynamics: Keratolytic activity.
CNS: Mental depression, mood changes.
Renal: Proteinuria, hematuria.
GI: Inflammatory bowel disease, regional ileitis.
Musculoskeletal: Hyperostosis.
Other: Hypertriglyceridemia, hyperuricemia.

Dosage/ Supplied as 10- to 40-mg tablets.
Concentrations:
Adult: 0.5–1 mg/kg/day in divided doses.

Contraindications: Hypertriglyceridemia and diabetes mellitus. Not for use in children.

Drug Interactions/ Excessive skin irritation with concurrent use of peel-
Allergy: ing, desquamating, or abrasive agents. Enhanced photo-sensitizing effects of vitamin A derivatives. Pseudotumor cerebri with tetracyclines.

LINDANE

Trade Names: Kwell, Bio-Well, G-Well, Kildane, Kwildane, Scabene, Thionex

Indications: Pediculosis capitis, pediculosis pubis, and scabies.

Pharmacokinetics: Absorption: through skin. $T_{1/2}$: 18 hr in infants and children.

LINDANE   *(continued)*

Pharmacodynamics:	Scabicidal and pediculicidal activity.
CNS:	Toxicity (convulsions).
Dosage/ Concentrations:	Available as cream, lotion, and shampoo.
Adult and Pediatric:	Apply 1% to skin or scalp.
Contraindications:	Convulsive disorders and irritated or broken skin.
Drug Interactions/ Allergy:	↑ Absorption with simultaneous application of skin, scalp, or hair preparations.

PERMETHRIN

Trade Name:	Nix Cream Rinse
Indications:	Pediculosis capitis.
Pharmacokinetics:	Absorption: 2% absorbed systemically. Metabolism: rapidly metabolized by ester hydrolysis to inactive metabolites. Elimination: in urine.
Pharmacodynamics:	Pediculicidal activity.
Dosage/ Concentrations:	
Adult:	Apply 1% lotion in a single application to hair and scalp.
Pediatric:	• >2 yr: same as adult dose.
	• <2 yr: not established.
Contraindications:	Acute scalp inflammation.
Drug Interactions/ Allergy:	Sensitivity to chrysanthemums, pyrethrins, or veterinary insecticides containing permethrin or synthetic pyrethoids.

PODOPHYLLUM

Trade Name:	Podofin
Indications:	Condylomatum acuminatum and multiple superficial epitheliomatosis.
Pharmacokinetics:	Absorption: systemic when applied to friable, bleeding, or recently biopsied warts.
Pharmacodynamics:	Keratolytic activity.

CNS:	Confusion, nervousness, excitement, irritability, autonomic neuropathy.
Pulmonary:	Difficulty in breathing.
GI:	Stomach pain, diarrhea, nausea, vomiting.
Musculoskeletal:	Muscle weakness.

Dosage/
Concentrations:

Adult and Pediatric: Apply (10%–25%) to warts once/week and to epitheliomatous lesions once/day.

Contraindications: Friable, bleeding, or recently biopsied warts.

Drug Interactions/   N/A.
Allergy:

PYRETHRINS, PIPERONYL BUTOXIDE

Trade Name: **A-200 Pediculocide Shampoo**

Indications: Pediculosis corporis, capitis, and pubis.

Pharmacokinetics: Absorption: poor; through intact skin when applied topically.

Pharmacodynamics: Pediculicidal activity.

Dosage/
Concentrations:

  Available as shampoo, gel, and topical solution.

Adult and Pediatric: Apply pyrethrins (0.18%–0.33%) and piperonyl butoxide (2.2%–4%) to hair and scalp in a single application; repeat in 1–2 weeks.

Contraindications: Acute inflammation of skin.

Drug Interactions/   Skin rash, sneezing.
Allergy:

PYRITHIONE ZINC

Trade Names: **Head & Shoulders, Head & Shoulders Dry Scalp Shampoo, Danex, DHS Zinc shampoo**

Indications: Seborrheic dermatitis (dandruff).

Pharmacokinetics: Topical application.

Pharmacodynamics: Antiseborrheic, antibacterial, and antifungal activity.

Dosage/
Concentration:

Adults and Pediatric: Apply 1%–2% cream or shampoo to scalp twice/wk.

PYRITHIONE ZINC   *(continued)*

Contraindications:	None.
Drug Interactions/ Allergy:	None.

RESORCINOL

Trade Name:	RA
Indications:	Acne vulgaris, seborrheic dermatitis, eczema, psoriasis, urticaria, and inflammatory skin disorders.
Pharmacokinetics:	Absorption: through skin or from ulcerated surfaces.
Pharmacodynamics:	Keratolytic activity.
CNS:	Dizziness, headache.
CVS:	↓ HR.
Pulmonary:	Shortness of breath.
GI:	Diarrhea, nausea, stomach pain, vomiting.
Other:	Methemoglobinemia in children.
Dosage/ Concentrations:	
Adult and Pediatric:	Apply lotion (2%–3%) or ointment (2%–20%) with or without sulfur (5%–8%) to skin.
Contraindications:	None.
Drug Interactions/ Allergy:	Excessive skin irritation from concurrent use of peeling, desquamating, or abrasive agents.

SELENIUM SULFIDE

Trade Names:	Exsel, Glo-Sel; Head & Shoulders Intensive Treatment Dandruff Shampoo, Selsun Blue
Indications:	Seborrheic dermatitis (dandruff) of the scalp; tinea versicolor
Pharmacokinetics:	Topical effect only.
Pharmacodynamics:	Antiseborrheic and antifungal activity.
Dosage/ Concentrations:	
Adult and Pediatric:	For dandruff: apply to scalp as 1%–2.5% lotion, twice/wk for 2 weeks, then once/wk.

For tinea versicolor, apply to body as 2.5% lotion once/day for 1 week.

Contraindications: Acute inflammation of skin.

Drug Interactions/ Allergy: None.

SULFAPYRIDINE

Trade Name: Dagenan

Indications: Dermatitis herpetiformis, pemphigoid, subcorneal pustular dermatitis, and pyoderma gangrenosum.

Pharmacokinetics: Absorption: incomplete. Peak concentration: 4–6 hr. Protein binding: ~ 50%. Vd: 0.4–1.2 L/kg. Biotransformation: hepatic. $T_{1/2}$: 6–14 hr. Elimination: in urine; 80% reabsorption in renal tubules.

Pharmacodynamics:
CNS: Headache.
Hepatic: Hepatic dysfunction.
GI: Diarrhea, anorexia, nausea, vomiting.
Musculoskeletal: Stevens-Johnson syndrome.
Other: Agranulocytosis, hemolytic anemia, porphyria.

Dosage/ Concentrations:
Adult: 0.25–1.0 g p.o. 2–4 times/day (500 = mg tablets <6 g/day).

Contraindications: Blood dyscrasias, G-6-PD deficiency, hepatic disorders, porphyria, renal function impairment, and sulfa allergy. Not to be used in children.

Drug Interactions/ Allergy: Anticoagulants, anticonvulsants, antidiabetic agents, methotrexate, phenylbutazone, and sulfin pyrazone displaced from protein-binding sites. Metabolism inhibited by sulfonamides. ↑ Potential toxicity of hemolytics. Hepatotoxic effects of other medications enhanced. Cross-sensitivity with other sulfonamides.

SULFUR

Trade Names: Fostex Medicated Cover-Up, Finac, Fostril Cream, Cuticura ointment, Sulpho-Lac

Indications: Acne vulgaris, seborrheic dermatitis, scabies, rosacea.

SULFUR   *(continued)*

Pharmacokinetics:	Topical effect.
Pharmacodynamics:	Antiseborrheic, keratolytic, and antibacterial activity.
Dosage/ Concentrations: Adults and Pediatric:	Cream or lotion, 2%; ointment, 0.5%–10%; bar soap, 5%–10%. Apply 1–3 times/day or p.r.n..
Contraindications:	Sensitivity to sulfur.
Drug Interactions/ Allergy:	Excessive irritation of skin from concurrent use of peeling, desquamating, or abrasive agents. Concurrent use of topical mercury compounds may cause a chemical reaction by releasing hydrogen sulfide.

TRETINOIN

Trade Name:	Retin-A
Indications:	Acne.
Pharmacokinetics:	Absorption: minimal (5% of topical dose recovered in urine).
Pharmacodynamics:	Keratolytic effect.
Dosage/ Concentrations:	Apply cream (0.025%–0.1%); gel (0.01%–0.025%); or topical solution (0.05%) to skin once/day.
Contraindications:	Eczema, sunburn.
Drug Interactions/ Allergy:	Excessive irritation of skin from concurrent use of peeling, desquamating, or abrasive agents. Physical incompatibility with benzoyl peroxide. Enhanced systemic absorption of topical minoxidil (may cause hypotension, arrhythmias, and impotence). ↑ Risk of photosensitization by isotretinoin.

TRIOXSALEN

Trade Name:	Trisoralen
Indications:	Vitiligo and increasing threshold of skin sensitivity to sunlight.
Pharmacokinetics:	Absorption: absorbed from GI tract. Activated by long wavelength ultraviolet light A (320–400 nm). Metabolism: in liver. Elimination: in urine.

Pharmacodynamics:
CNS: Dizziness, headache, mental depression.
GI: Nausea.
Other: Swelling in lower legs.

**Dosage/
Concentrations:**
Adult: 20–40 mg p.o. 2–4 hr before ultraviolet light A exposure 2–3 times/week.

Pediatric: • >12 yr: same as adult dose.

                    • <12 yr: not established.

Contraindications: Photosensitization conditions (e.g., albinism), aphakia, cataracts, and skin cancer.

**Drug Interactions/
Allergy:**   Additive phototoxicity with furocoumarin-containing foods and photosensitizing drugs.

21

Diuretics

Arnold S. Friedman, M.D.
Thomas Heiman, M.D.

ACETAZOLAMIDE

Trade Names:	AK-Zol, Dazamide, Diamox
Indications:	Open-angle and secondary glaucoma, preoperatively in acute angle-closure glaucoma, petit mal and centrencephalic seizures, edema, acute mountain sickness.
Pharmacokinetics:	$T_{1/2}$: 2.4–5.8 hr. Metabolism: 70%–100% excreted unchanged in urine within 24 hr. Protein binding: 90%. Onset: 1 hr (tablet), 2 hr (sustained-release), 2 min (IV). Duration: 8–12 hr (tablet), 18–24 hr (sustained-release), 4–5 hr (IV).

Pharmacodynamics:

CNS:	↓ Rate of CSF formation, inhibited epileptic seizures, drowsiness, paresthesias, confusion, taste alteration, hearing dysfunction, tinnitus, transient myopia, convulsions, ↓ rate of aqueous humor formation and IOP.
CVS:	↓ BP.
Pulmonary:	↑ Acidosis in pulmonary obstruction or emphysema.
Hepatic:	Hepatic insufficiency.
Renal:	Metabolic acidosis, electrolyte disturbances (especially hypokalemia), polyuria, hematuria, renal calculi.
GI:	Nausea, vomiting, diarrhea, anorexia, melena.
Other:	Urticaria, rash, teratogenicity, photosensitivity, hyperglycemia, bone marrow depression.

Dosage/ Concentrations:	Tablets: 125 or 250 mg; sustained-release tablets: 500 mg; IV: 500 mg, sterile powder.
Adult:	For open-angle or chronic simple glaucoma: p.o., 250 mg 1–4 times/day, or 500 mg sustained-release tablet b.i.d.
	For closed-angle or secondary and acute glaucoma: IV, 250–500 mg, repeat in 2–4 hr, maximum 1 g/day.
	For edema: p.o. or IV, 250–375 mg q.d. or q.o.d.
	For epilepsy: p.o., 8–30 mg/kg/day in divided doses (sustained-release tablets not recommended).
	For altitude sickness: p.o., 125–250 mg q 6 hr or 500 mg sustained-release tablets q 12–24 hr (initiate 24–48 hours prior to ascent).
Pediatric:	For glaucoma: 8–30 mg/kg/day p.o. divided q 6–8 hr. IM or IV, 20–40 mg/kg/day divided q 6 hr, maximum, 1 g/day.
	For edema: p.o., IM, or IV, 5 mg/kg q.d. or q.o.d.
	For epilepsy: p.o., 8–30 mg/kg/day in 2–4 divided doses, maximum 1 g/day.
	For hydrocephalus in infancy: p.o. or IV, 25 mg/kg/day divided t.i.d., maximum, 100 mg/kg/day.
	For urine alkalinization: p.o., 5 mg/kg/dose, 2–3 times/24 hr.

ACETAZOLAMIDE   *(continued)*

Contraindications: Hepatic or significant renal insufficiency, hyponatremia, hypokalemia, hyperchloremic acidosis, adrenocortical insufficiency, and COPD. Sustained-release tablets not recommended in epilepsy. Sensitivity to other sulfonamides.

Drug Interactions/   Salicylates associated with coma and death. ↓ Serum
Allergy: lithium and primidone. ↑ Serum cyclosporin, amphetamine, quinidine, and ephedrine.

AMILORIDE

Trade Name: Midamor

Indications: Counteracts potassium loss induced by potent kaliuretic diuretics in hypertensive or edematous states.

Pharmacokinetics: Oral absorption: 50%. Metabolism: excreted unchanged equally in urine and feces. Onset: 2 hr (p.o.). Duration: 24 hr (p.o.). $T_{1/2}$: 6–9 hr. Protein binding: 23%.

Pharmacodynamics:
CNS: Dizziness, headache, paresthesias, confusion, depression.
CVS: ↓ BP, ↓ HR, congestive heart failure, dyspnea, angina.
Hepatic: Precipitation of hepatic coma in patients with severe liver disease.
Renal: Hyperkalemia, hyponatremia, hypochloremia, polyuria.
GI: Nausea, vomiting, diarrhea, constipation, abdominal pain, GI bleeding.
Other: ↑ Hyperkalemia in patients with acidosis; impotence, pruritus, rash, alopecia, aplastic anemia, leukopenia.

Dosage/   Tablets: 5 mg.
Concentrations:
Adult: 5–10 mg/day, up to 20 mg/day.

Contraindications: Anuria, acute or chronic renal failure, hyperkalemia, severe hepatic disease, diabetic nephropathy. Do not give with K^+ supplements, other K^+-sparing diuretics, salt substitutes, indomethacin, or ACE inhibitors.

Drug Interactions/ K^+ supplements, other K^+-sparing diuretics, salt substi-
Allergy: tutes, indomethacin, or ACE inhibitors may cause toxic serum K^+ levels. ↑ Serum lithium and amantadine. NSAIDs ↓ diuretic effect.

BUMETANIDE

Trade Name:	Bumex
Indications:	Edema.
Pharmacokinetics:	Bioavailability: 80%. Serum peak (C_{max}): 1–2 hr. Vc: 3–6 L. $T_{1/2}$: 1–1.5 hr (adults), 2.5 hr (infants <6 months). Metabolism: primarily via oxidation of N-butyl side chain. 80% excreted in urine (45% as unchanged drug); 2% excreted in bile. Protein binding: 94%–96%. Onset: IV, within a few min; p.o., 30–60 min. Duration: 4–6 hr.

Pharmacodynamics:

CNS:	Ototoxicity after rapid IV injection, headache, dizziness, vertigo.
CVS:	Hypovolemia, orthostatic hypotension, thrombosis, embolism.
Hepatic:	Precipitation of hepatic coma, ↑ LFTs.
Renal:	Hyponatremia, hypokalemia, hypochloremia, alkalosis, hypomagnesemia, hypocalcemia.
GI:	Nausea, vomiting, diarrhea, constipation.
Other:	Hyperglycemia, hyperuricemia, ↑ cholesterol, thrombocytopenia, photosensitivity, hives, pruritus, impotence; may exacerbate lupus.

Dosage/ Concentrations:	Tablets: 0.5, 1, or 2 mg. IV: 2, 4, or 10 cc vials of 0.25 mg/cc injection.
Adult:	Oral: 0.5–2 mg; repeat q 4–5 hr; maximum 10 mg/day. IV: 0.5–1 mg; repeat q 2–3 hr, maximum 10 mg/day. Reduce dosage in hepatic disease.
Pediatric:	Oral (>6 mo): 0.015 mg/kg q.d. or q.o.d.; maximum, 0.1 mg/kg/day.
Contraindications:	Anuria, hepatic coma, severe electrolyte depletion, and sensitivity to sulfonamides.
Drug Interactions/ Allergy:	ACE inhibitors may produce hypotension and acute renal failure. ↑ Risk of digitalis toxicity. ↑ Serum lithium. ↑ Risk of ototoxicity with aminoglycosides. ↓ Diuretic and antihypertensive efficacy with indomethacin.

CHLOROTHIAZIDE

Trade Names:	Diuril
Indications:	Edema and hypertension.
Pharmacokinetics:	Absorption: oral: (10%–20%). $T_{1/2}$: 45–120 min. Metabolism: renal: 96% excreted unchanged in urine. On-

CHLOROTHIAZIDE *(continued)*

set: IV, 15 min; p.o., 2 hr. Duration: IV, 2 hr; p.o., 6–12 hr.

Pharmacodynamics:

CNS:	Lethargy, confusion, seizures, coma.
CVS:	Hypovolemia, ↓ BP.
Hepatic:	Precipitation of hepatic coma.
Renal:	Hyponatremia, hypokalemia, hypochloremia, alkalosis, hypomagnesemia, hypercalcemia.
GI:	Nausea, vomiting.
Other:	Hyperglycemia, hyperuricemia; ↑ triglycerides, ↑ cholesterol, photosensitivity; may exacerbate lupus.

Dosage/
Concentrations: Tablets: 250 and 500 mg. Dry, lyophilized, white powder: 500 mg, IV. Oral suspension: 250 mg/5 cc.

Adult: Oral or IV, 0.5–2 g/day in 2 divided doses.

Pediatric:
- <6 mo: oral: up to 30 mg/kg/day in 2 divided doses.

- >6 mo: oral: up to 20 mg/kg/day in 2 divided doses.

Contraindications: Anuria, hepatic coma, and sensitivity to other sulfonamides.

Drug Interactions/
Allergy: NSAIDs decrease diuretic and antihypertensive effects. ↑ Serum lithium. ↓ Vascular response to pressor amines. Exacerbates hypokalemia with ACTH and corticosteroids. ↑ Risk of digitalis toxicity.

ETHACRYNIC ACID

Trade Name: Edecrin

Indications: Edema, hypertension, and ascites.

Pharmacokinetics: Bioavailability: 100%. Protein binding: extensive. Metabolism: conjugated in liver to cysteine and excreted in bile and urine. Onset: IV, 5 min; p.o., 30 min. Duration: IV, 2 hr; p.o., 6–8 hr.

Pharmacodynamics:

CNS:	Headache, blurred vision, confusion, seizures, ototoxicity after rapid IV injection.
CVS:	Hypovolemia, orthostatic hypotension, thrombosis, embolism, arrhythmias.
Hepatic:	↑ LFTs, jaundice, precipitation of hepatic coma.
Renal:	Hyponatremia, hypokalemia, hypocalcemia, hypomagnesemia, hypochloremia, alkalosis, hematuria.

GI:	Nausea, vomiting, diarrhea, pancreatitis.
Other:	Hyperglycemia, hyperuricemia, ↑ triglycerides, ↑ cholesterol, thrombocytopenia, photosensitivity, fever, neutropenia.

Dosage/ Concentrations:	Tablets: 25 or 50 mg. IV: sterile, freeze-dried powder equivalent to 50 mg injection.
Adult:	Oral: 50–100 mg/day in 1–2 divided doses; may increase by 25–50 mg every several days; maximum, 200 mg/day. IV: 0.5–1 mg/kg, or 50 mg, maximum, 100 mg. Do not give repeated doses.
Pediatric:	Oral: 25 mg/day; may increase by 25 mg q 2–3 days p.r.n.; maximum 3 mg/kg/day. IV: 1 mg/kg/dose. Do not give repeated doses.
Contraindications:	Anuria, severe electrolyte imbalance, and watery diarrhea.
Drug Interactions/ Allergy:	↑ Serum lithium. Diuretic and antihypertensive effects decreased by NSAIDs. Renal effect decreased by probenecid. ↑ Risk of ototoxicity with aminoglycosides. Displaces warfarin from plasma protein, thus reducing the dosage of warfarin. ↑ Risk of digitalis toxicity. ↑ GI bleeding with steroids.

FUROSEMIDE

Trade Name:	Lasix
Indications:	Edema, hypertension, and hypercalcemia.
Pharmacokinetics:	Bioavailability: 60%–64%. $T_{1/2}$: 1–2 hr. Protein binding: 91%–99%. Metabolism: renal: 50% excreted unchanged in urine. Hepatic: 33% metabolized or excreted unchanged in bile. Onset: IV, 5 min; p.o., 30–60 min. Duration: IV, 2 hr; p.o., 6–8 hr.
Pharmacodynamics:	
CNS:	Headache, blurred vision, paresthesias, seizures, ototoxicity after rapid IV injection, ↓ ICP.
CVS:	Hypovolemia, orthostatic hypotension, thrombosis, embolism, peripheral vasodilation.
Hepatic:	Precipitation of hepatic coma, jaundice.
Renal:	Hyponatremia, hypokalemia, hypochloremia, alkalosis, hypocalcemia.
GI:	Nausea, vomiting, diarrhea, constipation, pancreatitis.
Other:	Hyperglycemia, hyperuricemia, anemia, leukopenia, thrombocytopenia, photosensitivity, rash, urticaria, pruritus, may exacerbate lupus.

FUROSEMIDE   *(continued)*

Dosage/	Tablets: 20, 40, or 80 mg.
Concentrations:	IV injection: 2, 4, or 10 cc vials of 10 mg/cc.
Adult:	Oral: 20–80 mg; increase by 20–40 mg q 6–8 hr.
	IV: 20–40 mg; increase by 20 mg q 1–2 hr
	until desired effect, to maximum of 600 mg/day.
Pediatric:	Oral: 2 mg/kg; increase by 1 mg, up to maximum of 6 mg/kg q 6–8 hr.
	IV: 1 mg/kg; increase by 1 mg, to a maximum of 6 mg/kg q 6–12 hr.
Contraindications:	Anuria and sensitivity to other sulfonamides.
Drug Interactions/	↑ Serum lithium. ↓ Arterial responsiveness to norepi-
Allergy:	nephrine. ↓ Diuretic and antihypertensive effects with indomethacin. ↓ Diuretic effect with Dilantin.
	↑ Risk of ototoxicity with aminoglycosides. Diuretic-induced hypokalemia increases risk of digitalis toxicity. ACE inhibitors may produce severe hypotension or acute renal failure. Prolonged neuromuscular blockade following d-tubocurarine or succinylcholine.

HYDROCHLOROTHIAZIDE (HCTZ)

Trade Names:	Esidrix, Ezide, HydroDIURIL, Hydro-Par, Oretic
Indications:	Edema and hypertension.
Pharmacokinetics:	Absorption: oral: 60%–80%. $T_{1/2}$: 5.6–14.8 hr. Metabolism: renal; rapid excretion unchanged in urine. Onset: p.o., 2 hr. Duration: p.o., 6–12 hr.
Pharmacodynamics:	
CNS:	Seizures, coma.
CVS:	Hypovolemia, ↓ BP.
Hepatic:	Precipitation of hepatic coma.
Renal:	Hyponatremia, hypokalemia, hypochloremia, alkalosis, hypomagnesemia, hypercalcemia.
GI:	Nausea, vomiting.
Other:	Hyperglycemia, hyperuricemia, ↑ triglycerides, ↑ cholesterol, photosensitivity; may exacerbate lupus.
Dosage/	Tablets: 25, 50, or 100 mg. Oral suspension:
Concentrations:	50 mg/5 cc.
Adult:	Oral: 25–50 mg/day in 1–2 doses, maximum 100 mg/day.
Pediatric:	• <6 mo: oral, 2–3 mg/kg/day in 2 divided doses.
	• >6 mo: oral, 2 mg/kg/day in 2 divided doses.

Contraindications:	Anuria, hepatic coma, and sensitivity to other sulfonamides.
Drug Interactions/ Allergy:	↑ Serum lithium. NSAIDs ↓ diuretic effect. ↓ Vascular response to pressor amines. Orthostatic hypotension potentiated with alcohol, barbiturates, and narcotics. Hypokalemia exacerbated with corticosteroids and ACTH. Diuretic-induced hypokalemia increases risk of digitalis toxicity.

MANNITOL

Trade Names:	Osmitrol, Resectisol
Indications:	High ICP, high IOP, oliguria in acute renal failure, promotion of excretion of toxic substances in urine, and use as irrigating solution in TURP.
Pharmacokinetics:	$T_{1/2}$: 1.1–1.6 hr. Metabolism: hepatic: minimal amounts metabolized to glycogen; renal: most excreted based on GFR. Onset: 1–3 hr (diuresis); 15 min (↓ ICP). Duration: 3–6 hr.
Pharmacodynamics:	
CNS:	↓ ICP (may ↑ ICP with disrupted blood-brain barrier), headache, blurred vision, dizziness, convulsions.
CVS:	Pulmonary edema in patients with myocardial dysfunction, hypovolemia.
Renal:	Hypernatremia, hyponatremia, hyperkalemia, hypokalemia.
GI:	Nausea, vomiting, diarrhea.
Other:	Hyperosmolar hyperglycemia, skin rash, skin necrosis, fever, urticaria.
Dosage/ Concentrations:	IV: 5%, 1000 cc; 10%, 500, 1000 cc; 15%, 150, 500 cc; 20%, 150, 250, 500 cc; 25%, 50, 500 cc.
Adult:	For diuresis: Test dose: 12.5 g over 3–5 min to produce urine > 30–50 cc/hr for 2–3 hr; then initial dose: 0.5–1 g/kg. Maintenance dose: 0.25–0.5 g/kg q 4–6 hr. For ICP/IOP: 1.5–2 g/kg as 15–20% solution over 30 min; maintain serum osmolality 310–320 mOsm/kg.
Pediatric:	For diuresis: Test dose: 200 mg/kg over 3–5 min to produce urine > 1 cc/kg/hr for 1–3 hr; then initial dose: 0.5–1 g/kg. Maintenance dose: 0.25–0.5 g/kg/hr q 4–6 hr.
Contraindications:	Severe renal disease, dehydration, electrolyte deple-

MANNITOL   *(continued)*

	tion, pulmonary edema, and active intracranial bleeding.
Drug Interactions/ Allergy:	Electrolyte-free mannitol solutions given concomitantly with blood may produce pseudoagglutination.

METOLAZONE

Trade Names:	Zaroxolyn, Mykrox
Indications:	Edema, mild to moderate hypertension, and induction of diuresis in patients not responsive to furosemide (Lasix).
Pharmacokinetics:	Bioavailability: 65% (Mykrox). $T_{1/2}$: 6–20 hr. Metabolism: small fraction metabolized; most excreted unchanged in urine. Protein binding: 95%. Onset: within 1 hr. Duration: 12–24 hr.
Pharmacodynamics:	
CNS:	Seizures, coma, dizziness, headache.
CVS:	Hypovolemia, dysrhythmias, orthostatic hypotension.
Renal:	Hyponatremia, hypokalemia, hypochloremia, alkalosis.
GI:	Nausea, vomiting.
Other:	Hyperglycemia, hyperuricemia, photosensitivity, may exacerbate lupus.
Dosage/ Concentrations:	Zaroxolyn, 2.5, 5, and 10 mg tablets; Mykrox, 0.5 mg tablet.
Adult:	For edema: Zaroxolyn, 5–20 mg q.d. For hypertension: Zaroxolyn, 2.5–5 mg q.d. Mykrox, 0.5 mg/day; may increase to a maximum 1.0 mg/day.
Contraindications:	Anuria, hepatic coma, and sensitivity to other thiazides or sulfonamide derivatives. Mykrox not to be used for edema.
Drug Interactions/ Allergy:	↑ Serum lithium. Diuretic-induced hypokalemia may increase the risk of digitalis toxicity. Synergistic effect with loop diuretics may result in large fluid or electrolyte loss. ↓ Vascular response to pressor amines.

SPIRONOLACTONE

Trade Name:	Aldactone
Indications:	Primary aldosteronism, essential hypertension, hypokalemia, edema, and precocious puberty.
Pharmacokinetics:	Protein binding: 91%–98%. Metabolism: hepatic; rapidly and extensively metabolized to sulfur-containing products, including canrenone (active metabolite). Elimination: excreted primarily in urine but some in bile. $T_{1/2}$: canrenone: 16.5 hr. Onset: 2–4 hr.

Pharmacodynamics:

CNS:	Drowsiness, confusion, headache, ataxia.
CVS:	↓ BP, ↓ HR.
Renal:	Hyperkalemia, hyperchloremic metabolic acidosis, hyponatremia.
GI:	Nausea, vomiting, diarrhea, constipation, gastritis, GI bleeding.
Other:	Drug fever, teratogenicity, gynecomastia, hirsutism, erectile dysfunction, agranulocytosis, rash, urticaria.

Dosage/ Concentrations:	Tablets: 25, 50 and 100 mg.
Adult:	For edema: 25–200 mg/day in 1–2 doses. For hypertension: 50–100 mg/day in 1–2 doses. For hypokalemia: 25–100 mg/day in 1–2 doses.
Pediatric:	• Neonate: 0.5–1 mg/kg/dose q 8 hr.
	• Child: 1–3.3 mg/kg/day in divided doses.
Contraindications:	Anuria, acute renal insufficiency, hyperkalemia.
Drug Interactions/ Allergy:	K^+ supplements, other K^+-sparing diuretics, salt substitutes, indomethacin, and ACE inhibitors may cause toxic K^+ levels. ↓ Vascular responsiveness to norepinephrine. ↑ Serum digoxin. ↓ Natriuretic effect with ASA.

TORSEMIDE

Trade Name:	Demadex
Indications:	Edema and hypertension.
Pharmacokinetics:	Bioavailability: 80%. Serum peak (C_{max}): 1 hr. Vd: 12–15 L; increased in cirrhosis. $T_{1/2}$: 3.5 hr. Clearance: hepatic metabolism, 80% (metabolized primarily to the inactive carboxylic acid derivative); renal excretion, 20%.

TORSEMIDE   *(continued)*

Protein binding: 99%. Onset: IV, 10 min; p.o., 30–60 min. Duration: IV or p.o., 6–8 hr.

Pharmacodynamics:
CNS: Seizures, ototoxicity.
CVS: Hypovolemia, orthostatic hypotension.
Hepatic: Precipitation of hepatic coma.
Renal: Hyponatremia, hypokalemia, hypochloremia, alkalosis, hypernatremia, hyperkalemia.
GI: Nausea, vomiting, diarrhea, constipation.

Dosage/   Tablets: 5, 10, 20, 100 mg; IV: 2 or 5 cc vials of 10
Concentrations: mg/cc injection.
               For congestive heart failure or chronic renal failure: 10–20 mg, up to 200 mg.
               For cirrhosis: 5–10 mg, up to 40 mg.
               For hypertension: 5 mg, up to 10 mg.

Contraindications: Anuria and sensitivity to other sulfonylureas.

Drug Interactions/   High-dose ASA predisposes to salicylate toxicity.
Allergy: NSAIDs may produce acute renal failure. ↑ Serum lithium.

TRIAMTERENE

Trade Name: Dyrenium

Indications: Edema.

Pharmacokinetics: Absorption: rapid. Metabolism: hepatic; primarily metabolized to hydroxytriamterene sulfate (active). Elimination: biliary (primary); renal: (secondary). Onset: 2–4 hr p.o. Duration: 7–8 hr p.o. $T_{1/2}$: 3 hr. Protein binding: 50%–67%.

Pharmacodynamics:
CNS: Dizziness, headache.
CVS: ↓ BP, ↓ HR.
Hepatic: ↑ LFTs, jaundice.
Renal: Renal stones, hyperkalemia, hypokalemia, azotemia.
GI: Nausea, vomiting, diarrhea.
Other: Hyperglycemia, hyperuricemia, metabolic acidosis, photosensitivity, rash, thrombocytopenia, megaloblastic anuria.

Dosage/   Tablets: 50, 100 mg.
Concentrations:

Adult:	100–200 mg/day in 2 daily doses; maximum 300 mg/day.
Pediatric:	2–4 mg/kg/day in 1–2 divided doses; maximum 300 mg/day.

Contraindications:	Anuria, acute or chronic renal failure, severe hepatic insufficiency, and ↑ serum K^+ levels.
Drug Interactions/ Allergy:	K^+ supplements, other K^+-sparing diuretics, salt substitutes, indomethacin, or ACE inhibitors may cause toxic serum K^+ levels. ↓ Arterial responsiveness to norepinephrine. NSAIDs may be associated with acute renal failure. ↑ Serum lithium. May potentiate effects of nondepolarizing muscle relaxants.

UREA

Trade Name:	Ureaphil
Indications:	High ICP, high IOP, promotion of diuresis.
Pharmacokinetics:	$T_{1/2}$: 1 hr. Metabolism: renal: excretion based on GFR. Onset: 1–2 hr (diuresis). Duration: 3–6 hr (diuresis up to 10 hr).
Pharmacodynamics:	
CNS:	↓ ICP (may ↑ ICP with disrupted blood-brain barrier), headache, syncope, disorientation.
CVS:	Venous thrombosis.
Renal:	Hyponatremia, hypokalemia.
GI:	Nausea, vomiting, ↑ ammonia in liver impairment.
Other:	Local irritation, tissue necrosis from IV extravasation.
Dosage/ Concentrations:	IV: 40 g/150 cc.
Adult:	IV: 1–1.5 g/kg over 1–2.5 hr; maximum, 120 g/24 hr.
Pediatric:	IV: slow infusion.
	• <2 yr: 0.1 g/kg/24 hr.
	• >2 yr: 0.5–1.5 g/kg/24 hr.
Contraindications:	Severe renal or hepatic disease, sickle cell anemia, active intracranial bleeding, dehydration, and electrolyte depletion.
Drug Interactions/ Allergy:	↓ Serum lithium.

22

Gastrointestinal Drugs

Jun Tang, M.D.

ACTIVATED CHARCOAL

Trade Names:	Actidose-Aqua/Sorbitol, Charcoaid, CharcoCaps, Insta-Char, Liqui-Char
Indications:	Nonspecific toxicity, diarrhea, and intestinal gas.
Pharmacokinetics:	Absorption: not absorbed from GI tract; sorbitol poorly absorbed from GI tract. Biotransformation: not metabolized. Elimination: intestinal.
Pharmacodynamics:	Detoxicant and antiflatulent effect.
GI:	Diarrhea or vomiting; swelling of abdomen.
Dosage/ Concentrations:	As antidote.
Adult and Geriatric:	25–100 g p.o.; with sorbitol, 48 g/120 ml.
Pediatric:	• <12 yr: 25–50 g p.o.
	• <1 yr: 1 g/kg p.o.
Contraindications:	Absence of bowel sounds, antidiarrheal use only (preparation without sorbitol only), dehydration, and acute and characterized dysentery.
Drug Interactions/ Allergy:	↓ Effectiveness of oral medications concurrently used with activated charcoal, especially acetylcysteine as antidote in acetaminophen overdose.

ATTAPULGITE

Trade Names:	Diar-Aid; Diasorb; Kaopectate; Kaopectate, Children's, Advanced Formula; Rheaban; St. Joseph Anti-Diarrheal for Children
Indications:	Diarrhea.
Pharmacokinetics:	Not absorbed.
Pharmacodynamics:	Constipation.
Dosage/ Concentrations:	
Adult, Children >12 yr, and Geriatric:	1.2–1.5 g p.o. (suspension) after each loose bowel movement (<9.0 g/24 hr).
Pediatric:	• <3 yr: (suspension) must be individualized.
	• 3–6 yr: 300 mg p.o. (suspension) after each loose bowel movement (<2.1 g/24 hr).
	• 6–12 yr: 600 mg p.o. (suspension) after each loose bowel movement (<4.2 g/24 hr).
Contraindications:	Dehydration in young children and elderly, acute dys-

ATTAPULGITE   *(continued)*

	entery, parasite-associated diarrhea, and bowel obstruction.
Drug Interactions/ Allergy:	Concurrent use with anticholinergics, antidyskinetics, digitalis glycosides, lincomycins, loxapine, phenothiazines, thioxanthenes, and xanthines may decrease their therapeutic effectiveness. May interfere with absorption of other oral drugs administered concurrently.

DIFENOXIN-ATROPINE

Trade Name:	Motofen
Indications:	Acute, nonspecific diarrhea and acute exacerbations of chronic diarrhea.
Pharmacokinetics:	Absorption: absorbed rapidly from GI tract. Biotransformation: hepatic. Peak serum concentration: 40–60 min. $T_{1/2}$: 12–24 hr. Elimination: renal or fecal route.
Pharmacodynamics:	
CNS:	Drowsiness, confusion.
Pulmonary:	Respiratory depression.
GI:	Paralytic ileus, toxic megacolon, nausea, vomiting, stomach cramps.
Musculoskeletal:	Muscle cramps.
Dosage/ Concentrations:	
Adult and Geriatric:	Difenoxin, 2 mg; atropine, 50 µg (2 tablets) p.o., then 1 tablet p.o. q 3–4 hr p.r.n. (maximum 8 mg/day).
Contraindications:	Severe colitis, diarrhea, dehydration from poisoning or dysentery, GI tract obstruction, and hepatic dysfunction.
Drug Interactions/ Allergy:	Alcohol use increases CNS depressant. Anticholinergic drugs may enhance the effects of atropine. MAOIs may raise BP and may block detoxification of atropine. Naltrexone may cause withdrawal symptoms.

DIPHENOXYLATE-ATROPINE

Trade Names:	Diphenatol, Logen, Lomanate, Lomotil, Lonox, Lo-Trol, Nor-Mil
Indications:	Diarrhea.
Pharmacokinetics:	Absorption: from GI tract. Onset: 45–60 min.

Duration: 3–4 hr. Biotransformation: hepatic; see also Difenoxin. $T_{1/2}$: 2½ hr. Elimination: fecal or renal route (<1% eliminated unchanged in urine).

Pharmacodynamics:

CNS: Nervousness, restlessness, irritability, unusual excitement, depression, headache.

CVS: Tachycardia.

Pulmonary: Respiratory depression

Renal: Urinary retention, especially in children.

GI: Paralytic ileus, toxic megacolon.

Musculoskeletal: Numbness of hands or feet.

Other: Dry skin and mucous membranes, flushing, hyperthermia.

Dosage/ Concentrations:

Adult, Geriatric, and Children >12 yr: Diphenoxylate, 2.5–5 mg; with atropine, 25 µg p.o. 3–4 times/day. Maintenance dose: 2.5 mg p.o. 2–3 times/day.

Pediatric (2–12 yr): Diphenoxylate, 0.3–0.4 mg/kg/day p.o.

Contraindications: Severe colitis, diarrhea following treatment with broad-spectrum antibiotics; dehydration in children, acute dysentery, GI tract obstruction, impaired hepatic function, and jaundice.

Drug Interactions/ Allergy: Alcohol or CNS depression may increase CNS depressant effects. Anticholinergics may enhance effects of atropine. MAOIs may precipitate hypertensive crisis and may block detoxification of atropine. Naltrexone may precipitate withdrawal symptoms.

KAOLIN, PECTIN

Trade Names: Kapectolin, K-C, K-P, K-Pek, Kaodene Non-Narcotic

Indications: Diarrhea.

Pharmacokinetics: Not absorbed (90% of pectin decomposed in GI tract).

Pharmacodynamics:

GI: Constipation.

Dosage/ Concentrations:

Adult: 60–120 ml oral suspension containing 5–6 g kaolin and 130–260 mg pectin/30 ml.

Pediatric:
- 0–3 yr: must be individualized.

- 3–6 yr: 15–30 ml oral suspension.

KAOLIN, PECTIN   *(continued)*

- 6–12 yr: 30–60 ml oral suspension.
- >12 yr: 45–60 ml oral suspension.

Contraindications: Dehydration (young children); acute dysentery; parasite-associated diarrhea

Drug Interactions/ Allergy: Concurrent use with anticholinergics, antidyskinetics, digitalis glycosides, lincomycins, loxapine, phenothiazines, thioxanthenes, and xanthines may decrease their therapeutic effectiveness. May interefere with absorption of other oral medications.

LAXATIVES

Trade Names: See Table.

Indications: Constipation and evacuation of bowel, laxative dependency, hyperacidity, hyperammonemia, biliary tract disorders, diarrhea, and irritable bowel syndrome.

Pharmacokinetics: Absorption: local; amount unknown. Elimination: fecal or renal route.

Pharmacodynamics:
Renal: Discoloration of urine (cascara, danthron, phenolphthalein, senna).
GI: Rectal irritation from rectal solutions, esophageal blockage, impaction (bulk-forming), discoloration of feces (phenolphthalein).
Other: Skin irritation, electrolyte imbalance.

Dosage/ Concentrations: See Table.

Generic Name	Trade Name	Dosage	
		Adult	*Pediatric*
Bulk-forming			
Psyllium	Cillium, Konsyl, Perdiem Plain, Siblin	2.5–8 g, 1–3 times/ day	>6 or 7 yr: 2.5–4 g, 1–3 times/day
Methylcellulose	Citrucel, Cologel	0.5–2 g, 1–3 times/ day	>6 yr: 0.5–1.0 g, 2–4 times/day
Psyllium hydrophilic mucilloid	Effer-Syllium, Hydrocil Instant, Konsyl-D, Metamucil Instant Mix	3–3.6 g, 1–3 times/ day	<6 yr: 1.6–1.8 g, 1–3 times/day
Calcium polycarbophil	FiberCon, Equalactin, Mitrolan, Fiberall	1.0 g, 1–4 times/day	2–6 yr: 0.5 g, 1–2 times/day 6–12 yr: 0.5 g, 1–3 times/day
Malt soup extract	Maltsupex, Syllamalt	3–32 g, 2–4 times/ day	3–16 g, 1–2 times/ day

		Dosage	
Generic Name	**Trade Name**	*Adult*	*Pediatric*
Bulk-forming *Continued*			
Psyllium seed husks	Naturacil, Syllact	3.3–3.4 g, 1–3 times/day	>6 yr: 1.7 g 1–3 times/day
Potassium bitartrate, sodium bicarbonate	Geo-Two	Rectal, 1 suppos.	Not recommended
Stool Softener			
Docusate sodium	Afko-lube, Colace (capsules, syrups, drops), Dialose	50–250 mg once/day	>6 yr: 50–100 mg once/day 3–6 yr: 20–60 mg/day <3 yr: 20 mg/day
Docusate potassium	Diocto-K, Kasof	100 mg 1–3 times/day	>6 yr: 100 mg once/day
Docusate calcium	Surfak Liquigels	60–240 mg once/day	50–150 mg once/day
Poloxamer 188	Alaxin	480 mg once/day	>6 yr: 240–480 mg once/day
Hyperosmotic			
Glycerin	Fleet Babylax (liquid)		>1 yr: entire contents of applicator (rectal)
Magnesium sulfate	Bilagog	300–600 mg once/day	
Magnesium citrate (liquid)		240 ml once/day	2–6 yr: 4–12 ml once/day 6–12 yr: 50–100 ml once/day
Magnesium hydroxide	Milk of Magnesia	1.8–14.4 g once/day	>6 yr: 0.9–7.2 g once/day
Magnesium oxide	Mag-Ox 400, Maox 420	2–4 g once/day	Not established
Lactulose	Cholac	10–20 g once/day	Not established
Sodium phosphate	Fleet Phospho-Soda, Fleet Enema, Fleet Pediatric Enema	10–20 g once/day	5–10 yr: 1.12–5.05 g once/day >10 yr: 2.25–10.1 g once/day
Lubricant or Emollient			
Mineral oil	Agoral Plain	2.1–8.4 g once/day	>6 yr: 1.4–5.6 g once/day
Mineral oil (heavy)	Kondremul	15–30 ml once/day	>6 yr: 5–10 ml once/day
Mineral oil (extra heavy)	Nujol	15–45 ml once/day	>6 yr: 5–15 ml once/day
Mineral oil (approx)	Milkinol	15–30 ml once/day	>6 yr: 5–10 ml once/day

Table continued on following page

LAXATIVES *(continued)*

Generic Name	Trade Name	Dosage	
		Adult	*Pediatric*
Stimulant			
Phenolphthalein	Alophen Pills No. 973	60–120 mg 1–2 times/day	>6 yr: 60 mg once/day
Phenolphthalein (yellow)	Espotabs, Evac-U-Lax, Ex-Lax, Medilax, Phenolax, Colax	65–194 mg once/day	>6 yr: 40–95 mg once/day
Castor Oil	Alphamul, Emulsoil	15–60 ml once/day	<2 yr: 1–5 ml once/day >2 yr: 5–15 ml once/day
Bisacodyl	Bisac-Evac, Bisco-Lax, Carter's Little Pills, Dulcolax, Fleet Bisacodyl	Oral, 5–15 mg once/day Rectal, 1 suppos once/day	6–12 yr: 5–10 mg once/day <2 yr: ½ supp >2 yr: 1 supp
Casanthranol	Black-Draught	30–90 mg once/day	<2 yr: 7.5–22.5 mg once/day 2–12 yr: 15–45 mg once/day
Senna equivalent	Tablets (OTC)	1200 mg once/day	>6 yr: 600 mg once/day
Senna	Fletcher's Castoria, Perdiem	N/A	1–6 months: 0.125–2.5 ml once/day 7–12 months: 2.5–5 ml once/day 1–5 yr: 5–10 ml once/day 6–12 yr: 10–15 ml once/day
Senna concentrate	Senexon, Senolax, Senokot	Oral, 374–434 mg once/day; rectal, 1 suppos.	>6 yr: 187–217 mg once/day >6 yr: ½ suppos.
Cascara sagrada	Nature's Remedy, Kondremul with Cascara, Caroid Laxative	150 mg once/day 5 g once/day	N/A >2 yr: 1–3 g once/day
Dehydrocholic acid	Cholan-HMB, Decholin	250–500 mg 3 times a day	Not established
Sennosides	Nytilax, Gentle Nature	12–40 mg once/day	>6 yr: 12–20 mg once/day

Contraindications: *All classes:* appendicitis, undiagnosed rectal bleeding, congestive heart failure, hypertension, diabetes mellitus, intestinal obstruction. *Bulk-forming:* dysphagia. *Hyperosmotic-saline:* dehydration, renal function impairment. *Hyperosmotic-saline and lubricant:* colostomy, ileostomy. *Lubricant:* dysphagia, bedridden patient in whom lipid pneumonia may develop from aspiration of mineral oil.

Drug Interactions/ Allergy:
All classes: ↓ Serum K$^+$ with potassium-sparing diuretics and potassium supplements. *Bulk-forming:* ↓ effects of anticoagulants, digitalis glycosides, and salicylates. ↓ effects with concurrent tetracycline use and calcium polycarbophil. *Hyperosmotic-saline: magnesium-containing:* anticoagulants, digitalis glycosides, and phenothiazines will reduce their effectiveness. Sodium polystyrene sulfonate may cause severe systemic alkalosis. Tetracyclines may cause formation of nonabsorbable complexes. *Lubricant:* effectiveness of anticoagulants, contraceptives, digitalis glycosides, and fat-soluble vitamins may be reduced. *Stimulant:* with antacids or histamine H$_2$-receptor antagonists, milk may cause gastric or duodenal irritation. *Stool softeners* may enhance the absorption of dantheon, mineral oil, phenolphthalein.

LOPERAMIDE

Trade Names:	Imodium, Kaopectate II
Indications:	Diarrhea.
Pharmacokinetics:	Absorption: poorly absorbed from GI tract (40%). Protein binding: 97%. Biotransformation: hepatic. Peak concentration: capsules, 5 hr; oral, 2.5 hr. Duration: up to 24 hr. T$_{1/2}$: 9–14 hr. Elimination: fecal or renal route.

Pharmacodynamics:
CNS: Drowsiness, dizziness.
GI: Toxic megacolon.

Dosage/ Concentrations:
Adult: 4 mg p.o. after first loose bowel movement, followed by 2 mg after each subsequent loose bowel movement. Total dose: 16 mg/day.
Pediatric: 80–240 μg/kg/day p.o. in 2 or 3 divided doses.

Contraindications: Severe colitis; diarrhea or dehydration related to dysentery; hepatic dysfunction; and previous allergic reaction to loperamide.

Drug Interactions/ Allergy: Opioid analgesics may increase risk of severe constipation. Skin rash.

OCTREOTIDE

Trade Name:	Sandostatin
Indications:	GI and pancreatic tumors, hypotension, acromegaly, and AIDS-associated diarrhea.
Pharmacokinetics:	Absorption: rapidly absorbed from injection site completely. Protein binding (65%). $T_{1/2}$: 1.5 hr. Time to peak concentration: ≤0.5 hr. Peak serum concentration: 5.5 ng/ml. Duration: up to 12 hr. Elimination: renal (32%).

Pharmacodynamics:
CNS:	Dizziness, headache.
GI:	Nausea, diarrhea, abdominal pain or discomfort, loose stools, vomiting, fat malabsorption.
Other:	Pain, stinging, tingling, or burning sensation at injection site, with redness and swelling.

**Dosage/
Concentrations:**
Adult and Geriatric:	Antidiarrheal (GI tumor): 50 μg IM q.d. or b.i.d. (limited 750 μg/day).
Pediatric:	1–10 μg/kg/day IM.
Contraindications:	Gallbladder disease, gallstones, diabetes mellitus, and severe renal function impairment.
Drug Interactions/ Allergy:	Antidiabetic agents, glucagon, growth hormone, and insulin may cause hypoglycemia or hyperglycemia.

OLSALAZINE

Trade Name:	Dipentum
Indications:	Inflammatory bowel disease in patients intolerant of sulfasalazine.
Pharmacokinetics:	Systemic bioavailability: <2% absorbed and rapidly acetylated. Peak concentration: olsalazine, 1 hr; 5-aminosalicylic acid, 4–8 hr. Protein binding: >99%. Absorbed olsalazine is converted to olsalazine-S, and unabsorbed olsalaze is converted to 5-aminosalicylic acid (slowly absorbed and acetylated in colon and liver). $T_{1/2}$: 0.9 hr. Elimination: 7 days required to eliminate metabolites; renal route (20%); fetal route (80%).

Pharmacodynamics:
CNS:	Anxiety, depression, drowsiness, dizziness, headache, insomnia.

Hepatic:	Hepatitis.
GI:	Exacerbation of ulcerative colitis, pancreatitis and GI disturbances.
Musculoskeletal:	Aching joints and muscle.
Other:	Blood dyscrasias.

Dosage/ Concentrations:

Adult and Geriatric:	500 mg p.o. b.i.d.
Pediatric:	N/A.

Contraindications: Renal function impairment.

Drug Interactions/ Allergy: None known.

OMEPRAZOLE

Trade Name: Prilosec

Indications: Gastroesophageal reflux, gastric hypersecretion, (Zollinger-Ellison syndrome, systemic mastocytosis, multiple endocrine adenoma, and duodenal and gastric ulcers).

Pharmacokinetics: Absorption: rapidly absorbed by gastric parietal cells. Protein binding: (95%). Onset: 1 hr. Time to peak concentration: 0.5–3.5 hr. Duration: >72 hr. Metabolism: hepatic. $T_{1/2}$: 0.5–1 hr; in chronic hepatic disease, 3 hr. Elimination: renal (70%–80%); fecal (20%–25%).

Pharmacodynamics:

CNS:	Dizziness, headache.
Hepatic:	Inhibited hepatic microsomal drug metabolism.
Renal:	Hematuria, proteinuria, UTI.
GI:	Abdominal pain, colic, GI disturbances.
Musculoskeletal:	Asthenia.
Other:	Anemia, eosinopenia, leukocytosis, neutropenia, pancytopenia, thrombocytopenia.

Dosage/ Concentrations:

Adult:	For gastroesophageal reflux: 20 mg p.o. q.d. 4–8 wk. For gastric hypersecretion: 60 mg p.o. q.d. For duodenal or gastric ulcer: 20–40 mg p.o. q.d.
Geriatric:	<20 mg/day.
Pediatric:	N/A.

Contraindications: Hepatic disease.

Drug Interactions/ Allergy: ↓ Absorption of ampicillin, iron salts, and ketoconazole. ↓ Metabolism of anticoagulants, diazepam, and

OMEPRAZOLE   *(continued)*

phenytoin in liver. ↑ Leukopenic or thrombocytopenic effects of chemotherapy.

PANCREATIN, PEPSIN, BILE SALTS, HYOSCYAMINE, ATROPINE, SCOPOLAMINE, PHENOBARBITAL

Trade Name:	Donnazyme
Indications:	Digestive disorders.
Pharmacokinetics:	Absorption: absorbed rapidly from GI tract. Protein binding: atropine, 50%; hyoscyamine, 26%; phenobarbital, 20%–45%; scopolamine, 10%. Biotransformation: hepatic. Duration: atropine, 4–6 hr; hyoscyamine, 4–6 hr; phenobarbital, 10–12 hr; scopolamine, 4–6 hr. $T_{1/2}$: atropine, 2.5 hr; hyoscyamine, 3.5 hr, phenobarbital, 53–118 hr; scopolamine, 8 hr.

Pharmacodynamics:

CNS:	Drowsiness, dizziness, hallucinations, nervousness, confusion, visual disturbances, headache, impairment of memory, ↑ IOP.
CVS:	↓ HR, ↑ HR in overdose.
Pulmonary:	Respiratory depression.
Hepatic:	Hepatitis, jaundice.
Renal:	Hyperuricemia, difficult urination.
GI:	Constipation, nausea, and vomiting.
Other:	Agranulocytosis, thrombocytopenia.

Dosage/ Concentrations:

Adult and Geriatric:	2 tablets (pancreatin, 300 mg; pepsin, 150 mg; bile salts, 150 mg; hyoscyamine, 52 μg; atropine, 10 μg; scopolamine, 3 μg; phenobarbital, 8 mg) p.o. after meals p.r.n.
Pediatric:	N/A.
Contraindications:	Cardiac disease, drug abuse, reflux esophagitis, GI tract obstruction or atony, glaucoma, acute hemorrhage, hiatal hernia associated with reflux esophagitis, myasthenia gravis, paralytic ileus, nonobstructive prostatic hypertrophy, tachycardia, severe ulcerative colitis, urinary retention, and uropathy.
Drug Interactions/ Allergy:	Alcohol, general anesthetics, MAOIs increase CNS depression. Antacids, adsorbent antidiarrheals, anticoagulants, digitalis glycosides, and ketoconazole decrease

therapeutic effects. ↑ GI lesions with KCl. Skin rash or hives.

PANCRELIPASE

Trade Names:	Cotazym; Ilozyme; Ku-Zyme HP; Pancrease; Pancrease MT 4, MT 10, MT 16; Protilase; Ultrase MT 12, MT 20, MT 24; Viokase; Zymase
Indications:	Pancreatic insufficiency, malabsorption, steatorrhea.
Pharmacokinetics:	Not absorbed.

Pharmacodynamics:

Pulmonary:	Respiratory difficulty (with inhalation of powder).
Renal:	Hyperuricemia, hyperuricosuria.
GI:	Irritation of the mouth, nausea, cramping, diarrhea.

Dosages:

Adult and Geriatric: 1–3 capsules (see Table).

		Lipase (USP Units)	Protease (USP Units)	Amylase (USP Units)
Capsules	Ku-Zyme HP	8,000	30,000	30,000
Delayed-release capsules	Pancrease MT 4	4,000	12,000	12,000
Tablet	Viokase	8,000	30,000	30,000
Powder	Viokase	16,800	70,000	70,000

Pediatric:	1–3 capsules.
Contraindications:	Acute pancreatitis and sensitivity to pork protein or pancreatin.
Drug Interactions/ Allergy:	Antacids (except calcium carbonate or magnesium hydroxide) can prevent inactivation of pancrelipase. ↓ Iron absorption. Skin rash or hives.

POLYETHYLENE GLYCOL-ELECTROLYTES SOLUTION

Trade Names:	Colovage, Colyte, GoLYTELY, NuLytely, OCL
Indications:	Preprocedural bowel evacuation.
Pharmacokinetics:	Absorption: negligible. Onset: 30–60 min. Elimination: renal route (<0.1%).

Pharmacodynamics:

GI:	Bloating, nausea, vomiting, abdominal cramps, anal irritation.

POLYETHYLENE GLYCOL-ELECTROLYTES SOLUTION *(continued)*

Dosage/ Concentrations:	
Adult and Geriatric:	Oral, 240 ml/10 min, up to 4 L or until fecal discharge is clear and free of solid matter.
Pediatric:	Oral, 25–40 ml/kg/hr until fecal discharge is clear and free of solid matter.
Contraindications:	Intestinal obstruction, paralytic ileus, perforated bowel, severe ulcerative colitis, toxic colitis, toxic megacolon, predisposition to regurgitation and aspiration, and unconscious or semiconscious state.
Drug Interactions/ Allergy:	Interference with absorption of concurrent oral medications. Skin rash.

SIMETHICONE

Trade Names:	Gas-X, Gas Relief, Mylicon, Phazyme
Indications:	Excess GI gas and adjunct in gastroscopy and bowel radiography.
Pharmacokinetics:	Elimination: fecal route (unchanged).
Pharmacodynamics:	Antiflatulent effect.
Dosage/ Concentrations:	
Adult and Geriatric:	Capsules: 125 mg p.o. q.i.d. p.c. and h.s. Suspension: 40 mg/0.6 ml p.o. q.i.d. p.c. and h.s. Tablets: 40–125 mg (<500 mg/24 hr) p.o. q.i.d. p.c. and h.s.
Contraindications:	None known.
Drug Interactions/ Allergy:	None known.

23

Hormones

Henry Huey, M.D.
Naomi M. Gonzales, Pharm.D.
Charles Louy, Ph.D., M.D.

ACETOHEXAMIDE, CHLORPROPAMIDE, TOLAZAMIDE, TOLBUTAMIDE, GLIPIZIDE, GLYBURIDE

Trade Names: Dymelor, Diabinese, Tolinase, Orinase, Glucotrol, Micronase, Diaβeta, Glynase PresTabs

Indications: Diabetes mellitus and non–insulin-dependent diabetes.

Pharmacokinetics:

	Equiv-alent Dose (mg)	Doses/ Day	Serum Half-Life (hr)	Time to Peak Concen-tration (hr)	Dura-tion of Action (hr)	Biotrans-formation (in Liver)	Elimi-nation (%)
First-generation							
Acetohexamide	500	1–2	6–8	1–3	12–24	Reduced to potent active metabolite	Renal (80) Biliary (10)
Chlorpropamide	250	1	36	2–4	24–48	80% metab-olized	Renal (80–90)
Tolazamide	250	1	7	3–4	10	Mildly active metabolites	Renal (85) Fecal (7)
Tolbutamide	1000	2–3	4.5–8.5	3–4	6–12	Inactive metabolites	Renal (75) Biliary (9)
Second-generation							
Glipizide	10	1–2	2–4	1–3	12–24	Inactive metabolites	Renal
Nonmicronized	5	1–2	10	4	24	Weakly active metabolites	Biliary (50)
Micronized	3	1–2	4	4	24		Renal (75)

Pharmacodynamics:

CNS: Drowsiness, coma, seizures due to SIADH.
CVS: Congestive heart failure (antidiuretic effect of chlor-propamide).
Hepatic: ↓ Hepatic glycogenolysis and gluconeogenesis, hepat-ic dysfunction.
Renal: ↑ Effect of ADH with central diabetes insipidus, SIADH (chlorpropamide only).
GI: Nausea, vomiting.
Endocrine: ↑ Release of insulin from pancreas.
Other: Bone marrow depression, aplastic anemia.

Dosage/   Tolbutamide: 250–3000 mg/day.
Concentrations: Tolazamide: 100–1000 mg/day.
                     Acetohexamide: 250–1500 mg/day.
                     Chlorpropamide: 100–750 mg/day.
                     Glyburide: 1.25–20 mg/day.

Glipizide: 2.5–40 mg/day.
Glynase: 0.75–12 mg/day.

Contraindications: Significant acidosis, severe burns, ketoacidosis, diabetic coma, severe infection, major surgery, and severe trauma.

Drug Interactions/ Allergy: Cross-sensitivity among oral antidiabetic agents. Disulfiram-like reaction with alcohol use. ↑ Effect of anticoagulants. Enhanced hypoglycemic effect of insulin.

CALCITONIN

Trade Names: Calcimar, Miacalcin, Cibacalcin

Indications: Bone pain, Paget's disease, osteoporosis, and hypercalcemia

Pharmacokinetics: Onset: 1 hr after single 0.5-mg SC dose. Metabolism: Rapidly converted to smaller inactive fragments. Elimination: A small amount of unchanged hormone and its active metabolites excreted in urine.

Pharmacodynamics:
Renal: ↑ Excretion of calcium, phosphate, and sodium by inhibition of tubular reabsorption.
GI: Diarrhea, anorexia, nausea, vomiting, abdominal pain
Musculoskeletal: Inhibition of bone resorption.

Dosage/ Concentrations:
Adult: Injection: Calcimar (calcitonin-salmon): 200 IU/ml solution (2-ml vial).
Miacalcin (calcitonin-salmon): 100 IU/ml (1-ml ampule).
Cibacalcin (calcitonin-human): 0.5 mg/vial (double-chambered).
For cancer bone pain: 10 U SC for 1 dose; if no side effects or reactions occur, 100 U SC each morning for 14 days.
Pediatric: N/A.

Contraindications: Allergy to proteins. Sensitivity to calcitonin more likely with salmon type.

Drug Interaction Allergy: Calcium-containing preparations or vitamin D may antagonize effects of calcitonin.

CHLOROTRIANISENE, DIETHYLSTILBESTROL, ESTRADIOL, ESTRADIOL CYPIONATE, ESTRADIOL VALERATE

Trade Names:	Tace, Stilphostrol, Estrace, Estraderm, Depo-Estradiol Cypionate, depGynogen, Depogen, Dura-Estrin, Estroject-L.A., Estra-D, Estro-Cyp, Valergen-10, Delestrogen, Dioval, Duragen-10, Estradiol L.A., Estraval
Indications:	Estrogen deficiency, atrophic vaginitis, hypogonadism in females, vulvar hyperplasia, primary ovarian failure, vasomotor symptoms of menopause, uterine bleeding, cancer of breast and prostate, prophylaxis for osteoporosis, and bleeding associated with renal failure.
Pharmacokinetics:	Onset: 1 hr. Absorption: oral; rapid. IM oils and suspension are immediately absorbed; activity continues for several days. Clearance: primarily metabolized in liver but also in kidneys, gonads, and muscle tissue. $T_{1/2}$: 13–27 hr. Protein binding: 50%–80%.

Pharmacodynamics:

CNS:	Mild dizziness, headache.
CVS:	Peripheral edema, ↑ risk of MI, pulmonary embolism, and thrombophlebitis in males taking large doses.
GI:	GI upset, cramping, bloating, nausea, anorexia.
Musculoskeletal:	Inhibited bone resorption.
Endocrine:	Hyperglycemia, hypercalcemia, gynecomastia.

Dosage/ Concentrations:	Estradiol cypionate (in oil): IV, 1–5 mg/dose. Estradiol valerate (in oil): IV, 10–30 mg/dose. Estradiol (transdermal): 0.05 mg/day. Estradiol (oral): 0.5 mg/day. Diethylstilbestrol: 1–15 mg/day. Diethylstilbestrol diphosphate: oral: 50–200 mg/dose; parenteral: 0.5–1 g/dose
Contraindications:	Breast cancer, vaginal bleeding, thrombophlebitis.
Drug Interactions/ Allergy:	↑ Therapeutic and toxic effects of glycocorticoids; interference with effects of bromocriptine, tamoxifen, and metabolism of cyclosporine; ↑ Risk of CVS side effects with smoking.

CLOMIPHENE CITRATE

Trade Names:	Clomid, Serophene, Milophene
Indications:	Anovulation or oligo-ovulation.
Pharmacokinetics:	Absorption: from rapidly absorbed GI tract. Duration:

6–12 hr. Clearance: biliary elimination. Metabolism: hepatic. $T_{1/2}$: 5 days.

Pharmacodynamics:

CNS: Vasomotor flushes, headache, irritability, depression, visual disturbance.

Renal: ↑ Urine output.

GI: Abdominal discomfort, nausea, vomiting.

Endocrine: ↑ Secretion of LH and FSH.

Dosage/ Concentrations: Tablet: 50 mg.

Adult: 50–100 mg p.o. daily.

Pediatric: N/A.

Contraindications: Pregnancy, uncontrolled thyroid or adrenal dysfunction, hepatic dysfunction, mental depression, intracranial lesion, thrombophlebitis, ovarian cyst (not related to polycystic ovarian syndrome).

Drug Interactions/ Allergy: None.

CORTISONE, HYDROCORTISONE, METHYLPREDNISOLONE, PREDNISOLONE, DEXAMETHASONE, BETAMETHASONE, TRIAMCINOLONE

Trade Names: Cortone Acetate, Solu-Cortef, Solu-Medrol, Delta-Cortef, Decadron

Indications: Adrenal insufficiency and anti-inflammatory and immunosuppressant effects.

	Relative Potency			Half-Life	
	Glucocorticoid Equivalent Dose (mg)	*Glucocorticoid Activity*	*Mineralocorticoid Activity*	*Plasma (hr)*	*Biologic (Tissue) (hr)*
Short-acting					
Cortisone	25	0.8	2+	0.5	8–12
Hydrocortisone	20	1	2+	1.5–2	8–12
Intermediate-acting					
Methylprednisolone	4	5	0	>3.5	18–36
Prednisolone	5	4	1+	2.1–3.5	18–36
Prednisone	5	4	1+	3.4–3.8	18–36
Triamcinolone	4	5	0	2–5	18–36
Long-acting					
Betamethasone	0.6	20–30	0	3–5	36–54
Dexamethasone	0.5–0.75	20–30	0	3–4.5	36–54
Paramethasone	2	10	0	3–4.5 hr	36–54

CORTISONE, HYDROCORTISONE, METHYLPREDNISOLONE, PREDNISOLONE, DEXAMETHASONE, BETAMETHASONE, TRIAMCINOLONE   *(continued)*

Pharmacokinetics:	Absorption: Readily absorbed in GI tract when taken orally. For most rapid onset, administer a water-soluble glucocorticoid ester IV. Vd: Hydrocortisone: reversibly bound to corticosteroid-binding globulin and corticosteroid-binding albumin. Only unbound drug is pharmacologically active, so that patients with low serum albumin concentrations may be more susceptible to glucocorticoid effects than those with normal concentrations. Glycocorticoids: cross placenta; may be distributed into breast milk. Metabolism and Excretion: Hydrocortisone: metabolized by liver (rate-limiting step in clearance). Synthetic glucocorticoids: similar. Prednisone: inactive, metabolized to prednisolone. Inactive metabolites: excreted by kidneys.

Pharmacodynamics:

CNS:	Inhibited hypothalamic-pituitary-adrenal axis, psychic disturbances.
CVS:	Degradation of connective tissue, ↑ vascular fragility and bruising, fluid retention, hypertension.
Pulmonary:	↑ Surfactant production.
Hepatic:	↑ Hepatic glycogen storage.
Renal:	Sodium reabsorption; water retention; excretion of potassium, calcium, and hydrogen.
GI:	GI irritation, nausea, peptic ulceration.
Musculoskeletal:	↑ Degradation of protein, muscle weakness, cramps, atrophy; ↓ bone formation; ↑ bone resorption and fractures.
Endocrine:	↓ Corticotropin secretion, ↓ adrenal androgen secretion, ↑ serum glucose, ↑ lipolysis, ↓ inflammatory process, ↓ immune response.
Other:	Hypernatremia, hypocalcemia, hypokalemia, metabolic alkalosis.

Dosage/ Concentrations:

	Cortisone:
Adult:	25–300 mg/day.
Pediatric:	0.5–10 mg/kg/24 hr (oral); 0.25–5 mg/kg/24 hr (injectable).
	Hydrocortisone:
Adult:	20–240 mg/day.
Pediatric:	0.5–8 mg/kg/dose.
	Hydrocortisone acetate:
Adult:	5–50 mg/dose.
Pediatric:	N/A.

	Hydrocortisone sodium succinate:
Adult:	100–500 mg/dose.
Pediatric:	0.2–4 mg/kg/dose.
	Prednisone:
Adult:	5–60 mg/day.
Pediatric:	0.5–2 mg/kg/day.
	Prednisolone:
Adult:	5–200 mg/day.
Pediatric:	0.1–2 mg/kg/day.
	Triamcinolone:
Adult:	4–100 mg/day.
Pediatric:	0.12–2 mg/kg/day.
	Triamcinolone acetonide:
Adult:	1–60 mg/dose.
Pediatric:	6–12 yr: 0.03–0.2 mg/kg/day.
	Methylprednisolone:
Adult:	4–250 mg/dose.
Pediatric:	0.16–2 mg/kg/day.
	Methylprednisolone sodium succinate:
Adult:	10–40 mg/dose.
Pediatric:	0.04–0.8 mg/kg/dose.
	Dexamethasone:
Adult:	0.75–9 mg/day (oral).
Pediatric:	0.03–0.3 mg/kg/day (oral).
	Dexamethasone acetate:
Adult:	0.8–16 mg/dose.
Pediatric:	N/A.
	Dexamethasone sodium phosphate:
Adult:	0.5–80 mg/day.
Pediatric:	0.0077–0.16 mg/kg/day.
	Betamethasone:
Adult:	0.6–7.2 mg/day.
Pediatric:	0.017–0.25 mg/kg/day.
	Betamethasone sodium phosphate:
Adult:	Limit: up to 9 mg/day.
Pediatric:	0.017–0.25 mg/kg/day

Contraindications: Coagulopathy, osteoporosis, congestive heart failure, hypertension, Cushing's syndrome, and sensitivity to porcine proteins.

Drug Interactions/ Allergy: With NSAIDs, GI ulceration or hemorrhage. With amphotericin B or carbonic anhydrase inhibitors, severe hypokalemia. With digitalis glycosides, arrhythmia. With ritodrine, maternal pulmonary edema and death.

DANAZOL

Trade Names: Danocrine, Cyclomen

Indications: Endometriosis, fibrocystic breast disease, hereditary angioedema, gynecomastia, amenorrhagia, and precocious puberty.

DANAZOL   *(continued)*

Pharmacokinetics:	Vd: highly concentrated in liver, kidneys, and adrenals. Clearance: excreted in urine and feces. $T_{1/2}$: > 15 hr.

Pharmacodynamics:

CNS:	Intracranial hypertension.
CV:	↑ BP (volume expansion).
Hepatic:	Cholestatic jaundice or hepatic dysfunction, ↑ AST (SGOT)
Renal:	↑ Creatine kinase (rhabdomyolysis), hematuria.
GI:	Acute pancreatitis.
Endocrine:	Breakthrough bleeding.
Other:	Thrombocytopenia.

Concentrations:	Capsule: 50, 100, 200 mg.
Dosage/ Concentrations:	Tablet: 50, 100, 200 mg.
Adult:	50–800 mg/day p.o.
Pediatric:	N/A.
Contraindications:	Cardiac disease, hepatic and renal dysfunction, and vaginal bleeding.
Drug Interactions/ Allergy:	May enhance effects of anticoagulants. Danazol may increase blood glucose level, resistance to insulin, and risk of nephrotoxicity. Danazol increases plasma cyclosporine level.

DESMOPRESSIN ACETATE, DDAVP

Trade Name:	Concentraid
Indications:	Diabetes insipidus, hemophilia A, von Willebrand disease (type I), factor VIII deficiency, primary nocturnal enuresis, and platelet dysfunction.
Pharmacokinetics:	Intranasal (antidiuretic effect). Onset: within 1 hr. Peak effect: 1–5 hr. Duration: 6–24 hr. IV (antihemorrhagic effect). Onset: within minutes. Peak effect: 15–30 min; increase in vWF occurs over 3 hr; increase in factor VIII occurs over 4–24 hr. Elimination: renal. $T_{1/2}$: 75 min.

Pharmacodynamics:

CNS:	Headache, mental status changes, seizures, coma.
CVS:	Hypertension (from smooth muscle contraction), hypotension (from peripheral vasodilation with rapid administration).

Renal:	↑ Water reabsorption (↓ urine output, ↑ urine osmolality, ↓ serum osmolality).
GI:	Smooth muscle contraction, abdominal cramps, nausea.
Musculoskeletal:	Smooth muscle contraction.
Other:	Hyponatremia, water intoxication, ↑ clotting factor VIII, ↑ vWF activity, platelet aggregation.

**Dosage/
Concentrations:**

Adult: IV: 4 μg/ml, 1-ml ampule from 0.3 to 0.5 μg/kg 30 min before surgery. Give over 15–30 min.
   Nasal solution: 0.1 mg/ml (0.1 mg = 400 IU arginine vasopressin). Dosages suitable for antihemorrhagic effect also result in antidiuresis. 0.1–0.4 cc daily

Pediatric: IV: 4 μg/cc, 1-ml ampule from 0.3 to 0.5 μg/kg 30 min before surgery.
   Nasal solution: 0.05–0.3 ml daily.

Contraindications: Infants < 3 months and patients with factor VIII concentrations of ≤ 5%; factor VIII antibodies, type IIB, severe, or classic von Willebrand disease (type III); severe coronary artery disease; hypertension; hypotension; renal failure; seizures, and migraine.

**Drug Interactions/
Allergy:**   ↑ Antidiuretic effect with carbamazepine, chlorpropamide and clofibrate. ↓ Antidiuretic effect with demeclocycline, lithium, and norepinephrine.

DEXTROTHYROXINE SODIUM

Trade Name: Choloxin

Indications: Primary hypercholesterolemia (type II hyperlipidemia) (now replaced by other antihyperlipidemic agents).

Pharmacokinetics: Absorption: 25% from GI tract. Clearance: some deiodinated drug (T_3 and monoiodothyronine) recovered in urine with unchanged drug. Metabolized in small amounts by liver. $T_{1/2}$ (plasma): 18 hr.

Pharmacodynamics:

CVS: ↑ Cardiovascular risk, ↑ mortality (coronary atherosclerosis).

Hepatic: ↑ Formation of LDL, ↑ catabolism of LDL.

Endocrine: Weak thyroid hormone effects due to levothyroxine (T4) contamination.

**Dosage/
Concentrations:**   Tablet: 1, 2, 4, 6 mg.

Adult: 1–8 mg/day.

DEXTROTHYROXINE SODIUM *(continued)*

Pediatric: 0.05–0.4 mg/kg/day or 4 mg/day.

Contraindications: Known or suspected heart disease, advanced liver or
                              kidney disease, and hypertension.

Drug Interactions/   ↓ Pharmacologic effect of β blockers. Digitalis glyco-
Allergy: sides ↓ therapeutic effectiveness of digoxin and may
                              exacerbate cardiac arrhythmias or congestive heart fail-
                              ure. TCAs ↑ CNS stimulation (irritability) and cardi-
                              ac arrhythmias. ↑ Effects of anticoagulants.
                              ↑ ↓ effect of antidiabetic agents. Cholestyramine, ur-
                              sodiol, and colestipol ↓ effects of dextrothyroxine.

DIAZOXIDE

Trade Name: Hyperstat

Indications: Malignant hypertension and hypertensive crisis.

Pharmacokinetics: Onset: 1 min. Peak effect: 2–5 min. Clearance: renal
                              elimination. Metabolism: hepatic. $T_{1/2}$: 21–45 hr (aver-
                              age 24 hr) (inversely proportional to creatinine clear-
                              ance). Protein binding: >90%. Duration: 4–12 hr.

Pharmacodynamics:
CNS: Tinnitus.
CVS: Arteriolar vasodilation, hypotension, tachycardia.
Renal: Sodium and water retention.
Endocrine: Hyperglycemia due to inhibition of insulin release
                              from pancreas, catecholamine-induced effects.
Other: Thrombocytopenia, thrombosis.

Dosage/   Injection: 15 mg/ml single-dose vial; 300 mg/20 ml
Concentrations: single-dose vial and ampule.
Adult: For hypertensive crisis: 1–3 mg/kg/dose q 5–15 min
                              IV.
                              For hyperinsulinemic hypoglycemia: 3–8 mg/kg/day
                              p.o.
Pediatric: For hypertensive crisis: 1–3 mg/kg/dose q 5–15 min
                              IV.
                              For hyperinsulinemic hypoglycemia: 8–15 mg/kg/day
                              p.o.

Contraindications: Aortic dissection, compensatory hypertension (aortic
                              coarctation and arteriovenous shunt), coronary or renal
                              insufficiency, diabetes mellitus, and uncompensated
                              congestive heart failure. Not effective for hypertension
                              from MAOI therapy or pheochromocytoma.

Drug Interactions/
Allergy:
Anticoagulants ↑ anticoagulant effects. Oral antidiabetic agents and insulin reverse hyperglycemic effect. NSAIDs, estrogens, and sympathomimetics antagonize hypertensive effects. β blockers prevent diazoxide-induced tachycardia and may increase hypotensive effects. Diuretics potentiate antihypertensive and hyperglycemic actions.

EPOETIN ALFA (HUMAN ALBUMIN)

Trade Names: Epogen, Procrit

Indications: Anemia.

Pharmacokinetics: Peak effect: 5–24 hr after SC administration. Clearance: not cleared by dialysis. $T_{1/2}$: after IV, 4–13 hr in patients with chronic renal failure (first-order kinetics)

Pharmacodynamics:
CNS: Seizures.
CVS: ↑ BP.
Renal: ↑ BUN, ↑ potassium, ↑ sodium, ↑ phosphorus, ↑ uric acid, ↑ creatinine.
Other: ↑ thrombosis, ↓ endogenous erythropoietin, ↓ serum ferritin, ↓ iron.

Dosage/
Concentrations:
Epogen (preservative-free). Injection: 2000, 3000, 4000, 10,000 U (1-ml vial). *Do not shake drug* (glycoprotein may be denatured, rendering it biologically inactive).
Adult: 25–100 U/kg/dose.
Pediatric: 25–100 U/kg/dose.

Contraindications: Sensitivity to mammalian cell–derived products, hypertension, hypercoagulable disorders, myelodysplastic syndromes, sickle cell anemia, vascular disease.

Drug Interactions/
Allergy:
None.

FLUDROCORTISONE

Trade Name: Florinef

Indications: Adrenocortical insufficiency, salt-losing forms of adrenogenital syndrome, and idiopathic orthostatic hypotension.

Pharmacokinetics: Peak effect: 1.7 hr. Absorption: readily absorbed by GI

FLUDROCORTISONE *(continued)*

tract. $T_{1/2}$: plasma, 3.5 hr, biologic, 18–36 hr. Biotransformation: hepatic. Elimination: renal.

Pharmacodynamics:

CVS:	Hypokalemic-induced arrhythmias, ↑ intravascular volume.
Renal:	↑ Potassium excretion, ↑ hydrogen ion excretion, ↑ sodium reabsorption, water retention.
GI:	Nausea, vomiting, anorexia.
Musculoskeletal:	Weakness of extremities and trunk, muscle cramps.
Other:	Hypokalemia, hypernatremia.

Dosage/ Concentrations: Tablet: 100 μg (0.1 mg).

Adult and Adolescent: For adrenocortical insufficiency: 0.1 mg/day p.o.
For adrenogenital syndrome: 0.1–0.2 mg/day p.o.
For antihypotensive (orthostatic) effect: 0.05–0.2 mg/day p.o.

Pediatric: 0.05–0.1 mg/day p.o.

Contraindications: Coronary artery disease, congestive heart failure, hypertension.

Drug Interactions/ Allergy: Digitalis glycosides may result in hypokalemic cardiac arrhythmias. Phenytoin and rifampin may accelerate hepatic metabolism. Lithium may antagonize mineralocorticoid effect.

GLUCAGON

Trade Name: N/A

Indications: Severe hypoglycemia, overdose of oral antidiabetic agents or insulin, promote relaxation of smooth musculature for GI radiology and endoscopy, relief of foreign body obstruction in esophagus, and treatment of toxicity from beta-adrenergic blocking and calcium-channel blocking agents.

Pharmacokinetics: Onset: 5–20 min. Clearance: Extensively degraded in liver, kidney, plasma and tissue receptor sites. $T_{1/2}$: 3–6 min. See Table p. 237.

Pharmacodynamics:

CVS:	Inotropic and chronotropic effects, arrhythmias.
Hepatic:	↑ Plasma, ↑ glucose.
GI:	↓ Peristalsis, nausea, vomiting.

Musculoskeletal:	Smooth muscle relaxation, muscle cramps, pain, weakness.
Other:	Hypokalemic syndrome, ↓ blood glucose (paradoxical effect).
Dosage/ Concentrations:	Powder for injection: 1 mg (1 unit) vial with 1 ml diluent; 10 mg (10-unit) vial with 10 ml diluent.
Adult:	0.25–5 mg/dose.
Pediatric:	0.03–0.1 mg/kg/dose.

Indication	Dose (mg)	Onset Time	Duration of Action
Hypoglycemia	1–5 mg SC, IM, or IV bolus	<20 min	Depends on liver glycogen
Cardiogenic shock or heart failure	1–5 mg IV bolus q 30–60 min or 1–10 mg/hr IV infusion	5–10 min	20–30 min for bolus
β-blocker overdose	1–5 mg IV bolus q 30–60 min or 1–10 mg/hr IV infusion	5–10 min	20–30 min for bolus
Esophageal impaction	1 mg IV bolus	5 min	30 min
Diverticular disease	1 mg IV bolus q 4 hr	3–12 hr	2–4 hr
Renal or biliary calculi	1 mg IV bolus q 4 hr	1–2 hr	2–4 hr

Contraindications:	Diabetes mellitus, insulinoma, and pheochromocytoma.
Drug Interactions/ Allergy:	None.

GROWTH HORMONE, HUMAN SOMATREM, SOMATROPIN

Trade Names:	Protropin, Humatrope, Nutropin
Indications:	Growth failure, pituitary growth hormone deficiency, and Turner's syndrome.
Pharmacokinetics:	Peak effect: 2–4 hr. Clearance: hepatic. $T_{1/2}$: 20–25 min.
Pharmacodynamics:	
Musculoskeletal:	↑ Long bone growth, ↑ size of muscle cells.
Endocrine:	Anabolic actions, ↑ cell growth, ↑ protein synthesis.
Other:	↑ RBC mass, ↑ erythropoietin stimulation.
Dosage/ Concentrations:	
Adult:	Somatrem powder for injection: 5 mg (~13 IU)/ vial; 10 mg (~26 IU)/vial. Somatropin powder for injection: 5 mg (~13 IU)/ vial. Limit: Up to 0.06 mg/kg (0.16 IU/kg/dose).
Pediatric:	Humatrope: 0.025–0.25 IU/kg/day.

GROWTH HORMONE, HUMAN SOMATREM, SOMATROPIN   *(continued)*

Contraindications:	Hypothyroidism, presence or growth of underlying tumor.
Drug Interactions/ Allergy:	ACTH or excessive adrenocorticoid hormones may inhibit growth response. Exogenous thyroid hormone may accelerate epiphyseal closure.

HUMAN CHORIONIC GONADOTROPIN (hCG)

Trade Names:	Glukor, A.P.L., Chorex-5, Chorex-10, Corgonject-5, Profasi, Profasi HP, Chorigon, Choron-10, Follutein, Gonic, Pregnyl
Indications:	Cryptorchidism and infertility.
Pharmacokinetics:	Onset: ~2 hr. Peak effect: within 6 hr. Vd: after IM, distributed mainly into male testes or female ovaries. Clearance: renal; 10%–12% excreted unchanged within 24 hr. $T_{1/2}$: (serum) biphasic, 11 and 23 hr.

Pharmacodynamics:

CNS:	Headache, irritability, mental depression, fatigue.
CVS:	↑ Vascular permeability, peripheral edema, thromboembolic events.
GI:	Abdominal pain, indigestion, nausea, vomiting, diarrhea.
Endocrine:	↑ Androgen production by testes; ↑ ovarian production of progesterone, ↑ estrogen.

Dosage/ Concentrations:	
Adult:	Powder for injection:

- 200 U/ml after reconstitution with diluent.
- 5000 U/vial with 10 ml diluent (makes 500 U/ml).
- 10,000 U/vial with diluent (makes 1000 U/ml).
- 20,000 U/vial with diluent (makes 2000 U/ml).
  Dose: 500–5000 U/dose. Reconstitute with diluent provided by manufacturer.

Pediatric:	500–5000 USP U/dose.
Contraindications:	Pituitary hypertrophy or tumor, precocious puberty, undiagnosed abnormal vaginal bleeding, fibroid uterine tumors, ovarian cyst or enlargement, thrombophlebitis, prostatic carcinoma, and androgen-dependent neoplasms.
Drug Interactions/ Allergy:	None.

INSULIN

Trade Names:	Regular Insulin, Semilente Insulin, NPH Insulin, Lente Insulin, Ultralente U	
Indications:	Diabetes mellitus and chronic pancreatitis.	
Pharmacokinetics:	$T_{1/2}$: 5 min, may be as long as 13 hr because hormone binding to antibodies after 2–3 months. Duration: longer because of tight binding to tissue receptors. Metabolism: degradation 80% in liver and kidneys.	

	Onset (hr)	Peak (hr)	Duration (hr)
Rapid-acting			
Regular Insulin	0.5–1	2–3	5–7
Prompt insulin zinc (Semilente)	0.5–1	4–7	12–16
Intermediate-acting			
Insulin-zinc (Lente)	1–2	8–12	18–24
Isophane insulin (NPH)	1–2	8–12	18–24
Long-acting			
Extended insulin zinc (Ultralente)	4–8	16–18	36
Protamine zinc insulin (PZI)	4–8	14–20	36

Pharmacodynamics:	Facilitation of glucose uptake and storage as glycogen by liver.
CNS:	Coma.
Hepatic:	Facilitates glucose uptake and storage as glycogen by liver, inhibited gluconeogenesis, ↑ conversion of free fatty acids to triglycerides (lipid). ↑ Risk of hypoglycemia if prolonged insulin effect in hepatic dysfunction.
Renal:	Prolonged hypoglycemic effect in renal dysfunction.
GI:	Oral dose more effective than IV in evoking insulin release.
Musculoskeletal:	↑ Skeletal muscle uptake of glucose and amino acids, ↑ protein biosynthesis
Other:	Movement of potassium into cells, ↓ plasma potassium; ↑ storage of fat in adipose cells; inhibited lipolysis.
Dosage/ Concentrations:	Insulin U-100 (100 U/cc) most commonly used commercial preparation (SC or IV). Regular Insulin in 40 U or 100 U is the only type suitable for IV.
Adult:	0.1–1 U/kg/day (IV or SC).
Pediatric:	0.1–1 U/kg/day (IV or SC).
Drug Interactions/ Allergy:	Glucagon, estrogens, and corticosteroids can potentiate glucose-induced stimulation of insulin secretion. Release of insulin occurs in response to hyperglycemia, glucagon, β stimulation, or release of acetylcholine.

INSULIN   *(continued)*

Release inhibited by hypoglycemia, α agonists, β blockade, somatostatin, diazoxide, thiazide diuretics, and volatile anesthetics. Systemic allergic reaction to insulin requires a change to insulin derived from a different species (e.g., porcine insulin is less antigenic than bovine product).

LEVOTHYROXINE (L-THYROXINE), LIOTHYRONINE, LIOTRIX

Trade Names:	Levoid, Levothroid, Levoxine, Synthroid, Cytomel, Thyrolar, Euthroid
Indications:	Thyroid hormone deficiency, simple goiter, and chronic lymphocytic thyroiditis.
Pharmacokinetics:	Levothyroxine: deiodinated in peripheral tissues to T_3; small amounts metabolized in liver. Liothyronine (levorotatory isomer of T_3): 2.5–3 times more potent than levothyroxine. Liotrix: a mixture of T_3 and T_4.

	$T_{1/2}$ (Days)			Time to	Duration
	Euthyroid	*Hypothyroid*	*Hyperthyroid*	**Peak Effect**	**of Action**
Levothyroxine	6–7	9–10	3–4	3–4 wk	1–3 wk
Liothyronine	1	1.4	0.6	48–72 hr	<72 hr

Pharmacodynamics:

CNS:	Hand tremors, headache, irritability, nervousness.
CVS:	↑ Intrinsic contractile state of cardiac muscle, ↓ cardiac cholinergic receptors, ↑ HR, arrhythmias, angina.
Pulmonary:	Dyspnea with ↑ oxygen consumption.
Hepatic:	↑ Hepatic blood flow, ↑ drug detoxification.
Renal:	↑ Renal blood flow, ↑ GFR.
GI:	↑ Appetite, ↑ GI motility.
Musculoskeletal:	Muscle cramps and weakness.
Metabolic/Endocrine:	Catabolic (calorigenic) and anabolic effects, hyperglycemia, ↑ free fatty acids, ↑ basal metabolism, ↑ oxygen consumption, ↑ heat production.
Other:	↑ Erythropoiesis, ↑ RBC turnover, anemia.

Dosage/ Concentrations:	Liothyronine sodium (T3) (Cytomel): 5–50 μg tablet. Levothyroxine (T_4) (Synthroid, Levoxine, Levothroid): 0.025–0.3 mg tablet. Liotrix (Thyrolar): 12.5–150 μg levothyroxine/tablet and 3.1–37.5 μg liothyronine/tablet.
Adult:	Liothyronine: 5–100 μg/day.

| Pediatric: | Liotrix: 12.5–100 μg levothyroxine and 3.1–25 μg liothyronine/dose.
Liotrix: 12.5–100 μg levothyroxine and 3.1–25 μg liothyronine/dose. |

Contraindications: Adrenocortical insufficiency, cardiovascular disease, hyperthyroidism, and pituitary insufficiency.

Drug Interactions/
Allergy: ↓ Metabolic clearance of adrenocorticoids with hypothyroidism, ↑ with hyperthyroidism. ↑ Anticoagulant effect. TCAs increase therapeutic and toxic effects of both drugs. ↑ Requirement of antidiabetic agents: β blockers decrease peripheral conversion of T_4 and T_3. Ketamine increases hypertension and tachycardia.

LYPRESSIN

Trade Name: Diapid

Indications: Diabetes insipidus (inadequate ADH).

Pharmacokinetics: A synthetic analog of the posterior pituitary hormone arginine vasopressin (ADH). Intranasal: onset, within 1 hour; peak effect, 30–120 min. Duration: 3–4 hr. Biotransformation: hepatic. Elimination: renal. Absorption: affected by nasal congestion, allergic rhinitis, and upper respiratory infection. Vd: Extracellular fluid. Metabolism: metabolized by liver and kidney to inactive metabolites. $T_{1/2}$: (plasma): ~15 min.

Pharmacodynamics:
CNS: Headache.
Pulmonary: Persistent coughing, chest tightness, shortness of breath.
Renal: ↑ Water reabsorption by kidney, ↓ urine output, ↑ urine osmolality, ↓ serum osmolality.
GI: Abdominal cramps, nausea, heartburn.
Other: Hyponatremia, water intoxication.

Dosage/
Concentrations:
Adult and Pediatric: 1–2 sprays/dose (intranasal).

Contraindications: Allergy to vasopressin. Use caution in hypertensive cardiovascular disease.

Drug Interactions/
Allergy: ↑ Antidiuretic effect with carbamazepine, chlorpropamide, and clofibrate. ↓ Antidiuretic effect with demeclocycline, lithium, and norepinephrine.

MENOTROPINS

Trade Name:	Pergonal
Indications:	Infertility (stimulation of ovarian follicle development and spermatogenesis); ovulation and implantation in women; and testosterone production and full masculinization in men.
Pharmacokinetics:	Clearance: renal; 8% unchanged. $T_{1/2}$: α, 4 hr and 20 min; terminal, 70 hr and 4 hr.
Pharmacodynamics:	
Endocrine:	Ovarian follicular growth and maturation, spermatogenesis.
Dosage/ Concentrations:	75 IU FSH and 75 IU LH ampule; 150 IU FSH and 150 IU LH ampule (dissolve in 2 ml normal saline solution).
Adult:	For induction of ovulation: 75 U FSH and 75 U LH q.d. IM. For assisted reproduction: 150 U FSH and 150 U LH q.d. IM. For male infertility: 75 U FSH and 75 U LH q.o.d.
Pediatric:	N/A.
Contraindications:	Abnormal vaginal bleeding (undiagnosed), ovarian cyst or enlargement (not associated with polycystic ovarian syndrome).
Drug Interactions/ Allergy:	None.

NANDROLONE DECANOATE, OXANDROLONE, OXYMETHOLONE, STANOZOLOL

Trade Names:	Deca-Durabolin, Hybolin, Neo-Durabolic, Androlone-D, Oxandrin, Anadrol-50, Winstrol
Indications:	Chronic infections, extensive surgery, severe trauma, anemia, breast cancer, prophylaxis of hereditary angioedema.
Pharmacokinetics:	Time to peak effect: 0.5–1.5 hr (oxandrolone); 6–14 hr (nandrolone). Metabolism: hepatic. $T_{1/2}$: β, 9 hr (oxandrolone); β, 6–8 days (nandrolone).
Pharmacodynamics:	
CVS:	↑ Risk of atherosclerosis.
Hepatic:	Hepatic dysfunction, jaundice, hepatocellular carcinoma.

Renal:	Bladder irritability (postpubertal males), prostatic hypertrophy or carcinoma (elderly men).
GI:	Gastric irritation, nausea, vomiting.
Musculoskeletal:	Muscle cramps.
Other:	↑ Protein anabolism and positive nitrogen balance, ↑ hypoglycemia, ↑ hypercalcemia in females, breast soreness, ↑ erythropoietin, ↑ hemoglobin, ↑ RBC volume, iron-deficiency anemia, suppression of clotting factors.

Dosage/ Concentrations:	Nandrolone decanoate:
Adult:	25–200 mg/dose.
Pediatric:	25–50 mg/dose.
	Oxandrolone:
Adult:	2.5–20 mg/day.
Pediatric:	≤0.1 mg/kg/day.
	Oxymetholone:
Adult:	1–5 mg/kg/day.
Pediatric:	0.175 mg/kg/day.
	Stanozolol:
Adult:	4–16 mg/day.
Pediatric:	1–2 mg/day.

Contraindications:	Breast cancer, hepatic dysfunction, hypercalcemia, nephrosis; prostate cancer, and pregnancy.
Drug Interactions/ Allergy:	↑ Anticoagulant effect. May worsen hypoglycemia with use of insulin.

PROGESTERONE, MEDROXYPROGESTERONE, HYDROXYPROGESTERONE CAPROATE, MEGESTROL, NORETHINDRONE, NORETHINDRONE ACETATE, NORGESTREL

Trade Names:	Provera, Megace, Norlutin, Delalutin, Duralutin, Hylutin, Hypergest, Amen, Curretab, Cycrin, Depo-Provera, Progestaject, Pro-Depo, Aygestin, Norlutate
Indications:	Amenorrhea, functional uterine bleeding, endometriosis, carcinoma; a test for endogenous estrogen production, and contraception.
Pharmacokinetics:	Time to peak effect: 0.5–4 hr. Metabolism: hepatic. $T_{1/2}$: β, 5–14 hr.
Pharmacodynamics: *CNS:*	↑ Thermogenesis, hypnotic effect (↓ inhalation anesthetic requirement in pregnancy).

PROGESTERONE, MEDROXYPROGESTERONE, HYDROXYPROGESTERONE CAPROATE, MEGESTROL, NORETHINDRONE, NORETHINDRONE ACETATE, NORGESTREL *(continued)*

CVS:	Risk of thrombophlebitis, thromboembolism (with estrogen/progestin).
Pulmonary:	↑ Respiratory stimulation, respiratory alkalosis.
Hepatic:	↑ Glycogen storage, ↑ ketogenesis, ↑ cholestasis.
Renal:	Competition with aldosterone, ↓ sodium reabsorption.
GI:	Nausea.
Musculoskeletal:	Unusual tiredness or weakness.
Endocrine:	↑ Lipoprotein lipase, ↑ fat deposition, ↑ basal insulin, ↑ insulin response to glucose, breast tenderness.
Other:	
Dosage/ Concentrations:	Hydroxyprogesterone caproate (Delalutin, Duralutin, Hylutin, Hypergest, Pro-Depo): 125–375 mg/dose IV. Medroxyprogesterone acetate (Provera, Amen, Curretab, Cycrin, Depo-Provera): 5–10 mg/day p.o. Megestrol (Megace): 400–800 mg/day p.o. Norethindrone (Micronor, Nor-Q.D.): 5–20 mg/day p.o. Norethindrone acetate (Aygestin, Norlutate): 2.5–15 mg/day p.o. Norgestrel (Ovrette): 2.5–15 mg/day p.o. Progesterone (Progestaject): 5–10 mg/day IV.
Contraindications:	Carcinoma of breast or reproductive organs, hepatic dysfunction, incomplete abortion, suspected pregnancy, and vaginal bleeding.
Drug Interactions/ Allergy:	Interference with effects of bromocriptine.

TESTOSTERONE, METHYLTESTOSTERONE, FLUOXYMESTERONE

Trade Names:	Delatest, Andro L.A. 200, Testone LA, Testred, depAndro, Depotest, Duratest, Depo-Testosterone, Testex, Halotestin
Indications:	Androgen deficiency, delayed male puberty, and breast cancer.
Pharmacokinetics:	Peak serum concentration: 1 hr after buccal dose; 2 hr after oral dose. Clearance: 44% of drug metabolized first pass in liver. $T_{1/2}$: longer with synthetics (fluoxymesterone, methyltestosterone).
Pharmacodynamics: *CNS:*	Headache, dizziness, confusion, mental depression.

CVS:	Pedal edema.
Hepatic:	Hepatic dysfunction, jaundice, hepatocellular carcinoma.
Renal:	Bladder irritability in males, possible prostatic hypertrophy or carcinoma.
GI:	Nausea, vomiting.
Musculoskeletal:	Fatigue, muscle cramps.
Other:	Hypoglycemia, hypercalcemia, ↑ erythropoietin and RBC production, leukopenia.

Dosage/
Concentrations: Fluoxymesterone:
Adult: 5–50 mg/day.
Pediatric: 2.5–10 mg/day.
        Methyltestosterone:
Adult: 5–200 mg/day.
Pediatric: 2.5–25 mg/day.
        Testosterone:
Adult: 25–400 mg/dose.
Pediatric: 25–100 mg/dose.

Contraindications: Breast and prostate cancer.

Drug Interactions/   With anticoagulants, androgen dose may need to be
Allergy: adjusted. Insulin may worsen hypoglycemia.

VASOPRESSIN TANNATE

Trade Name: Pitressin Tannate

Indications: Diabetes insipidus.

Pharmacokinetics: Absorption: poor with nasal dose. Peak effect: 30–120 min. Vd: throughout extracellular fluid. Clearance: metabolized and rapidly destroyed in liver and kidney. SC dose: 5% of drug excreted unchanged in urine after 4 hr. dose: 5%–15% of drug excreted in urine. $T_{1/2}$: 10–20 min. Protein binding: none. Duration: 2–8 hr after SC or IM dose.

Pharmacodynamics:
CVS: Hypertension.
Renal: ↑ Water reabsorption (↑ permeability of collecting ducts).
Musculoskeletal: Necrosis, gangrene.
Other: Water intoxication.

Dosage/   Injection: Synthetic: 20 pressor U/ml (0.5 or 1 ml ampule). Tannate in oil: 5 pressor U/ml (1 ml ampule).
Concentrations:
Adult: 10–40 U/day SC or IM.

VASOPRESSIN TANNATE   *(continued)*

Pediatric: 5–40 U/day SC or IM (no IV formulation).

Contraindications: Asthma, seizure, heart failure, migraine, coronary ar-
                      tery disease, hypertension, renal failure, and IV admin-
                      istration for children.

Drug Interactions/   ↑ Antidiuretic effect with carbamazepine, chlorpro-
Allergy: pamide, and clofibrate. ↓ Antidiuretic effect with
                      demeclocycline, lithium, and norepinephrine.

24

Inhalation Anesthetics

Ian Smith, B.Sc., M.B.B.S., F.R.C.A.

DESFLURANE

Trade Name:	Suprane
Indications:	Maintenance of general anesthesia and agent of choice when rapid emergence or precise control of anesthetic depth is required.
Pharmacokinetics:	Blood:gas solubility: 0.42. Boiling point: 23.5°C. Saturated vapor pressure (at 20°C): 664 mmHg. MAC (in 60% N_2O): 18–30 yr, 7.25% (4.0%); 31–65 yr, 6.0% (2.8%); >65 yr, 5.2% (1.7%). Resistant to metabolism.

Pharmacodynamics:

CNS:	Generalized depression of CNS function, extremely rapid emergence from anesthesia, ↑ ICP.
CVS:	↓ Vascular resistance, ↓ MAP, ↑ HR with deep anesthesia, tachycardia with rapid change in concentration.
Pulmonary:	↓ TV, ↑ respiratory rate, airway irritant.
GI:	Nausea
Musculoskeletal:	Muscle relaxation.
Dosage/ Concentrations:	Supplied in 250-ml bottles. Pressurized, electrically heated vaporizer required for delivery. Usual inspired concentration: 2%–8%.
Contraindications:	Trigger to malignant hyperpyrexia and inhalation induction in children (because of airway irritation)
Drug Interactions/ Allergy:	Potentiates effects of muscle relaxants. ↓ MAC with opioids, N_2O, and benzodiazepines.

ENFLURANE

Trade Name:	Ethrane
Indications:	Maintenance of general anesthesia.
Pharmacokinetics:	Blood:gas solubility: 1.9. Boiling point: 56°C. Saturated vapor pressure (at 20°C): 175 mmHg. MAC (in 60% N_2O): 18–30 yr, 2% (0.68%); 31–65 yr, 1.68% (0.57%); >65 yr, 1.3% (0.45%). Metabolism: 2%, hepatic.

Pharmacodynamics:

CNS:	Generalized depression of CNS function, epileptiform paroxysmal spike activity at concentrations >3%; rapid emergence from anesthesia, ↑ ICP (similar to isoflurane).

CVS:	Myocardial depressant, ↓ vascular resistance, ↓↓ MAP, ↑ HR, arrhythmias (low incidence).
Pulmonary:	Moderately irritant, respiratory depression.
Renal:	Renal dysfunction.
GI:	Nausea.
Musculoskeletal:	Muscle relaxation.

Dosage/ Concentrations: Supplied in 250-ml bottles. Maximum vaporizer setting of 5% may be inadequate for induction of anesthesia. Usual inspired concentration: 0.4%–1.6%.

Contraindications: Epilepsy, trigger to malignant hyperpyrexia, prolonged cases, and renal failure.

Drug Interactions/ Allergy: Potentiates effects of muscle relaxants. ↓ MAC with opioids, N_2O, and benzodiazepines.

HALOTHANE

Trade Name: Fluothane

Indications: Maintenance of general anesthesia and induction agent of choice for difficult airway.

Pharmacokinetics: Blood:gas solubility: 2.5. Boiling point: 50°C. Saturated vapor pressure (at 20°C): 243 mmHg. MAC (in 60% N_2O): 18–30 yr, 0.9% (0.35%); 31–65 yr, 0.75% (0.29%); >65 yr, 0.6% (0.23%).

Pharmacodynamics:

CNS:	Generalized depression of CNS function, cerebral vasodilatation causing ↑ ICP.
CVS:	↓ HR from vagal stimulation, moderate depression of cardiac output, small ↓ MAP, arrhythmias.
Pulmonary:	↓ TV, ↑ respiratory rate, potent bronchodilator, nonirritant, ↓ secretions.
Hepatic:	Fulminant hepatic failure (halothane hepatitis).
GI:	↓ Motility.
Uterus:	Uterine relaxation.
Musculoskeletal:	Muscle relaxation.

Dosage/ Concentrations: Supplied in 250 ml bottles. Induction: 2%–3%. Usual inspired concentration: 0.5%–1%. Induction: up to 5%.

Contraindications: Trigger to malignant hyperpyrexia and recent previous halothane exposure.

Drug Interactions/ Allergy: Potentiates effects of muscle relaxants. ↓ MAC with opioids, N_2O, and benzodiazepines.

ISOFLURANE

Trade Name:	Forane

Indications: Maintenance of general anesthesia.

Pharmacokinetics: Blood:gas solubility: 1.4. Boiling point: 49°C. Saturated vapor pressure (at 20°C): 250 mmHg. MAC (in 70% N_2O): 18–30 yr, 1.28% (0.56%); 31–55 yr, 1.15% (0.50%); >55 yr, 1.05% (0.37%). Metabolism: 0.2%.

Pharmacodynamics:
CNS: Generalized depression of CNS function, rapid emergence from anesthesia, ↑ ICP.
CVS: ↓ cardiac output, ↓ vascular resistance, ↓ MAP, ↑ HR.
Pulmonary: Airway irritant, respiratory depression.
GI: Nausea.
Musculoskeletal: Muscle relaxation

Dosage/ Concentrations: Supplied in 250-ml bottles. Usual inspired concentration: 0.5%–1.5%.

Contraindications: Trigger to malignant hyperpyrexia.

Drug Interactions/ Allergy: Potentiates effects of muscle relaxants, ↓ MAC with opioids, N_2O, and benzodiazepines.

NITROUS OXIDE

Trade Name:	N/A

Indications: Analgesia and carrier gas for other anesthetics to reduce MAC.

Pharmacokinetics: Blood:gas solubility: 0.47. Boiling point: −88°C. Critical temperature: 36.5°C. Critical pressure: 72.6 Bar. MAC: ≈105%.

Pharmacodynamics:
CNS: Concentration-dependent generalized depression of CNS function
CVS: Depression of CO, ↑ HR, ↑ vascular resistance.
Pulmonary: Nonirritant, mild respiratory depressant
GI: Nausea, vomiting.
Other: Diffusion hypoxia on discontinuation, megaloblastic anemia, agranulocytosis, fetal abnormalities with chronic exposure.

Dosage/ Concentrations:	Supplied as a liquid in cylinders. (Pressure gauge does not reflect contents of cylinder.) Usual inspired concentration: 40%–70% in oxygen.
Contraindications:	Pneumothorax (if not drained), recent pneumoencephalography, middle ear surgery, and bowel obstruction.
Drug Interactions/ Allergy:	MAC of volatile anesthetics reduced by 1% per 1% administered.

SEVOFLURANE

Trade Name:	Ultane, Sevorane
Indications:	Excellent induction agent for rapid emergence and precise control of anesthetic depth.
Pharmacokinetics:	Blood:gas solubility: 0.69. Boiling point: 58.6°C. Saturated vapor pressure (at 20°C): 160 mmHg. MAC (in 60% N_2O): Child, 2.6% (2.0%). Adult, 1.71% (0.66%). Metabolized to hexafluoroisopropanol (nontoxic); yields free fluoride ions.
Pharmacodynamics: *CNS:*	Generalized depression of CNS function, rapid emergence from anesthesia, ↑ ICP.
CVS:	↓ Vascular resistance, ↓ MAP.
Pulmonary:	Respiratory depression; nonirritant.
GI:	Nausea.
Musculoskeletal:	Muscle relaxation.
Dosage/ Concentrations:	Supplied in 250-ml bottles. Uses conventional vaporizer technology. Usual inspired concentration: 0.5%–2%. Induction: 5%–8%.
Contraindications:	Trigger to malignant hyperpyrexia, prolonged cases (fluoride), and closed-circuit anesthesia.
Drug Interactions/ Allergy:	Potentiates effects of muscle relaxants, ↓ MAC with opioids, N_2O, and benzodiazepines.

25

Intravenous Anesthetics

Ronald L. Harter, M.D.

ELTANOLONE (PREGNANOLONE)*

Trade Name:	N/A

Indications: Induction and maintenance of general anesthesia, sedation during local and regional anesthesia, and sedation in the ICU.

Pharmacokinetics: Rapid distribution ($T_{1/2}$: α, 0.04 hr), redistribution ($T_{1/2}$: β, 0.5 hr), and elimination. Vd: 0.1–0.4 L/kg; steady-state, 1.2–2.3 L/kg. Clearance: 1.4–1.9 L/kg/hr. Metabolism: primarily hepatic. Elimination: excreted in urine as gluconide conjugate. Protein binding >98%; lipid emulsion. $T_{1/2}$: γ, 3–4 hr.

Pharmacodynamics:

CNS: Dose-dependent depression, sedation, drowsiness, dizziness.

CVS: Hypotension, tachycardia, ↓ cardiac output.

Pulmonary: ↓ TV, ↓ $\dot{V}_E$.

Hepatic: ↓ Liver blood flow with ↓ cardiac output.

GI: Nausea, vomiting.

Musculoskeletal: Tremor, muscle twitching (myoclonia).

Other: Glucocorticoid-like effects (pregnanolone), ↓ cortisol, ↑ ACTH with surgical stress, ↑ temperature, pain on injection.

Dosage/ Concentrations: 4 mg/ml in a vial containing 20 ml of drug in a 10% egg lecithin emulsion. Refrigerate at 2–8°C.
Induction: 0.3–0.75 mg/kg IV (decreases with age).
Maintenance: 0.15–0.3 mg/kg IV, bolus injections.

Contraindications: Allergy to soybeans, eggs, and intralipid-type emulsions.

Drug Interactions/ Allergy: Synergistic interactions with other sedative-hypnotics, volatile anesthetics, and opioid analgesics. Rash and urticaria.

ETOMIDATE

Trade Name:	Amidate

Indications: IV induction of anesthesia or sedation, in patients with coronary artery or cerebrovascular disease, unstable cardiovascular status, or depleted intravascular volume.

---

*Investigational drug.

ETOMIDATE *(continued)*

Pharmacokinetics:	Adult	Geriatric
Vd (L/kg):	2.2–4.5	2.9–5.5
Clearance (ml/kg/min):	10–20	7–15
$T_{1/2}$: α, *fast (min):*	2.6–3.9	—
$T_{1/2}$: α, *slow (min):*	7.4–13.4	—
$T_{1/2}$: β *(hr):*	2–5	3–7

Pharmacodynamics:

CNS:	↓ CBF, ↓ $CMRO_2$, seizures, ↑ SSEP amplitude.
CVS:	↓ MAP, ↓ SVR.
Pulmonary:	↓ TV, ↓ respiratory rate, apnea after rapid IV bolus.
GI:	Postoperative nausea and vomiting.
Musculoskeletal:	Myoclonus at induction; hiccoughs.
Other:	Dose-dependent adrenocortical suppression, ↑ mortality when used for prolonged sedation in critically ill patients, pain on injection.

Dosage/ Concentrations: 2 mg/ml.

	IV Bolus (mg/kg)	IV Infusion (mg/min)
Adult:	0.3	5–10
Pediatric:	0.3–0.4	—
Geriatric:	0.15–0.25	—

Contraindications: Use caution with seizure disorders or adrenocortical pathology.

Drug Interactions/ Allergy: None.

KETAMINE

Trade Names:	Ketalar, Ketaject
Indications:	Rapid induction of general anesthesia, especially as IM route in patients without IV access; sedation; and analgesia.

Pharmacokinetics:	Adult	Pediatric
Vd (L/kg):	2.5–3.5	1.2–3.0
Clearance (ml/kg min):	16–18	25–35
$T_{1/2}$: α *(min):*	10–15	—
$T_{1/2}$: β *(hr):*	1–2	0.5–1

Pharmacodynamics:

CNS:	Cerebral vasodilation (≤60% ↑ CBF); abolishes EEG α activity; EEG theta dominance; ↑ cortical ampli-

	tude of SSEP; ↓ response of BAER and VER, nystagmus, delirium.
CVS:	↑ Systemic and pulmonary arterial pressures, (↑ HR, ↑ cardiac output), ↑ myocardial oxygen consumption, ↓ BP and ↓ cardiac output in depleted catecholamine stores.
Pulmonary:	↓ Respiratory rate, apnea, ↑ tracheobronchial mucous gland secretions, bronchodilation.
GI:	↑ Salivary gland secretion.
Musculoskeletal:	Hypertonus, purposeful skeletal movements.

Dosage/Concentrations: 10, 50, or 100 mg/ml.

	IV bolus (mg/kg)	IV infusion (µg/kg/min)
Adult:	1–3	20–60
Pediatric:	2–4	—

Contraindications: High ICP, systemic or pulmonary hypertension, severe coronary artery disease, and some ophthalmologic procedures due to nystagmus.

Drug Interactions/Allergy: Ketamine's sympathomimetic effects may be blunted or eliminated by concomitant use of benzodiazepines, barbiturates, or a potent inhalational agent. Inhalational agents prolong ketamine's duration of action. Enhanced nondepolarizing neuromuscular blockade. Plasma cholinesterase activity inhibited. In combination with aminophylline, ketamine lowers seizure threshold. Allergic reaction: Erythema, rash.

METHOHEXITAL

Trade Name:	Brevital
Indications:	Rapid induction and maintenance of general anesthesia.
Pharmacokinetics:	Vd: 1.1–2.2 L/kg. Clearance: 10.9–12.1 ml/kg/min. $T_{1/2}$: α, rapid; 5.6–6.2 min. α, slow; 58.3 min. β, 1.6–3.9 hr.

Pharmacodynamics:

CNS:	Postoperative seizures.
CVS:	Pain on injection.
Pulmonary:	↓ Respiration, apnea followed by spontaneous ventilation.
Renal:	↓ RBF, ↓ GFR.
Musculoskeletal:	Involuntary movements (myoclonic activity), hiccoughs.

METHOHEXITAL *(continued)*

Dosage/ Concentrations:	IV: 1%; for rectal use: 2%–10%		
	IV Bolus (mg/kg)	**IV Infusion (µg/kg/min)**	**Rectal (mg/kg)**
Adult:	1–1.5	80–100	—
Pediatric:	1–2	—	15–30
Geriatric:	1	—	—

Contraindications:	Acute intermittent porphyria.
Drug Interactions/ Allergy:	Anaphylactic or anaphylactoid reaction.

PROPOFOL

Trade Name:	Diprivan
Indications:	IV induction and maintenance of anesthesia, and sedation during anesthesia.

Pharmacokinetics:	**Adult**	**Pediatric**
Vd (L/kg):	3.5–4.5	5.0–10.9
Clearance (ml/kg/min):	30–60	30–40
$T_{1/2}$ α, *fast (min):*	1.8–8.3	1.5–4.1
$T_{1/2}$ α, *slow (min):*	34–64	—
$T_{1/2}$ β *(min):*	30–90	24–56

Pharmacodynamics:

CNS:	↓ Cerebral perfusion pressure, ↓ CBF, ↓ ICP, ↑ latency, ↓ amplitude of SSEP.
CVS:	↓ BP, direct myocardial depression.
Pulmonary:	Profound ventilatory depressant effect, apnea.
GI:	Antiemetic effect.
Musculoskeletal:	Hypertonus, tremor, hiccoughs.
Other:	Pain on injection, infection.

Dosage/ Concentrations:	10 mg/ml.	
	Induction (mg/kg)	**Maintenance (µg/kg/min)**
Adult:	2.0–2.5	75–150
Pediatric:	2.5–3.5	150–250
Elderly:	1.0–1.5	50–100

Contraindications:	Hypovolemia and allergy to intralipid-type compounds

and soybeans, and compromised LV function in the elderly.

Drug Interactions/   Skin rash.
Allergy:

THIAMYLAL

Trade Name: Surital

Indications: Rapid induction of general anesthesia, treatment of convulsions and elevated ICP, and possible cerebral protection prior to ischemic events.

Pharmacokinetics:	**Adult/Geriatric**	**Pediatric**
Vd (L/kg):	1.5–2.5	2.1
Clearance (ml/kg/min):	3.4–3.6	6.6
$T_{1/2}$: α, rapid (min):	2.5–8.5	6.3
$T_{1/2}$: α, slow (min):	46.4–62.7	43
$T_{1/2}$: β (hr):	5.1–11.6	6.1

Pharmacodynamics:
CNS: ↓ CBF, ↓ ICP, ↓ $CMRO_2$, ↑ low-voltage, fast-wave (1–5 Hz) activity, ↓ frequency to isoelectricity.
CVS: ↓ BP, ↑ HR, minimal direct myocardial depression, ↓ venous return.
Pulmonary: ↓ Respiration, apnea followed by spontaneous ventilation.
Hepatic: ↓ Hepatic blood flow, induction of microsomal enzymes, ↑ glucuronyl transferase activity.
Renal: ↓ RBF, ↓ GFR.
Musculoskeletal: Transient skeletal muscle relaxation.
Other: Peak umbilical vein concentration within 1 min of maternal IV administration.

Dosage/   20 mg/ml (2.0%). Stable for up to 6 days if refrigerated; ≤24 hr at room temperature.
Concentrations:
Adult: 3–5 mg/kg.
Pediatric: 4–7 mg/kg.

Contraindications: Acute intermittent porphyria.

Drug Interactions/   Anaphylactic or anaphylactoid reaction.
Allergy:

THIOPENTAL SODIUM

Trade Name:	Pentothal
Indications:	Rapid induction of general anesthesia, treatment of convulsions and elevated ICP, and possible cerebral protection prior to ischemic events.

Pharmacokinetics:	Adult/Geriatric	Pediatric
Vd (L/kg):	1.5–2.5	2.1
Clearance (ml/kg/min):	3.4–3.6	6.6
$T_{1/2}$: α, rapid (min):	2.5–8.5	6.3
$T_{1/2}$: α, slow (min):	46.4–62.7	43
$T_{1/2}$: β (hr):	5.1–11.6	6.1

Pharmacodynamics:

CNS:	$\downarrow$ CBF, $\downarrow$ ICP, $\downarrow$ CMRO$_2$, $\uparrow$ low-voltage, fast-wave (1–5 Hz) activity, $\downarrow$ frequency to isoelectricity, nerve injury with inadvertent intra-arterial injection.
CVS:	$\downarrow$ BP, $\uparrow$ HR, minimal direct myocardial depression, $\downarrow$ venous return.
Pulmonary:	$\downarrow$ Respiration, apnea followed by spontaneous ventilation.
Hepatic:	$\downarrow$ Hepatic blood flow, induction of microsomal enzymes; $\uparrow$ glucuronyl transferase activity.
Renal:	$\downarrow$ RBF, $\downarrow$ GFR.
Musculoskeletal:	Transient skeletal muscle relaxation.
Other:	Peak umbilical vein concentration within 1 min of maternal IV administration, distal gangrene with inadvertent intra-arterial injection.

Dosage/ Concentrations:	25 mg/ml (2.5%); stable at room temperature $\geq$2 wk.
Adult:	3–5 mg/kg^{-1}.
Pediatric:	4–7 mg/kg^{-1}.
Geriatric:	2–3 mg/kg^{-1}.
Contraindications:	Acute intermittent porphyria. Inadvertent intra-arterial injection may cause distal gangrene or permanent nerve injury.
Drug Interactions/ Allergy:	Anaphylactic or anaphylactoid reaction.

26

Local Anesthetics

Noor M. Gajraj, M.B.B.S., F.R.C.A.

BUPIVACAINE

Trade Name:	Marcaine
Indications:	Infiltration, peripheral nerve blocks, and extradural and spinal anesthesia.
Pharmacokinetics:	Onset: slow. Duration: long (240–480 min after infiltration). Vd: 73 L. Clearance: 0.58 L/min. $T_{1/2}$: 2.7 hr. pKa: 8.1. Relative potency: 8. Protein binding: 95%.

Pharmacodynamics:

CNS:	Anxiety, restlessness, disorientation, confusion, tremors, shivering, seizures, tinnitus.
CVS:	Bradycardia, refractory ventricular fibrillation, myocardial depression, hypotension, cardiovascular collapse.
Pulmonary:	Respiratory arrest.
GI:	Nausea, vomiting.

Dosage/Concentrations:	0.25% to 0.75% solutions. Maximum: 2 mg/kg. (0.75% concentration not recommended for epidural anesthesia in obstetrics.)
Contraindications:	Hypersensitivity to para-aminobenzoic acid or parabens.
Drug Interactions/Allergy:	In patients receiving antiarrhythmic drugs with local anesthetic activity (e.g., lidocaine), toxic effects may be additive.

2-CHLOROPROCAINE

Trade Name:	Nesacaine
Indications:	Peripheral and epidural anesthesia.
Pharmacokinetics:	Rapidly hydrolyzed by plasma cholinesterase. $T_{1/2}$: 45 sec. Onset: fast. Duration: short (30–45 min after infiltration). pKa: 9.1. Relative potency: 1. Low systemic toxicity.

Pharmacodynamics:

CNS:	Anxiety, restlessness, circumoral paresthesia, disorientation, confusion, tonic-clonic convulsions, seizures, drowsiness, unconsciousness, tinnitus, blurred vision, sensory deficit (intrathecal injection).
CVS:	Myocardial depression, hypotension, bradycardia, refractory ventricular fibrillation, cardiovascular collapse.
Pulmonary:	Respiratory arrest.
Musculoskeletal:	Motor deficit (intrathecal injection).
Other:	Urticaria, transient stinging or burning at injection site.

Dosage/ Concentrations:	1%, 2%, and 3% solutions. Maximum dose 800–1000 mg.
Contraindications:	Myasthenia gravis and concurrent use of bupivacaine.
Drug Interactions/ Allergy:	One of the metabolites, 4-amino-2-chloroprocaine, may impair subsequent action of bupivacaine.

EUTECTIC MIXTURE OF LOCAL ANESTHETICS (LIDOCAINE, PRILOCAINE)

Trade Name:	Emla Cream
Indications:	Venipuncture, venous cannulation, and minor skin surgery.
Pharmacokinetics:	N/A.

Pharmacodynamics:

CNS:	Anxiety, restlessness, confusion, tremors, shivering, seizures, drowsiness, unconsciousness, tinnitus.
CVS:	Bradycardia, myocardial depression, cardiovascular collapse, hypotension.
Pulmonary:	Respiratory arrest.
GI:	Nausea, vomiting.
Other:	Methemoglobinemia.
Dosage/ Concentrations:	1–2 g/10 cm² area of skin.
Contraindications:	Congenital or idiopathic methemoglobinemia, infants under age 12 months who are receiving methemoglobin-inducing drugs (e.g., sulfonamides), hypersensitivity to prilocaine or lidocaine, and patients receiving class I antiarrhythmic drugs (e.g., tocainide, mexiletine).
Drug Interactions/ Allergy:	↑ Serum concentration of lignocaine with concomitant use of cimetidine or propranolol.

ETIDOCAINE

Trade Name:	Duranest
Indications:	Infiltration, peripheral nerve blockade, and extradural anesthesia.
Pharmacokinetics:	Onset: fast. Duration: long (240–480 min after infiltration). $T_{1/2}$: 2.7 hr. Vd: 134 L. Clearance: 1.11

ETIDOCAINE   *(continued)*

L/min. pKa: 7.7. Relative potency: 6. Protein binding: 95%.

Pharmacodynamics:
CNS: Anxiety, restlessness, disorientation, confusion, trem-
                    ors, shivering, seizures, drowsiness, unconsciousness,
                    tinnitus, predominant motor block (epidural).
CVS: Bradycardia, myocardial depression, hypotension, car-
                    diovascular collapse.
Pulmonary: Respiratory arrest.
GI: Nausea, vomiting.

Dosage/   0.5%–1.5% solutions. Maximum: 4.0 mg/kg.
Concentrations:

Contraindications: None.

Drug Interactions/   None.
Allergy:

LIDOCAINE

Trade Name: Xylocaine

Indications: Topical anesthesia, infiltration, peripheral nerve blocks,
                         spinal and extradural anesthesia, IV regional anesthe-
                         sia, and treatment of ventricular arrhythmias.

Pharmacokinetics: Onset: fast. Duration: moderate (60–120 min after in-
                         filtration). $T_{1/2}$: 1.6 hr. Vd: 91 L. Clearance: 91
                         L/min. pKa: 7.9. Relative potency: 2. Protein binding:
                         65%.

Pharmacodynamics:
CNS: Lethargy, coma, paresthesia, agitation, slurred speech,
                         muscle twitching, seizures, anxiety, euphoria, hallucina-
                         tions, double vision.
CVS: Bradycardia, hypotension, heart block, arrhythmias, car-
                         diovascular collapse.
Pulmonary: Respiratory depression or arrest.
GI: Nausea, vomiting.

Dosage/   0.5%–4.0% solutions, 2.0% viscous jelly, 2.5%, 5.0%
Concentrations: ointment. Maximum: 4–7 mg/kg.

Contraindications: Heart block.

Drug Interactions/   ↑ Serum concentration with concomitant use of cimeti-
Allergy: dine or propanolol.

MEPIVACAINE

Trade Name:	Carbocaine
Indications:	Infiltration, peripheral nerve block, and epidural anesthesia.
Pharmacokinetics:	Onset: fast. Duration: moderate (90–120 min after infiltration). Longer duration than lidocaine when used without epinephrine. $T_{1/2}$: 1.9 hr. Vd: 84 L. Clearance: 0.78 L/min. pKa: 7.7. Relative potency: 2. Protein binding: 75%.

Pharmacodynamics:

CNS:	Anxiety, restlessness, disorientation, confusion, tremors, shivering, seizures, drowsiness, unconsciousness, tinnitus.
CVS:	Bradycardia, myocardial depression, hypotension, cardiovascular collapse.
Pulmonary:	Respiratory arrest.
GI:	Nausea, vomiting.
Dosage/ Concentrations:	1.0%, 1.5%, 2.0% solutions. Maximum: 4–7 mg/kg.
Contraindications:	Allergy to sodium bisulfate.
Drug Interactions/ Allergy:	Bupivacaine may decrease binding of mepivacaine to α_1-acid glycoprotein and may increase risk of systemic toxicity.

PRILOCAINE

Trade Name:	Citanest
Indications:	Infiltration, peripheral nerve blockade, extradural anesthesia, IV regional anesthesia.
Pharmacokinetics:	Rapid hepatic metabolism to *o*-toluidine. Onset: fast. Duration: moderate (60–120 min after infiltration). $T_{1/2}$: 1.6 hr. Vd: 191 L. Clearance: 2.37 L/min. pKa: 7.9. Relative potency: 2. Protein binding: 55%.

Pharmacodynamics:

CNS:	Anxiety, restlessness, disorientation, confusion, tremors, shivering, seizures, drowsiness, unconsciousness, tinnitus.
CVS:	Bradycardia, myocardial depression, hypotension, cardiovascular collapse.
Pulmonary:	Respiratory arrest.

PRILOCAINE   *(continued)*

GI:	Nausea, vomiting.
Other:	Methemoglobinemia (>600 mg).

**Dosage/
Concentrations:**

0.25–3.0% solutions. Maximum: 7–8 mg/kg.
For methemoglobinemia, treat with IV methylene blue,
1–2 mg/kg.

Contraindications:

Anemia and congenital or acquired methemoglobinemia.

**Drug Interactions/
Allergy:**

None known.

PROCAINE

Trade Name: Novocain

Indications: Spinal and epidural anesthesia, diagnostic differential
spinal blocks, peripheral nerve block.

Pharmacokinetics: Onset: slow. Duration: short (45–60 min after infiltration). Rapidly hydrolyzed by plasma cholinesterase to
para-aminobenzoic acid. pKa: 8.9. Relative potency: 1.
Protein binding: 6%.

Pharmacodynamics:
CNS: Anxiety, restlessness, circumoral paresthesia, disorientation, confusion, tonic-clonic convulsions, seizures,
drowsiness, unconsciousness, miosis, tinnitus.
GI: Nausea, vomiting.
Other: Skin discoloration, burning sensation at site of
injection, pain, tissue irritation.

**Dosage/
Concentrations:**   1%, 2%, 10% solutions. Maximum: 11–14 mg/kg.

Contraindications: Hypersensitivity to para-aminobenzoic acid.

**Drug Interactions/
Allergy:**   Antagonized pharmacologic action of sulfonamides
and aminosalicylic acid. Potentiated effects of succinylcholine, anticholinesterase, and digitalis.

ROPIVACAINE

Trade Name: Naropin

Indications: Local and regional anesthesia for surgical procedures
and acute pain management.

Pharmacokinetics:	Absorption: slow from epidural space. $T_{1/2}$: α, 4 hr; β, 4.2 hr (epidural). Vd at steady state: 47 L; 94% protein bound (α_1-acid glycoprotein); hepatic metabolism (P_{450} 1A) to less active hydroxy metabolites. Clearance: 440 ml/min; Elimination: urinary. Onset: similar but of shorter duration of motor blockade compared to bupivacaine.

Pharmacodynamics:

CNS:	Restlessness, tremors, paresthesias, shivering, convulsions, coma, respiratory arrest.
CVS:	Cardiac conduction ($\downarrow$ HR), excitability, refractoriness (AV block), and contractility ($\downarrow$ cardiac output, $\downarrow$ BP); ventricular arrhythmias, minimal peripheral vasodilation.
GI:	Nausea, vomiting (<5%).
Musculoskeletal:	Back pain (<5%).

Dosage/ Concentrations:	2–10 mg/ml (0.2%–1%). For major nerve block: up to 250 mg (50 ml). For cesarean delivery: up to 150 mg (30 ml of 0.5%) epidurally in 3- to 5-ml increments.
Contraindications:	Hypersensitivity to amide-type (bupivacaine) local anesthetics.
Drug Interactions/ Allergy:	Potential interaction with other P_{450} metabolized drugs (e.g., theophylline, acetaminophen, imipramine).

TETRACAINE

Trade Name:	Pontocaine
Indications:	Spinal anesthesia and local anesthesia of the eye.
Pharmacokinetics:	Onset: slow. Duration: long (60–180 min after infiltration). pKa: 8.4. Relative potency: 8. Protein binding: 85%.

Pharmacodynamics:

CNS:	Anxiety, apprehension, nervousness, disorientation, seizures, drowsiness, unconsciousness, tinnitus, lacrimation, photophobia, corneal epithelial erosion, keratitis, corneal opacification, miosis.
CVS:	Cardiac arrest, bradycardia, myocardial depression, cardiac arrhythmias, hypotension.
Pulmonary:	Respiratory arrest.
GI:	Nausea, vomiting.
Other:	Urticaria, contact dermatitis (topical form).

TETRACAINE   *(continued)*

Dosage/ Concentrations:	1%, 2% solutions; 0.5% for ophthalmic anesthesia. Maximum: 1.0–1.5 mg/kg.
Contraindications:	Ophthalmic secondary bacterial infection.
Drug Interactions/ Allergy:	Antagonizes effects of aminosalicylic acid and sulfonamides.

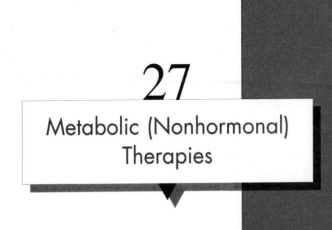

27

Metabolic (Nonhormonal) Therapies

Ahmed F. Ghouri, M.D.
Eugene Y. Lai, M.D.

ALGLUCERASE

Trade Name: Ceredase

Indications: Palliative treatment in type I Gaucher disease.

Pharmacokinetics: $T_{1/2}$: 3.6–10.4 min. Peak concentration: 60 min after
                          IV infusion of 0.6–234 U/kg over 4 hr. Vd: 49–282
                          ml/kg.

Pharmacodynamics:
GI: Abdominal discomfort, nausea, vomiting.
Other: Burning and swelling at injection site, IgG antibody
                          formation with chronic use, low-grade fever, and
                          chills.

**Dosage/
Concentrations:**
Adult and Pediatric: 30–60 U/kg monthly in divided doses, each IV over 4
                          hr (optimal dosing controversial).

Contraindications: N/A.

Drug Interactions/   Hypersensitivity rare.
Allergy:

ALLOPURINOL

Trade Names: Lopurin, Zyloprim

Indications: Gouty arthritis, hyperuricemia associated with neoplas-
                          tic disease or chemotherapy, uric acid nephropathy,
                          and prophylaxis for calcium oxalate renal calculi.

Pharmacokinetics: Absorption: 80%–90% from GI tract. Biotransforma-
                          tion: primarily hepatic to oxipurinol (active metabo-
                          lite). $T_{1/2}$: allopurinol, 1–3 hr; oxipurinol, 12–30 hr.
                          Elimination: renal; 10% as allopurinol, 70% as oxipuri-
                          nol.

Pharmacodynamics:
CNS: Drowsiness, headache.
Hepatic: Hepatotoxicity, ↑ transaminase and alkaline phospha-
                          tase levels.
Renal: Renal insufficiency or failure, xanthine calculus.
GI: Nausea, vomiting, diarrhea, anorexia.
Other: Gout, leukopenia, thrombocytopenia, rash, fever, vascu-
                          litis, Stevens-Johnson syndrome, peripheral neuritis.

Dosage/ Concentrations: Adult:	Tablet: 100 and 300 mg. Initial: 100 mg/day p.o.; increase dosage weekly until desired serum urate level. Dosages exceeding 300 mg/day should be administered in divided dosage. For mild gout: 200–300 mg/day. For severe gout: 400–600 mg/day.
Contraindications:	None.
Drug Interactions/ Allergy:	Potentiated effects of coumarin, azathioprine, or mercaptopurine. ↓ Clearance of theophylline and chlorpropamide.

BROMOCRIPTINE

Trade Name:	Parlodel
Indications:	Antihyperprolactinemic, antiparkinsonian, and anti-amenorrheic agent.
Pharmacokinetics:	Oral dosing: only 6% systemic absorption due to first-pass effect. $T_{1/2}$: α, 4 hr; β, 15 hr. Duration: antiprolactin effect, 2 hr; antiparkinsonian effect, 30–60 min.
Pharmacodynamics: CNS:	Psychiatric disorders, confusion, dyskinesia, hallucinations, headaches, dizziness, fainting, sedation, CSF rhinorrhea in patients with pituitary macroadenomas.
CVS:	Orthostatic hypotension, MI, angina.
Pulmonary:	Pulmonary infiltrates, pleural thickening, pleural effusion.
Hepatic:	↑ LFT values.
Renal:	Urinary frequency, incontinence, retention.
GI:	Nausea, vomiting, GI hemorrhage, peptic ulceration, retroperitoneal fibrosis.
Other:	↑ Raynaud's phenomenon, fetal hypoprolactinemia.
Dosage/ Concentrations: Adult:	1.25–30 mg p.o. daily.
Pediatric:	Safety and efficacy not established.
Contraindications:	Routine use in suppression of postpartum lactation; uncontrolled hypertension; pre-eclampsia; and use of ergot alkaloids.
Drug Interactions/ Allergy:	Use with ergot alkaloids may precipitate MI or coronary spasm. ↓ Alcohol tolerance. Use carefully with antihypertensives.

CHENODEOXYCHOLIC ACID, CHENODIOL

Trade Name:	Chenix
Indications:	Oral dissolution of cholesterol gallstones.
Pharmacokinetics:	Absorption: well absorbed from GI tract. Biotransformation: hepatic; metabolized to taurine and glycine conjugates, which are secreted in bile. Elimination: 80% fecal; 20% reabsorbed and converted in liver to sulfolithocholyl conjugates. Time to peak concentration: 50–120 min.

Pharmacodynamics:
CVS: ↑ Atherosclerosis, ↑ serum cholesterol, ↑ LDL cholesterol.
Hepatic: Mild transient hypertransaminasemia.
GI: Constipation, anorexia, nausea, vomiting, abdominal cramps, possible dehydration from diarrhea.

Dosage/ Concentrations: Tablet: 250 mg.

Adult: 250 mg/day for first 1–2 wk; thereafter titrate dose upward until daily dose of 13–16 mg/kg/day in 2 divided doses. Overweight patients may require up to 20 mg/ kg/day. Dissolution of stones may require 3 months to 2 yr. Discontinue therapy if no response after 18 months.

Contraindications: Pregnancy, hepatic function impairment, bile duct abnormalities (primary biliary cirrhosis, cholangitis, cholestasis), and gallstone complications (biliary fistulas and obstruction, cholecystitis, pancreatitis).

Drug Interactions/ Allergy: ↓ Absorption of chenodiol with antacids, cholestyramine, or colestipol. Effect of chenodiol with clofibrate, estrogens, neomycin, or progestins.

CHOLESTYRAMINE

Trade Names:	Cholybar, Questran, Questran Light
Indications:	Adjunctive therapy for primary hypercholesterolemia; pruritus associated with partial biliary obstruction; digitalis overdose; steatorrhea due to ileal resection; and hyperoxaluria.
Pharmacokinetics:	No oral absorption; 100% eliminated in feces. Onset: 24–48 hr. Peak effect: 2–4 wk.

Pharmacodynamics:
CNS: Headache, dizziness, anxiety.
CVS: ↑ Triglycerides, ↓ serum cholesterol, ↓ LDL.
Pulmonary: Aspiration of cholestyramine granules.
Hepatic: ↑ Transaminase and alkaline phosphatase levels.
GI: Constipation, fecal impaction, nausea, vomiting, diarrhea, pancreatitis, GI bleeding, gallstones, malabsorption syndrome.
Other: Hypochloremic acidosis, hyponatremia, hyperphosphatemia, hypocalcemia, osteoporosis, Schilling test affected, hypoprothrombinemia, vitamin K deficiency, bleeding tendency.

Dosage/
Concentrations:
Adult: 1 packet or 1 scoop = 5 g.

                15–30 g/day p.o. in 2–4 divided doses; mix with water.

Contraindications: Complete biliary obstruction, children < 2 yr. of age, and phenylketonuria (Questran Light contains phenylalanine).

Drug Interactions/   ↓ Absorption of fat-soluble vitamins, propranolol,
Allergy: chlorothiazide, warfarin, digitalis, ursodiol, thyroid hormones, tetracycline, penicillin G, vancomycin, phenobarbital, phenylbutazone, and folic acid. Administer medications 2 hr before or 4 hr after cholestyramine dose (warfarin, 6 hr, and digitalis, 8 hr, after cholestyramine dose). Sudden discontinuation of cholestyramine may increase absorption of medications (↑ risk of toxicity).

CLOFIBRATE

Trade Names: Abitrate, Atromid-S

Indications: Adjunctive therapy for type III primary hyperlipidemia, pancreatitis associated with hypertriglyceridemia, and partial central diabetes insipidus.

Pharmacokinetics: De-esterification in GI tract and hepatic metabolism to clofibric acid (active form). Absorption: virtually 100%. Onset: 2–5 days. $T_{1/2}$: normal, 6–25 hr; anuria, 113 hr. Elimination: renal (95%–99%).

Pharmacodynamics:
CNS: Headache, dizziness, fatigue.
CVS: Cardiac dysrhythmias, angina.
Hepatic: Cholelithiasis, cholecystitis, liver function abnormalities.

CLOFIBRATE   *(continued)*

Renal:	Direct renal toxicity (dysuria, hematuria, proteinuria, oliguria), acute renal failure associated with rhabdomyolysis.
GI:	Stomatitis, gastritis, nausea, vomiting, diarrhea.
Musculoskeletal:	Myalgia, myositis, myopathy, flu-like syndrome, rhabdomyolysis, ↑ risk of myopathy associated with renal dysfunction.
Other:	Impotence, decreased libido, anemia, leukopenia, hypoglycemia.
Dosage/ Concentrations:	500 mg/capsule.
Adult:	2 g/day p.o. in divided doses.
Contraindications:	Pregnancy, nursing women, children < 2 yr of age, clinically significant hepatic or renal dysfunction, and primary biliary cirrhosis. Use caution with coronary artery disease.
Drug Interactions/ Allergy:	↑ Effects of coumarin, oral hypoglycemic agents (especially tolbutamide), and phenytoin (decrease coumarin dose and monitor protime). ↓ Renal clearance with probenecid (↑ risk of toxicity).

COLCHICINE

Trade Name:	ColBenemid
Indications:	Gouty arthritis, Mediterranean fever, calcium pyrophosphate deposition disease, amyloidosis, Paget disease of bone, and dermatitis herpetiformis.
Pharmacokinetics:	Biotransformation: hepatic. $T_{1/2}$: α, 20 min; β, 1 hr. Onset: IV, 6–12 hr; p.o. 12 hr. Duration of pain relief: 24–48 hr after oral administration. Elimination: slow over days; primarily biliary; 10%–20% renal.
Pharmacodynamics:	
CNS:	Depressed medullary ventilatory center.
CVS:	Myocardial injury, ↓ contractility, profound shock.
Pulmonary:	Respiratory failure.
Hepatic:	Hepatocellular damage.
Renal:	Renal failure, hematuria, oliguria.
GI:	Abdominal pain, nausea, vomiting, diarrhea, hemorrhagic gastroenteritis, burning pain in throat and stomach.
Musculoskeletal:	Myopathy, muscle weakness and paralysis.
Other:	Agranulocytosis, aplastic anemia, thrombocytopenia,

coagulopathy, DIC, hyponatremia, hypokalemia, metabolic acidosis, teratogenic effects.

**Dosage/
Concentrations:**
Adult:

Ampules: 2 cc vials (0.5 mg/cc).

IV: loading dose, 2 mg, followed by 0.5 mg every 6 hr for acute attacks. Not to exceed 4 mg/day.

Contraindications: Serious cardiac, hepatic, GI, or renal disorders.

**Drug Interactions/
Allergy:**

↑ Risk of toxicity with alcohol, anticoagulants, phenylbutazone, antineoplastic agents, and radiation therapy. Enhanced effects produced by CNS depressants and sympathomimetics.

COLESTIPOL

Trade Name: Colestid

Indications: Adjunctive therapy for primary hypercholesterolemia, pruritus associated with partial biliary obstruction, digitalis overdose, and steatorrhea due to ileal resection.

Pharmacokinetics: No oral absorption. Elimination: feces (100%). Onset: 24–48 hr. Peak effect: 1 month.

Pharmacodynamics:
CNS: Headache, dizziness, anxiety.
CVS: Triglycerides.
Pulmonary: Aspiration of colestipol granules.
Hepatic: Transaminase and alkaline phosphatase levels.
GI: Constipation, fecal impaction, nausea, vomiting, diarrhea, GI bleeding, gallstones, malabsorption syndrome.
Other: Possible hypochloremic acidosis, hyponatremia, hyperphosphatemia, hypoprothrombinemia, vitamin K deficiency, bleeding tendency.

**Dosage/
Concentrations:**
Adult:

1 packet or 1 scoop = 5 g.

15–30 g/day p.o. in 2–4 divided doses; mix with water.

Contraindications: Complete biliary obstruction and children <2 yr of age.

**Drug Interactions/
Allergy:**

Absorption of fat-soluble vitamins, propranolol, chlorothiazide, warfarin, digitalis, ursodiol, thyroid hormones, tetracycline, furosemide, penicillin G, gemfibrozil, and vancomycin. Administer medications 2 hr before or 4 hr after colestipol dose. (For warfarin, 6 hr, and digitalis, 8 hr, after colestipol dose.) Sudden

COLESTIPOL *(continued)*

discontinuation of colestipol may increase absorption of medications (↑ risk of toxicity).

DIMERCAPROL, DIMERCAPTOPROPANOL

Trade Names:	BAL (British antilewisite), BAL in Oil
Indications:	Arsenic (nongaseous), gold, inorganic mercury, and lead toxicity.
Pharmacokinetics:	Peak concentrations: 30–60 min after IM injection. Duration: ~ 4 hr. 50% eliminated as metal-dimercaprol (BAL) complex in urine and bile, 50% metabolized to inactive compounds.

Pharmacodynamics:

CNS:	Drowsiness, convulsions, blepharospasm, ↑ lacrimation, conjunctivitis.
CVS:	↑ Increased HR, ↑ BP.
Hepatic:	↑ SGPT, ↑ SGOT.
Renal:	Nephrotoxicity.
GI:	Nausea; vomiting; burning in lips, mouth, and throat; abdominal pain.
Musculoskeletal:	Tightness of hands.
Other:	↓ ^{131}I thyroid uptake in diagnostic testing, neutropenia, fever, rhinorrhea, diaphoresis, hemolysis in G-6-PD deficiency.

Dosage/ Concentrations:	For IV/IM use only: 10% solution in peanut oil. Dosing depends on plasma sampling of BAL–metal complex and varies according to individual metal. Toxicity pronounced at >5 mg/kg doses; may limit therapy.
Contraindications:	Arsine gas (AsH$_3$) poisoning, hepatic or renal impairment, and allergy to peanuts or peanut products.
Drug Interactions/ Allergy:	CNS distribution and encephalopathy in methylmercury or organic mercury intoxication. Do not take with iron supplements.

EDETATE DISODIUM

Trade Names:	Disotate, Endrate
Indications:	Emergent treatment of acute hypercalcemia and digitalis glycoside toxicity.

Pharmacokinetics:	Biotransformation: none. Elimination: renal (95% of dose in urine within 24 hr); principally eliminated as calcium chelate; change in urine flow or pH does not affect excretion.
Pharmacodynamics:	Increased urinary potassium excretion.
CNS:	Hypocalcemia (seizures, anxiety, delirium, psychosis, confusion).
CVS:	Hypocalcemia (hypotension, prolonged QT interval, arrhythmias), hypokalemia (T-wave inversion, depressed ST segments), prolonged QT interval, U waves, atrial and ventricular arrhythmias, postural hypotension.
Pulmonary:	Hypocalcemia (respiratory fatigue, dyspnea, laryngeal stridor).
Renal:	Nephrotoxicity.
GI:	Abdominal pain and cramps, diarrhea
Musculoskeletal:	Hypocalcemia (muscle spasms, tetany, hypokalemia muscle weakness).
Other:	Thrombophlebitis, hypoglycemia, hypomagnesemia, febrile reactions.
Dosage/ Concentrations:	150 mg/cc vials, diluted in D_5W; final concentration < 30 mg/cc.
Adult:	50 mg/kg IV over 24 hr.
Pediatric:	40 mg/kg IV over 24 hr.
Contraindications:	Hypocalcemia, anuria, and renal failure. Use cautiously in renal insufficiency.
Drug Interactions/ Allergy:	Possible chelation of zinc in insulin. Hypocalcemia caused by edetate disodium antagonizes inotropic and chronotropic effects of digitalis. ↑ Effects of muscle relaxants.

ETIDRONATE DISODIUM

Trade Names:	Didronel, EHDP
Indications:	Paget's disease, heterotopic ossification, and hypercalcemia of malignancy.
Pharmacokinetics:	Bioavailability: IV (100%), oral dosing variable (1% at 5 mg/kg/day to 6% at 20 mg/kg/day). Clearance: 50% of absorbed or infused drug renally cleared. $T_{1/2}$: 6 hr; remainder absorbed by bone. Not metabolized.
Pharmacodynamics:	
Renal:	Worsened renal function.
GI:	Metallic or altered taste, diarrhea, nausea.
Musculoskeletal:	Bone pain, poor healing of fractures.

ETIDRONATE DISODIUM *(continued)*

Other:	Mild hypocalcemia, hyperphosphatemia, overhydration with IV dose and hydration therapy.
Dosage/ Concentrations:	IV: 7.5 mg/kg/day in 250 cc normal saline over 2 hr for 3 days. Oral: (200 mg tablets): Paget's disease and heterotopic ossification 5–20 mg/kg/day, depending on disease and duration of treatment. Reduce dose if serum creatinine level is 2.5–4.9 mg/dl.
Contraindications:	Serum creatinine > 5 mg/dl. Use caution in elderly and in cardiac failure.
Drug Interactions/ Allergy:	Allergic reactions: angioedema; swelling of larynx, glottis, tongue, lips, and face; urticaria; pruritus. Bioavailability with mineral supplements and antacids.

GALLIUM NITRATE

Trade Name:	Ganite
Indications:	Adjunct to IV hydration therapy for hypercalcemia of malignancy.
Pharmacokinetics:	$T_{1/2}$: α, 1 hr; β, 24 hr (72–115 hr with prolonged infusions). Duration: 6 days. Metabolism: none. Clearance: renal (100%).
Pharmacodynamics:	
CNS:	Hypocalcemia and hypophosphatemia (anxiety, delirium, psychosis, paresthesias, ataxia, seizures, confusion).
CVS:	Hypocalcemia (hypotension, prolonged QT interval, arrhythmias).
Pulmonary:	Mild asymptomatic respiratory alkalosis, laryngeal stridor.
Renal:	Renal insufficiency.
GI:	Nausea, vomiting, diarrhea, metallic taste, hypocalcemia (abdominal cramps).
Musculoskeletal:	Hypocalcemia (muscle spasms, tetany), hypophosphatemia (muscle weakness).
Other:	Anemia, hemolysis, platelet dysfunction.
Dosage/ Concentrations:	500 mg in 20 cc vials (25 mg/cc).
Adult:	100–200 mg/m² of body surface area/day IV; infuse over 24 hr daily for up to 5 days.
Contraindications:	Serum creatinine > 2.5 mg/dl and breast-feeding.

| Drug Interactions/ Allergy: | Additive nephrotoxicity with nephrotoxic medications. Calcium preparations and vitamin D may antagonize effect of gallium nitrate. ↓ Uptake of gallium citrate ^{67}Ga scintigraphy for localizing tumor or abscess. |

GEMFIBROZIL

Trade Name	Lopid
Indications:	Adjunctive therapy for primary hyperlipidemia and pancreatitis associated with hypertriglyceridemia.
Pharmacokinetics:	Absorption: Well absorbed from GI tract. Biotransformation: hepatic. $T_{1/2}$: single dose, 1.5 hr; multiple doses, 1.3 hr. Elimination: renal (70%, largely unchanged); fecal (6%).

Pharmacodynamics:

CNS:	Headache, dizziness, somnolence, depression.
Hepatic:	Cholelithiasis, cholecystitis, liver function abnormalities.
Renal:	Direct renal toxicity (dysuria, hematuria, proteinuria, oliguria), acute renal failure associated with rhabdomyolysis.
GI:	Abdominal pain, nausea, vomiting, diarrhea.
Musculoskeletal:	Myalgia, myositis, myopathy, flu-like syndrome, rhabdomyolysis
Other:	Impotence; decreased libido, anemia, leukopenia.

Dosage/ Concentrations:	Tablet: 600 mg.
Adult:	600 mg p.o. b.i.d.
Contraindications:	Clinically significant hepatic or renal impairment, primary biliary cirrhosis, children < 2 yr of age, and gallbladder disease.
Drug Interactions/ Allergy:	↑ Effects of coumarin. ↑ Risk of rhabdomyolysis with concurrent use of lovastatin.

GOLD SODIUM THIOMALATE

Trade Name:	Myochrysine
Indications:	Adult and juvenile rheumatoid arthritis.
Pharmacokinetics:	Absorption: GI tract (25%). $T_{1/2}$: β, 21–31 days (blood); 42–128 days (tissues). Duration: may take

GOLD SODIUM THIOMALATE   *(continued)*

3–6 months for therapeutic effects. Elimination: 60%–90% renal excretion.

Pharmacodynamics:
CNS: Confusion, convulsions, encephalitis, hallucinations.
CVS: Angioedema, anaphylaxis.
Pulmonary: Intersitial pneumonitis, "gold" bronchitis.
Hepatic: Toxic hepatitis with jaundice, cholestasis.
Renal: Nephrotic syndrome, glomerulitis, hematuria.
GI: Glossitis, gingivitis, stomatitis, nausea, diarrhea.
Other: Leukopenia, thrombocytopenia, inhibited phagocytic mechanisms, altered collagen biosynthesis, dermatitis, urticaria, vesicular lesions.

**Dosage/
Concentrations:**
Adult: 10–50 mg IM/wk. Limit: 50 mg/dose.
Pediatric: 1 mg/kg IM/wk.

Contraindications: Breast-feeding. Avoid with penicillamine (see below). Use caution in blood dyscrasias, vascular disease, SLE, or Sjögren's syndrome.

**Drug Interactions/
Allergy:**   Cross-sensitivity to other gold-containing substances. Sesame and paraben formulation may precipate allergy in sensitive persons. Additive nephrotoxicity with nephrotoxic medications. Use with penicillamine causes marked hematotoxicity and nephrotoxicity. Dimercaprol (BAL) chelates gold in overdose.

LOVASTATIN

Trade Name: Mevacor

Indications: Antihypercholesterolemic agent

Pharmacokinetics: Peak plasma concentration: within 2–6 hr after oral dose. Steady-state plasma concentrations achieved within 2–3 days. Therapeutic response: 2 wk; maximal response within 4–6 wk. $T_{1/2}$: 1–2 hr. Elimination: renal (80%) and biliary excretion of inactive metabolites. Hydrolyzed in vivo to mevalonic acid.

Pharmacodynamics: Decreased production of cholesterol precursors.
CNS: Fever, unusual tiredness or weakness, blurred vision.
Hepatic: ↑ Liver function enzymes.
Renal: Rhabdomyolysis leading to renal failure
GI: Constipation, diarrhea, cramping, nausea.

Musculoskeletal:	Myalgia.
Other:	Impotence.

**Dosage/
Concentrations:**
Adult: 20–80 mg/day/p.o.
Pediatric: Safety not established.

Contraindications: Pregnant and breast-feeding women and children < 2 yr of age.

**Drug Interactions/
Allergy:**   Rhabdomyolysis in patients treated with immunosuppressants, gemfibrozil, erythromycin, and niacin.

MESNA

Trade Name: Mesnex

Indications: Prophylaxis against ifosfamide-induced hemorrhagic cystitis.

Pharmacokinetics: Plasma $T_{1/2:}$ mesna 0.36 hr; dimesna 1.17 hr. Terminal $T_{1/2}$: approx 7 hr. Elimination: renal (rapid). Vd: 0.65 L/kg.

Pharmacodynamics: Detoxifying effect of ifosfamide (an antineoplastic agent) in GU tract.
CNS: Headache, fatigue.
Renal: False-positive test for urinary ketones.
GI: Nausea, vomiting, diarrhea.

**Dosage/
Concentrations:**   Ampules (100 mg/cc): 2, 4, 10 cc vials.
Adult: 20% of ifosfamide dosage IV at time of ifosfamide administration and 4 and 8 hr after each dose of ifosfamide.

Contraindications: None.

**Drug Interactions/
Allergy:**   Not compatible in formulation with cisplatin.

METHIMAZOLE

Trade Name: Tapazole

Indications: Antithyroid agent.

Pharmacokinetics: Absorption: GI tract (rapid); bioavailability: 93%. Peak plasma concentration: 1 hr. Crosses placenta and

METHIMAZOLE   *(continued)*

distributed into maternal milk. $T_{1/2}$: β, 5–13 hr. Elimination: Urinary excretion. Duration: effect requires 4–7 wk.

Pharmacodynamics:

CNS:	Headache, drowsiness, vertigo, paresthesias, encephalopathy.
CVS:	Periarteritis due to SLE-like syndrome.
Hepatic:	Jaundice, fulminant hepatitis and necrosis.
GI:	Nausea, vomiting, loss of taste.
Musculoskeletal:	Peripheral neuritis, arthralgias, myalgia.
Other:	Rash, urticaria, pruritus, hair loss, pigmentation, agranulocytosis, pancytopenia, fetal hypothyroidism and goiter if given during pregnancy.

Dosage/ Concentrations:	Use lowest effective dose (risk of agranulocytosis dose-related).
Adult:	5–20 mg p.o. t.i.d.
Pediatric:	0.4 mg/kg p.o. daily in divided doses.

Contraindications:	Acute hyperthyroid state and exogenous thyrotoxicosis (not effective); co-administration of thyroid hormone advised during pregnancy.

Drug Interactions/ Allergy:	As patients become euthyroid, reduce doses of methylxanthines and digitalis. Potassium iodide, amiodarone, and iodine decrease response. ↑ or ↓ Effects of coumarin.

METYRAPONE

Trade Name:	N/A
Indications:	Short-term treatment of cortisol excess (Cushing syndrome).
Pharmacokinetics:	Absorption: oral (rapid). Biotransformation: hepatic to active alcohol (metyrapol). $T_{1/2}$: β, 20–26 min. Duration: <4 hr after oral administration. Elimination: 40% renal excretion as glucuronide metabolites in 72 hr.

Pharmacodynamics:

CNS:	Nervousness, confusion, loss of consciousness (in acute adrenal insufficiency with overdose).
CVS:	Hypotension, ↑ HR, dysrhythmias, cardiovascular collapse (in acute adrenal insufficiency with overdose).

GI:	Nausea, vomiting, diarrhea, cramping.
Musculoskeletal:	Muscle weakness.
Other:	Adrenal insufficiency or addisonian crisis, hirsutism, bone marrow suppression, hypokalemic alkalosis, edema, weight gain, alopecia, diaphoresis, acne.

**Dosage/
Concentrations:**

Adult:	750 mg p.o. q 4 hr.
Pediatric:	15 mg/kg p.o. q 4 hr.

Contraindications: Adrenocortical insufficiency, hypopituitarism, pre-eclampsia, or in patients at risk for hypertensive crises (e.g., pheochromocytoma).

**Drug Interactions/
Allergy:** ↓ Efficacy with phenytoin, estrogens, progestins, corticosteroids, phenothiazines, chlordiazepoxide, chlorpromazine, amitriptyline, phenobarbital, and methysergide. Allergic reaction: skin rash.

PEGADEMASE

Trade Name: Adagen

Indications: Treatment of adenosine deaminase deficiency in patients with SCID who are not candidates for bone marrow transplantation or who have not had a successful transplant.

Pharmacokinetics: $T_{1/2}$: 3–6 days. Peak plasma concentration: 2–3 days after 15 U/kg IM injection. Duration: 2–6 months for clinical improvement in immune status.

Pharmacodynamics:

CNS:	Headache.
Musculoskeletal:	Pain at injection site.

**Dosage/
Concentrations:**

Adult and Pediatric: 10–20 U/kg IM for first 3 wk. Maintenance 20 U/kg IM/wk. Monitoring of serum levels necessary. Weekly maintenance therapy required.

Contraindications: Severe thrombocytopenia.

**Drug Interactions/
Allergy:** Vidarabine (substrate for adenosine deaminase) causes altered responses. Bovine preparations may cause antibody formation and allergy.

PENICILLAMINE

Trade Names:	Cuprimine, Depen
Indications:	Chelating agent in Wilson's disease, heavy metal toxicity, rheumatoid arthritis, rheumatoid vasculitis, Felty's syndrome, cystinuria, and renal calculi.
Pharmacokinetics:	Biotransformation: Hepatic. Onset: Wilson's disease, 1–3 months; rheumatoid arthritis, 2–3 months. Elimination: Renal and fecal.
Pharmacodynamics:	Reduction of IgM rheumatoid factor and immune complexes.
CNS:	Optic neuritis, peripheral neuropathy, diplopia, myasthenia gravis–like syndrome.
Pulmonary:	Obliterative bronchiolitis, Goodpasture's syndrome.
Hepatic:	Intrahepatic cholestasis, toxic hepatitis, jaundice.
Renal:	Membranous glomerulopathy (proteinuria, hematuria, nephrosis).
GI:	Oral ulcers, aphthous stomatitis, nausea, vomiting, diarrhea, cheilosis, glossitis, gingivostomatitis, peptic ulcer, pancreatitis.
Musculoskeletal:	Muscle weakness.
Other:	Skin friability, small white papules at venipuncture and surgical sites, delayed wound healing, leukopenia, thrombocytopenia, aplastic anemia, agranulocytosis.
Dosage/ Concentrations:	Tablet and capsule: 250 mg.
Adult:	125 mg–1.5 g/day in divided doses depending on disease. Limit dose to 250 mg/day during surgery.
Pediatric:	30 mg/kg/day.
Contraindications:	Penicillamine-related agranulocytosis, aplastic anemia, rheumatoid arthritis with renal insufficiency, and breast-feeding.
Drug Interactions/ Allergy:	Risk of toxicity with gold therapy, antimalarials, cytotoxic drugs, oxyphenbutazone, and phenylbutazone (avoid concomitant therapy with these drugs). Allergic reactions. Drug fever, rash, lymphadenopathy, arthralgias.

POTASSIUM IODIDE, KI

Trade Names:	Pima, SSKI
Indications:	Antihyperthyroid agent; however, SSKI does not completely control manifestations of hyperthyroidism.

Pharmacokinetics:	Rapid GI absorption of ions. Duration: antithyroid effects usually observed within 24 hr; maximal after 10–15 days of continual therapy, then subside. Readily crosses placenta.

Pharmacodynamics:

CNS:	Metallic taste, severe headache (iodism due to overdose).
Pulmonary:	Laryngeal inflammation, productive cough, pulmonary edema (iodism).
GI:	Diarrhea, dyspepsia, burning in mouth and throat, pharyngeal inflammation, salivary gland hypersecretion and tenderness (iodism).
Other:	Angioedema, mucosal hemorrhage, fever, arthralgias, adenopathy, eosinophilia, SLE, fatal TTP, arteritis, hypocomplementemic vasculitis, autoimmune thyroid disease, paradoxical thyrotoxicosis in low doses, goiter, hypothyroidism in adult (with prolonged therapy) and in neonate.

Dosage/ Concentrations:

Adult and Pediatric:	Syrup or solution, 50–500 mg p.o. 3–6 times daily.
Contraindications:	Acute bronchitis. Use cautiously in tuberculosis.
Drug Interactions/ Allergy:	Lithium greatly enhances effect. Use with potassium supplements may cause hyperkalemia and dysrhythmias.

PROBENECID

Trade Names:	Benemid, Probalan
Indications:	Gouty arthritis, hyperuricemia associated with tumor lysis, and adjunct to antibiotic therapy (penicillins and some cephalosporins).
Pharmacokinetics:	Absorption: rapid and complete. Protein binding: very high. Biotransformation: hepatic, rapid; metabolites have uricosuric activity. Dose-dependent $T_{1/2}$: 3–8 hr after 500 mg, 6–12 hr with larger doses. Elimination: primarily hepatic, with renal excretion of metabolites; 5%–10% excreted unchanged renally (alkalinization of urine increases excretion).

Pharmacodynamics:

CNS:	Dizziness, headache.
Hepatic:	Hepatic necrosis.
GI:	Nausea, vomiting, anorexia, sore gums.
Renal:	Urate nephropathy, renal colic, nephrotic syndrome.

PROBENECID   *(continued)*

Other:	Aplastic anemia, leukopenia, hemolytic anemia (associated with G-6-PD deficiency), blood dyscrasias, anaphylaxis, fever, urticaria, pruritus.
Dosage/ Concentrations:	Tablet: 500 mg. For hyperuricemia: 250 mg p.o. b.i.d. for 1 wk; maintenance dose: 500 mg p.o. b.i.d. As antibiotic therapy adjunct (penicillin or cephalosporin): 500 mg p.o. q.i.d. For sexually transmitted diseases: 1 g p.o. concurrently with appropriate antibiotic. For neurosyphilis: 500 mg p.o. q.i.d. with 2.4 million units of penicillin G per day
Contraindications:	Blood dyscrasias, uric acid stones, children < 2 yr of age.
Drug Interactions/ Allergy:	↓ Induction dose of thiopental; prolonged effects of ketamine and thiopental. ↑ Plasma half-life (toxicity) of heparin, lorazepam, oxazepam, temazepam, NSAIDs, chlorpropamide, sulfonamides, furosemide, penicillins, cephalosporins, ciprofloxacin, acetaminophen, rifampin, nitrofurantoin, and sulfinpyrazone. Additive antihyperuricemic effects with allopurinol. ↓ Risk of urate nephropathy with antineoplastic agents.

PROBUCOL

Trade Name:	Lorelco
Indications:	Antihyperlipidemic agent.
Pharmacokinetics:	Absorption: GI tract (7%); accumulates in fat with prolonged therapy. Peak concentrations: steady state at 4 months. $T_{1/2}$: >6 wk after cessation of therapy (slow biliary elimination).
Pharmacodynamics:	
CNS:	Paresthesias.
CVS:	Prolonged QT interval.
GI:	Diarrhea, flatulence, abdominal pain, nausea.
Other:	Angioneurotic edema, eosinophilia.
Dosage/ Concentrations: Adult:	500 mg p.o. b.i.d.

Contraindications:	Recent MI, known ventricular irritability, pregnancy, breast-feeding, or children < 2 yr of age.
Drug Interactions/ Allergy:	Possible interaction with antiarrhythmics that prolong QT interval (amiodarone, bretylium, disopyramide, encainide).

PROPYLTHIOURACIL, PTU

Trade Name:	Propyl-Thyracil
Indications:	Antithyroid agent (thyroid storm).
Pharmacokinetics:	Absorption: oral (rapid). Bioavailability: 75%. Readily crosses placenta. Distributed into mother's milk. $T_{1/2}$: 1–2 hr. Glucuronide excreted into urine. Vd: 0.4 L/kg. Peak antithyroid effect requires average of 17 wk.

Pharmacodynamics:	
CNS:	Headaches, drowsiness, vertigo, encephalopathy, paresthesias.
CVS:	Periarteritis due to SLE-like syndrome.
Pulmonary:	Interstitial pneumonitis.
Hepatic:	Jaundice, fulminant hepatitis and necrosis.
Renal:	Nephritis.
GI:	Nausea, vomiting, loss of taste.
Musculoskeletal:	Peripheral neuritis, arthralgias, myalgias.
Other:	Rash, urticaria, pruritus, hair loss, pigmentation, agranulocytosis, pancytopenia, fetal hypothyroidism and goiter if given during pregnancy.

Dosage/ Concentrations:	Use lowest effective dose (risk of agranulocytosis dose-related).
Adult:	100–400 mg p.o. t.i.d.
Pediatric:	• Neonate: 5–10 mg/kg/day p.o.
	• Child: 15–100 mg/kg/day p.o. in divided doses.

Contraindications:	Acute hyperthyroid state and exogenous thyrotoxicosis (not effective). Co-administration of thyroid hormone advised during pregnancy.
Drug Interactions/ Allergy:	As patients become euthyroid, reduce doses of methylxanthines and digitalis. Potassium iodide, amiodarone, and iodine decrease response. ↑ or ↓ coumarin's effects.

SODIUM POLYSTYRENE SULFONATE

Trade Name:	Kayexalate
Indications:	Antihyperkalemic agent.
Pharmacokinetics:	Absorption: not absorbed from GI tract. Onset: hours to days; use dialysis in emergencies. Resin exchange efficiency: 33%.

Pharmacodynamics:

CNS:	Confusion, irritability (if hypokalemia present).
CVS:	Dysrhythmias (if hypokalemia), congestive heart failure (if fluid retention due to increased sodium).
Pulmonary:	Pulmonary edema with sodium retention in congestive heart failure.
Renal:	Fluid retention.
GI:	Fecal impaction, cramping of abdominal muscles (if hypocalcemia), colonic necrosis due to sorbitol in enema.
Musculoskeletal:	Hypocalcemia, hypokalemia (tetany, weakness).

Dosage/ Concentrations:

Adult:	Oral, 15 g powder 1 to 4 times daily in 10–20 ml 70% sorbitol syrup to prevent constipation. Rectal, 25–100 g via enema p.r.n.
Pediatric:	Oral and rectal, 1 g/kg 1 to 4 times daily; follow rectal dose with cleansing non–sodium-containing enema after 1–4 hr.
Contraindications:	Low K^+, Ca^{2+}, or Mg^{2+} levels. Use caution in congestive heart failure, edematous conditions, or severe hypertension due to sodium retention.
Drug Interactions/ Allergy:	Use with magnesium- or calcium-containing laxatives can lead to systemic alkalosis. Potassium-sparing diuretics and K^+ supplementation counter effects.

SULFINPYRAZONE

Trade Name:	Anturane
Indications:	Gouty arthritis and hyperuricemia associated with chronic gout.
Pharmacokinetics:	Absorption: rapid, complete. Protein binding: very high. Biotransformation: hepatic; metabolites have uricosuric and antiplatelet effects. $T_{1/2}$: 1–5 hr. Elimination: primarily renal; 5% excreted in feces.

Pharmacodynamics:

CNS:	Convulsions, coma.
Hepatic:	Jaundice.
Renal:	Urate nephropathy, renal colic.
GI:	↑ Peptic ulcer disease, nausea, vomiting, diarrhea.
Other:	Anemia, leukopenia, thrombocytopenia, aplastic anemia, hypoglycemia, bleeding tendency.

**Dosage/
Concentrations:**   Tablet: 100 mg. Capsule: 200 mg.

Adult: Initial dose 200–400 mg/day p.o. in 2 divided doses.
Maintenance: 400–800 mg/day p.o. in 2 divided doses.

Contraindications: Blood dyscrasias, peptic ulcer disease.

**Drug Interactions/
Allergy:**   ↑ Effects of sulfonamides and insulin (possible hypoglycemia). ↑ Bleeding effects of coumarin, heparin, thrombolytic agents, and NSAIDs. ↑ Effects of verapamil and phenytoin by protein-binding displacement. ↑ Risk of urate nephropathy with antineoplastic agents. Additive antihyperuricemic effects with allopurinol.

TIOPRONIN

Trade Names: Capen, Thiola, Thiosol, Vincol

Indications: Antiurolithic agent for cystine calculi in severe homozygous cystinuria.

Pharmacokinetics: $T_{1/2}$: 4 hr. Elimination: renal.

Pharmacodynamics:

Hepatic:	Hepatotoxicity.
Renal:	Renal dysfunction.
Other:	Bone marrow suppression, leukopenia, thrombocytopenia.

**Dosage/
Concentrations:**   Tablet: 100 mg. Adjust doses to urinary cysteine concentrations.

Adult: 800 mg/day p.o. in 3 divided doses.

Pediatric:
- \> 9 yr: 15 mg/kg/day p.o. divided t.i.d.
- \< 9 yr: Safety not established.

Contraindications: Preexisting agranulocytosis, aplastic anemia, thrombocytopenia, hepatic or renal dysfunction.

**Drug Interactions/
Allergy:**   Avoid with concurrent use of hepatotoxic, nephrotoxic, or bone marrow suppressing medications.

TRIENTINE

Trade Name:	Syprine
Indications:	Copper chelating agent in Wilson's disease.
Pharmacokinetics:	Elimination: renal and biliary.

Pharmacodynamics:
Pulmonary: Bronchitis, asthma.
Other: Iron chelation and anemia, SLE-like syndrome (fever, malaise, arthralgias, rash, adenopathy).

**Dosage/
Concentrations:**
Adult and Adolescent: 750–1250 mg/day p.o. in divided doses.
Pediatric: 500–750 mg/day p.o. in divided doses.

Contraindications: Preexisting iron deficiency anemia, copper deficiency states, cystinuria, rheumatoid arthritis, and primary biliary cirrhosis.

**Drug Interactions/
Allergy:** Ineffective if taken with copper or iron supplements.

URSODIOL

Trade Name:	Actigall
Indications:	Anticholelithic agent (cholesterol gallstones only).

Pharmacokinetics: Absorption: oral (90%) from small intestine. Peak effect: 1–3 hr. Elimination: fecal. First-pass hepatic clearance with metabolism to taurine and glycine (secreted into bile).

Pharmacodynamics:
Hepatic: ↑ SGPT.

**Dosage/
Concentrations:**
Adult: 8–10 mg/kg/day p.o. in divided doses with meals.
Pediatric: Safety not established.

Contraindications: Not efficacious in calcified cholelithiasis (radiopaque stones) or unresolved stones after 12 months of therapy. Avoid if surgery is indicated (obstruction, pancreatitis, cholecystitis).

**Drug Interactions/
Allergy:** ↑ Sensitivity to bile acids. ↓ Efficacy with progestins, estrogens, cholestyramine, colestipol, aluminum-containing antacids, clofibrate, and neomycin.

28
Miscellaneous Compounds

Michael W. Jopling, M.D.

ALPROSTADIL, PGE₁, **PROSTAGLANDIN E₁**

Trade Name:	Prostin VR Pediatric
Indications:	Palliative therapy for temporary maintenance of patency of a patent ductus arteriosus and pulmonary vasodilator (non-FDA approved).
Pharmacokinetics:	Metabolism: very rapid; as much as 80% metabolized by lung in first pass. Elimination: metabolites excreted by kidney (81%–99% protein bound to albumin). $T_{1/2}$:β, 5–10 min.

Pharmacodynamics:

CVS:	Systemic and pulmonary vasodilation.
Pulmonary:	Apnea in $\sim$ 12% of neonates (most often <2 kg) with congenital heart disease.
GI:	↑ Stimulation of intestinal smooth muscle, gastric outlet obstruction secondary to antral hyperplasia in neonates.
Other:	↑ Stimulation of uterine smooth muscle, inhibited platelet aggregation, inhibited activation of coagulation factor X via increasing cAMP, ↑ fibrinolysis.

Dosage/ Concentrations:	Packaged as 500 μg/1-ml ampule.
Adult:	0.03–0.15 μg/kg/min continuous infusion. Up to 1.0 μg/kg/min of norepinephrine via left atrial line also needed to offset systemic vasodilation.
Pediatric:	0.05–0.40 μg/kg/min continuous infusion. Starting dose: 0.1 μg/kg/min.
Contraindications:	None.
Drug Interactions/ Allergy:	None.

DANTROLENE

Trade Name:	Dantrium
Indications:	Malignant hyperthermia and clinical spasticity from upper motor neuron disorders.
Pharmacokinetics:	$T_{1/2}$: β, 12 hr.

Pharmacodynamics: Skeletal muscle relaxation.

CNS:	Drowsiness, dizziness, fatigue, general malaise.
Renal:	Diuresis.
GI:	Diarrhea.
Musculoskeletal:	Significant muscular weakness.

Dosage/
Concentrations:
IV: vials, each containing 20 mg lyophilized dantrolene and 3000 mg mannitol. Reconstitution is difficult and is to be *only* with 60 ml sterile water (nonbacteriostatic).

Oral: Capsules: 25, 50, and 100 mg.

For preoperative prophylaxis of malignant hyperthermia: Oral: 4–8 mg/kg/day dantrolene in 3 or 4 divided doses for 1 or 2 days prior to surgery. IV: 2.5 mg/kg over 1 hr ~ 1.25 hr prior to planned surgery.

For malignant hyperthermia crisis: rapid IV push of 1 mg/kg dantrolene; repeat until symptoms subside or a maximum cumulative dose of 10 mg/kg has been reached.

After malignant hyperthermia crisis: Oral: 4–8 mg/kg/day dantrolene in 3–4 divided doses for 1–3 days to prevent recurrence.

Contraindications: None.

Drug Interactions/
Allergy:
None.

DINOPROST

Trade Name: Prostin F2 alpha*

Indications: Vasodilating agent in angiographic procedures and induction of labor.

Pharmacokinetics: $T_{1/2}$: IV, <1 min. Metabolism: undergoes enzymatic after dehydrogenation primarily in maternal lungs and liver. Elimination: kidneys; only 5% excreted in feces.

Pharmacodynamics:
CNS: Faintness, feeling of panic, paresthesia, double vision.
CVS: Peripheral vasoconstriction; tachycardia, bradycardia; second-degree heart block, hypertension.
Pulmonary: Bronchoconstriction.
Renal: Dysuria, hematuria, urinary retention.
GI: Nausea, vomiting, adynamic ileus.
Musculoskeletal: Abdominal, leg, back, chest, or shoulder pain.
Other: Anaphylaxis, endometritis, uterine bleeding and pain.

Dosage/
Concentrations:
Available as 5 mg base/ml. For induction of labor, starting dose is 2.5 μg/min IV; dose is doubled every hour, if necessary, to a maximum of 20 μg/min.

Contraindications: None.

---

*Available in Canada. Manufacture discontinued in 1991 in United States.

DINOPROST *(continued)*

Drug Interactions/ Allergy:	None.

METHYLERGOMETRINE, METHYLERGONOVINE

Trade Name:	Methergine
Indications:	Postpartum and postabortal uterine hemorrhage.
Pharmacokinetics:	Absorption: rapid after IM (78%) or oral (60%) dose. Onset: oral, 5–10 min; IM, 2–5 min. Duration (uterine contraction): 3 hr oral/IM; ~ 45 min IV. Metabolism: extensive first-pass biotransformation. Elimination: principally renal excretion of metabolites.
Pharmacodynamics:	Agonist and antagonist activity at some CNS serotonin and dopamine receptors.
CNS:	Hallucinations, dizziness.
CVS:	Arterial vasoconstriction, bradycardia, coronary vasospasm, hypertension, ventricular arrhythmias, severe peripheral vasospasm.
GI:	Nausea and vomiting.
Musculoskeletal:	↑ Uterine contraction.
Dosage/ Concentrations:	0.2 mg/1-ml ampule and 0.2 mg tablets. IV/IM: 0.2 mg after delivery, then q 2–4 hr p.r.n. Oral: 0.2 mg 3 or 4 times a day for a maximum of 1 wk.
Contraindications:	Except in severe life-threatening hemorrhage, do not give to patients with hypertension, MI, pre-eclampsia, eclampsia, CVA, occlusive peripheral vascular disease, or Raynaud's phenomenon.
Drug Interactions/ Allergy:	Use extreme caution in administering vasoactive substances (e.g., ephedrine) after treatment.

NITRIC OXIDE

Trade Name:	Investigational drug
Indications:	Pulmonary hypertension after cardiac surgery, adult respiratory distress syndrome, and neonatal pulmonary hypertension.
Pharmacokinetics:	Inhalation as hemoglobin inactivates the compound almost instantaneously.

Pharmacodynamics:
Pulmonary: Pulmonary vasodilation.
Other: Prolonged bleeding time, water intoxication.

Dosage/   Inspired concentration: 6–40 ppm.
Concentrations:

Contraindications: N/A.

Drug Interactions/   N/A.
Allergy:

29

Muscle Relaxants

Dori Ann McCulloch, M.D.

ATRACURIUM BESYLATE

Trade Name:	Tracrium
Indications:	Endotracheal intubation and skeletal muscle relaxation during surgery or mechanical ventilation.
Pharmacokinetics:	Onset: 2–2.5 min. ED_{95}: 200 μg/kg. Vd: 0.2 L. Duration: intermediate. Clearance: 5.5 ml/kg/min. $T_{1/2}$: 20 min. Protein binding: high. Metabolism: ester hydrolysis and Hofmann elimination; metabolites include laudanosine (convulsant properties in large doses). Excretion: renal and biliary; < 10% (unchanged).

Pharmacodynamics:

CVS:	Tachycardia, hypotension, vasodilation secondary to histamine release.
Pulmonary:	Bronchospasm secondary to histamine release.

Dosage/ Concentrations:	10 mg/ml.
Adult:	0.4–0.5 mg/kg.
Pediatric:	• Infant: 0.3–0.4 mg/kg.
	• Child and adolescent: 0.4–0.5 mg/kg.
Contraindications:	None.
Drug Interactions/ Allergy:	Prolonged action with inhalation agents. Inconsistent duration with combinations of other nondepolarizing agents. Probable prolonged effects with some antibiotics and anticonvulsants.

CISATRACURIUM

Trade Name:	Nimbex
Indications:	Endotracheal intubation and skeletal muscle relaxation during surgery or mechanical ventilation.
Pharmacokinetics:	Onset: 1.5–2 min. Peak effect: 3–3.5 min. ED_{95}: 50 μg/kg. Vd at steady-state: 145 ml/kg. Clearance; 5 ml/kg/min (Hofmann degradation). $T_{1/2}$: Children, 22 min; elderly, 26 min. Duration: intermediate–long.

Pharmacodynamics:

CVS:	Lack of histamine release.
Musculoskeletal:	Muscle weakness.

Dosage/ Concentration:	2 mg/ml in 10-ml vial.
Adult:	0.15–0.2 mg/kg.
Pediatric:	0.1 mg/kg.

CISATRACURIUM *(continued)*

Contraindications:	None.
Drug Interactions/ Allergy:	Prolonged action with inhalation agents. Inconsistent duration with combinations of other nondepolarizing agents. Probable prolonged effects with some antibiotics and anticonvulsants.

DOXACURIUM CHLORIDE

Trade Name:	Nuromax
Indications:	Endotracheal intubation and skeletal muscle relaxation during surgery or mechanical ventilation.
Pharmacokinetics:	Onset: 4–5 min. ED_{95}: 25 μg/kg. Vd: 0.2 L/kg. Duration: long. Clearance: 2.5 ml/kg/min. $T_{1/2}$: 120 min. Protein binding: 30%. Metabolism: minimal. Excretion: primarily via renal and biliary pathways (unchanged).
Pharmacodynamics:	
Hepatic:	Prolonged duration in hepatic failure.
Renal:	Prolonged duration in renal disease.
Other:	Prolonged duration in elderly.
Dosage/ Concentrations:	1 mg/ml.
Adult:	0.05 mg/kg.
Pediatric:	• Child, 0.05 mg/kg.
	• Adolescent, 0.05 mg/kg.
Contraindications:	None.
Drug Interactions/ Allergy:	Prolonged action with inhalation agents. Inconsistent duration with combinations of other nondepolarizing agents. Probable prolonged effects with some antibiotics, anticonvulsants, and calcium channel blockers.

METOCURINE IODIDE

Trade Name:	Metubine Iodide
Indications:	Endotracheal intubation and skeletal muscle relaxation during surgery or mechanical ventilation.
Pharmacokinetics:	Onset: 3–5 min. ED_{95}: 0.28 mg/kg. Vd: 0.4 L/kg. Duration: long. Clearance: 1.3 ml/kg/min. $T_{1/2}$: 220 min.

Protein binding: moderate. Metabolism: hepatic. Excretion: 50% renal (unchanged).

Pharmacodynamics:
CVS: Tachycardia, hypotension secondary to histamine release.
Pulmonary: Bronchospasm secondary to histamine release.
Renal: Prolonged duration in renal disease.

Dosage/ 2 mg/ml.
Concentrations:
Adult: 0.3 mg/kg.
Pediatric: • Child 0.2–0.3 mg/kg.

• Adolescent: 0.2–0.3 mg/kg.

Contraindications: Hypersensitivity to iodine.

Drug Interactions/ Prolonged action with inhalation agents. Inconsistent
Allergy: duration with combinations of other nondepolarizing agents. Probable prolonged effects with some antibiotics and anticonvulsants.

MIVACURIUM CHLORIDE

Trade Name: Mivacron

Indications: Endotracheal intubation and skeletal muscle relaxation during surgery or mechanical ventilation.

Pharmacokinetics: Onset: 2–2.5 min. ED_{95}: 80 µg/kg. Vd: 0.2 L/kg. Duration: short. Clearance: 4.2 ml/kg/min. $T_{1/2}$: 2–3 min. Protein binding: minimal. Metabolism: hydrolysis by plasma cholinesterase. Excretion: renal and biliary pathways (minor).

Pharmacodynamics:
CVS: Tachycardia, hypotension, vasodilation secondary to histamine release.
Pulmonary: Bronchospasm secondary to histamine release.
Hepatic: Prolonged duration (300%) in hepatic failure.
Renal: Prolonged duration (50%) in renal failure.
Other: Prolonged duration in elderly.

Dosage/ 2 mg/ml vials; also premixed flexible container of 50
Concentrations: or 100 ml (0.5 mg/ml in 5% dextrose).
Adult: 0.15–0.2 mg/kg.
Pediatric: • Infant: 0.2 mg/kg.

• Child and adolescent: 0.2 mg/kg.

Contraindications: Use extreme caution in patients with abnormal or atypical plasma cholinesterase activity.

MIVACURIUM CHLORIDE *(continued)*

Drug Interactions/ Allergy:	Prolonged action with inhalation agents. Possible prolonged effect with combinations of other nondepolarizing agents. Probable prolonged effects with some antibiotics and anticonvulsants.

PANCURONIUM BROMIDE

Trade Name: Pavulon

Indications: Endotracheal intubation and skeletal muscle relaxation during surgery or mechanical ventilation.

Pharmacokinetics: ED_{95}: 50 μg/kg. Vd: 0.3 L/kg. Duration: long. Clearance: 1–2 ml/kg/min. $T_{1/2}$: 100–130 min. Protein binding: 80%. Metabolism: hepatic, 25% as 3 hydroxy ($^1/_2$ as potent as pancuronium). Excretion: renal, 80% (unchanged); bile, 10% (unchanged).

Pharmacodynamics:
CVS: Tachycardia, ↑ BP, cardiac output secondary to vagolytic effects.
Hepatic: Prolonged duration in hepatic failure.
Renal: Prolonged duration in renal failure.

Dosage/
Concentrations: 1 or 2 mg/ml.
Adult: 0.06–0.1 mg/kg.
Pediatric:
- Neonate: 0.02 mg/kg (as test dose).
- Infant: 0.06–0.1 mg/kg.
- Child and adolescent: 0.06–0.1 mg/kg.

Contraindications: None.

Drug Interactions/
Allergy: Prolonged action with inhalation agents. Inconsistent duration with combinations of other nondepolarizing agents. Probable prolonged effects with some antibiotics, anticonvulsants, and TCAs. ↓ Effect with steroid treatment.

PIPECURONIUM BROMIDE

Trade Name: Arduan

Indications: Endotracheal intubation and skeletal muscle relaxation during surgery or mechanical ventilation

Pharmacokinetics: Onset: 3 min. ED_{95}: 50 μg/kg Vd: 0.3 L/kg. Duration long. Clearance: 2.4 ml/kg/min. $T_{1/2}$: 140 min. Metabolism: metabolites include active 3-decacetyl. Excretion: primarily renal.

Pharmacodynamics:
Hepatic: Probable prolonged duration in hepatic failure.
Renal: Prolonged duration in renal failure.

Dosage/   Powder for reconstitution.
Concentrations:
Adult: 0.07–0.085 mg/kg.
Pediatric: • Infant: 0.04 mg/kg (ED_{95}).

                    • Child and adolescent: 0.05 mg/kg (ED_{95}).

Contraindications: None.

Drug Interactions/   Prolonged action with inhalation agents. Inconsistent
Allergy: duration with combinations of other nondepolarizing
                         agents. Possible prolonged effects with some antibiotics and anticonvulsants.

ROCURONIUM BROMIDE

Trade Name: Zemuron

Indications: Endotracheal intubation and skeletal muscle relaxation during surgery or mechanical ventilation

Pharmacokinetics: Onset 1–3 min (dose dependent). ED_{95}: 300 µg/kg.
                        Vd: 0.3 L/kg. Duration: intermediate. Clearance: 4.0
                        ml/kg/min. $T_{1/2}$: 130 min. Protein binding: 30%. Metabolism: primarily hepatic. Excretion: primarily hepatic.

Pharmacodynamics:
CVS: Transient tachycardia in children.
Hepatic: Prolonged duration (50%) in hepatic failure.
Renal: Variable duration in renal failure.

Dosage/   10 mg/ml.
Concentrations:
Adult: 0.6–1.2 mg/kg.
Pediatric: • Infant: 0.6 mg/kg.

                    • Child and adolescent: 0.6 mg/kg.

Contraindications: None.

Drug Interactions/   Prolonged action with inhalation agents. Possible pro-
Allergy: longed effect with combinations of other nondepolarizing agents. Probable prolonged effects with some antibiotics and anticonvulsants.

SUCCINYLCHOLINE

Trade Names:	Anectine, Quelicin
Indications:	Rapid sequence inductions, endotracheal intubation, and skeletal muscle relaxation during surgery.
Pharmacokinetics:	Onset: 1–2 min, 3–5 min IM. ED$_{95}$: 300 μg/kg. Vd: N/A. Duration: ultrashort. Clearance: N/A. T$_{1/2}$: 2–4 min. Metabolism: hydrolyzed by plasma cholinesterase. Excretion: renal; 10% (unchanged).

Pharmacodynamics:

CNS:	↑ ICP, ↑ intraocular pressure, ↑ K$^+$ in patients with denervation, e.g., burns, tetanus, paraplegia, spinal cord transection, crush injury, neuromuscular disease, stroke, prolonged immobility.
CVS:	Bradycardia, asystole, nodal or ventricular escape related to vagal stimulation, possible cardiac arrest in patients with denervation.
GI:	↑ Intragastric pressure clinically balanced by ↑ esophageal sphincter tone.
Musculoskeletal:	Fasciculations, myalgia, jaw muscle spasm, phase II block.
Dosage/ Concentrations:	20, 50, 100 mg/ml.
Adult:	1–1.5 mg/kg; 3–4 mg/kg (IM).
Pediatric:	• Infant: 2–3 mg/kg (+atropine 10–20 μg/kg); 5 mg/kg (IM). • Child and adolescent: 2 mg/kg; 3–4 mg/kg (IM).
Contraindications:	History or family history of malignant hyperthermia or with genetic or induced disorders of plasma cholinesterase. Use extreme caution in patients with myopathies (especially Duchenne's)
Drug Interactions/ Allergy:	Block antagonized by nondepolarizing neuromuscular blocking agents. Effect potentiated by cholinesterase inhibitors, inhalational anesthetics, and lithium. Concomitant use of digitalis glycosides may cause arrhythmias.

TUBOCURARINE CHLORIDE

Trade Name:	N/A
Indications:	Defasciculating agent prior to succinylcholine administration. Endotracheal intubation and skeletal muscle relaxation during surgery or mechanical ventilation.

Pharmacokinetics:	Onset: 2–5 min. ED$_{95}$: 0.5 µg/kg. Vd: 0.3 L/kg. Duration: long. Clearance: 1–3 ml/kg/min. T$_{1/2}$: 84–120 min. Protein binding: moderate. Metabolism: hepatic. Excretion: renal, 40% (unchanged); biliary, 12% (unchanged).

Pharmacodynamics:

CNS:	Blocked autonomic ganglia.
CVS:	Tachycardia, hypotension secondary to histamine release.
Pulmonary:	Bronchospasm secondary to histamine release.
Hepatic:	Prolonged duration in hepatic disease.
Renal:	Prolonged duration in renal disease.

Dosage/ Concentrations:	3 mg/ml.
Adult:	0.3–0.5 mg/kg.
Pediatric:	• Infant: 0.25–0.5 mg/kg.
	• Child and adolescent: 0.5 mg/kg.

Contraindications:	None.
Drug Interactions/ Allergy:	Prolonged action with inhalation agents. Inconsistent duration with combinations of other nondepolarizing agents. Probable prolonged effects with some antibiotics and anticonvulsants.

VECURONIUM BROMIDE

Trade Name:	Norcuron
Indications:	Endotracheal intubation and skeletal muscle relaxation during surgery or mechanical ventilation
Pharmacokinetics:	Onset: 2.5–3 min. ED$_{95}$: 50 µg/kg. Vd: 0.3–0.4 L/kg. Duration: intermediate. Clearance: 3–4.5 ml/kg/min. T$_{1/2}$: 65–75 min. Protein binding: 60%–80%. Metabolism: 5%–10% hepatic. Excretion: 30%–35% renal (unchanged); 25%–50% in bile.

Pharmacodynamics:

Hepatic:	Prolonged duration in hepatic disease.
Renal:	Prolonged duration in renal failure.

Dosage/ Concentrations:	Powder for reconstitution.
Adult:	0.08–0.1 mg/kg.
Pediatric:	• Infant: 0.1 mg/kg.
	• Child and adolescent: 0.1 mg/kg.

VECURONIUM BROMIDE   *(continued)*

Contraindications: None known.

Drug Interactions/   Prolonged action with inhalation agents. Inconsistent
Allergy: duration with combinations of other nondepolarizing
                        agents. Probable prolonged effects with some antibiot-
                        ics and anticonvulsants.

30

Nonsteroidal Anti-inflammatory Drugs

Andrew J. Souter, M.B., Ch.B.

ACETAMINOPHEN

Trade Names:	Tylenol, Panadol
Indications:	Mild to moderate pain and fever.
Pharmacokinetics:	Vd: 0.94 L/kg. Clearance: 19.3 L/hr. $T_{1/2}$: β, 2.8 hr.

Pharmacodynamics:

CNS:	Analgesic and antipyretic effects.
GI:	Nausea, vomiting, and hepatotoxicity in overdose.
Other:	Agranulocytosis, thrombocytopenia.

Dosage/ Concentrations:	Oral solution: 100 mg/ml. Tablet: 120–500 mg. Suppository: 120–650 mg.
Adult (oral):	350–1000 mg q 3–6 hr; maximum daily dose, 4 g.
Pediatric (oral):	• 0–3 months, 40 mg q 4 hr
	• 4–12 months, 80 mg q 4 hr
	• 1–2 yr, 120 mg q 4 hr
	• 2–4 yr, 160 mg q 4 hr
	• 4–6 yr, 240 mg q 4 hr
	• 6–9 yr, 320 mg q 4 hr
	• 9–12 yr, 320–480 mg q 4 hr

Contraindications:	Viral hepatitis, hepatocellular disease, phenylketonuria, severe renal impairment, and alcoholism.
Drug Interactions/ Allergy:	↑ Risk of hepatotoxicity with alcohol, hepatic enzyme–inducing, and hepatotoxic medications. ↑ Prothrombin time with anticoagulants. ↑ Risk of nephropathy with NSAIDs.

ASPIRIN (ACETYLSALICYLIC ACID)

Trade Name:	Anacin
Indications:	Mild to moderate pain, fever, inflammation, rheumatic conditions, and thromboembolic prophylaxis.
Pharmacokinetics:	Vd: 0.15 L/kg. Clearance: 3.9 L/hr. $T_{1/2}$: β, 0.25 hr; β of active metabolite, salicylate: 2–30 hr.

Pharmacodynamics:

CNS:	Analgesic, anti-inflammatory, and antipyretic effects; tinnitus.
Respiratory:	Bronchospasm.
GI:	Peptic mucosal damage; ulceration and bleeding.
Other:	Irreversible inhibition of platelet aggregation, angioneurotic edema.

Dosage/ Concentrations:	Tablet: 80–650 mg. Suppository: 60–650 mg.
Adult (oral):	325–1000 mg q 3–6 hr; maximum daily dose, 4 g.
Pediatric (oral):	• 0–6 yr: safety not established
	• > 6 yr: 325 mg q 4–6 hr
Contraindications:	Peptic ulceration or bleeding, moderate to severe renal impairment, angioneurotic edema, and asthma.
Drug Interactions/ Allergy:	↑ Risk of GI and renal side effects with alcohol, other NSAIDs, and acetaminophen. ↑ Anticoagulant effect with other anticoagulants, heparin, and thrombolytic agents. ↑ Plasma levels of anticonvulsants and antidiabetic medications can lead to toxicity.

DICLOFENAC SODIUM

Trade Name:	Voltaren
Indications:	Pain, inflammation, and rheumatic conditions.
Pharmacokinetics:	Vd: 0.15 L/kg. Clearance: 15.6 L/hr. $T_{1/2}$: β, 1.5 hr.
Pharmacodynamics:	
CNS:	Analgesic, anti-inflammatory and antipyretic effects.
Respiratory:	Bronchospasm.
GI:	Mucosal damage; ulceration and bleeding.
Other:	Reversible inhibition of platelet aggregation.
Dosage/ Concentrations:	Tablet: 25, 50, 75 mg.
Adult:	25–100 mg q 8–12 hr; maximum daily dose, 200 mg.
Pediatric:	Dosage not established.
Contraindications:	Peptic ulceration, GI bleeding, and asthma.
Drug Interactions/ Allergy:	↓ Excretion of methotrexate, lithium, and digoxin can cause toxicity. Sodium and water retention can cause decreased effect of diuretics and antihypertensive medication. Concurrent use of other NSAIDs or acetaminophen increases risk of nephropathy or GI side effects.

DIFLUNISAL

Trade Name:	Dolobid
Indications:	Pain, inflammation, and rheumatic conditions.
Pharmacokinetics:	Vd: 0.11 L/kg. Clearance: 0.35–0.49 L/hr. $T_{1/2}$: β, 10.8 hr.

DIFLUNISAL   *(continued)*

Pharmacodynamics:
CNS: Analgesic, anti-inflammatory, and antipyretic effects.
Respiratory: Bronchospasm.
GI: Mucosal damage; ulceration and bleeding.
Other: Reversible inhibition of platelet aggregation.

Dosage/   Tablet: 250 mg, 500 mg.
Concentrations:
Adult: 250–500 mg q 8–12 hr; maximum daily dose, 1.5 g.
Pediatric: Dosage not established.

Contraindications: Peptic ulceration, GI bleeding, and asthma.

Drug Interactions/   ↓ Excretion of methotrexate, lithium, and digoxin can
Allergy: cause toxicity. Sodium and water retention can cause
                          decreased effect of diuretics and antihypertensive medi-
                          cation. Concurrent use of other NSAIDs or acetamino-
                          phen increases risk of nephropathy or GI side effects.

FLURBIPROFEN

Trade Name: Ansaid

Indications: Pain, inflammation, and rheumatic conditions.

Pharmacokinetics: Vd: 0.1 L/kg. Clearance: 1.3 L/hr. $T_{1/2}$: β, 3.5 hr.

Pharmacodynamics:
CNS: Analgesic, anti-inflammatory, and antipyretic effects.
Respiratory: Bronchospasm.
GI: Mucosal damage; ulceration and bleeding.
Other: Reversible inhibition of platelet aggregation.

Dosage/   Tablet: 50, 100 mg.
Concentrations:
Adult: 50–100 mg q 6–12 hr; maximum daily dose, 300 mg.
Pediatric: Dosage not established.

Contraindications: Peptic ulceration, GI bleeding, and asthma.

Drug Interactions/   ↓ Excretion of methotrexate, lithium, and digoxin can
Allergy: cause toxicity. Sodium and water retention can cause
                          decreased effect of diuretics and antihypertensive medi-
                          cation. Concurrent use of other NSAIDs or acetamino-
                          phen increases risk of nephropathy or GI side effects.

IBUPROFEN

Trade Names:	Motrin, Nuprin
Indications:	Mild to moderate pain, inflammation, fever, and rheumatic conditions.
Pharmacokinetics:	Vd: 0.14 L/kg. Clearance: 3.5 L/hr. $T_{1/2}$: β, 2.5 hr.

Pharmacodynamics:

CNS:	Analgesic, anti-inflammatory, and antipyretic effects.
Respiratory:	Bronchospasm.
GI:	Peptic mucosal damage; ulceration and bleeding.
Renal:	Inhibition of prostaglandin-mediated autoregulation.
Other:	Reversible inhibition of platelet aggregation.

Dosage/ Concentrations:	Oral suspension: 100 mg/5 ml. Tablet: 200–400 mg.
Adult:	300–800 mg q 4–6 hr; maximum daily dose, 3.2 g.
Pediatric:	• 0–12 months: safety and efficacy not established
	• 1–12 yr: 30–40 mg/kg per 24 hr in 3–4 divided doses
Contraindications:	Asthma, peptic ulceration, bleeding, and renal impairment.
Drug Interactions/ Allergy:	↓ Excretion of methotrexate, lithium, and digoxin can cause toxicity. Sodium and water retention can cause decreased effect of diuretics and antihypertensive medication. Concurrent use of other NSAIDs or acetaminophen increases risk of nephropathy or GI side effects.

INDOMETHACIN

Trade Name:	Indocin
Indications:	Pain, inflammation, rheumatic conditions in which less toxic NSAIDs are ineffective, and ankylosing spondylitis.
Pharmacokinetics:	Vd: 0.2 L/kg. Clearance: 6.3 L/hr. $T_{1/2}$: β, 6 hr.

Pharmacodynamics:

CNS:	Analgesic, anti-inflammatory, and antipyretic effects.
Respiratory:	Bronchospasm.
GI:	Peptic mucosal damage; ulceration and bleeding.
Renal:	Inhibition of prostaglandin-mediated autoregulation.
Other:	Reversible inhibition of platelet aggregation.

Dosage/ Concentrations:	Tablet: 25, 50 mg.

INDOMETHACIN *(continued)*

Adult:	25–50 mg q 6–12 hr; maximum daily dose, 200 mg.
Pediatric:	1.5–2.5 mg/kg per 24 hr in 3 or 4 divided doses.

Contraindications: Asthma, peptic ulceration or bleeding, moderate to severe renal impairment, pregnancy, and breast-feeding.

Drug Interactions/ Allergy: ↓ Excretion of methotrexate, lithium, and digoxin can cause toxicity. Sodium and water retention can cause decreased effect of diuretics and antihypertensive medication. Concurrent use of other NSAIDs or acetaminophen increases risk of nephropathy or GI side effects.

KETOPROFEN

Trade Name: Orudis

Indications: Pain, inflammation, and rheumatic conditions.

Pharmacokinetics: Vd: 0.11 L/kg. Clearance: 5.2 L/hr. $T_{1/2}$: β, 1.4 hr.

Pharmacodynamics:
CNS: Analgesic, anti-inflammatory, and antipyretic effects.
Respiratory: Bronchospasm.
GI: Mucosal damage; ulceration and bleeding.
Other: Reversible inhibition of platelet aggregation.

Dosage/ Concentrations: Tablet: 25, 50, 75 mg.

Adult:	50–75 mg q 6–8 hr; maximum daily dose, 300 mg.
Pediatric:	Dosage not established.

Contraindications: Peptic ulceration, GI bleeding, and asthma.

Drug Interactions/ Allergy: ↓ Excretion of methotrexate, lithium, and digoxin can cause toxicity. Sodium and water retention can cause decreased effect of diuretics and antihypertensive medication. Concurrent use of other NSAIDs or acetaminophen increases risk of nephropathy or GI side effects.

KETOROLAC TROMETHAMINE

Trade Name: Toradol

Indications: Moderate to severe postoperative pain.

Pharmacokinetics: Vd: 0.11–0.25 L/kg. Clearance: 0.35–0.55 L/hr. $T_{1/2}$: β, 5.4 hr.

Pharmacodynamics:
CNS: Analgesic, anti-inflammatory, and antipyretic effects.
Respiratory: Bronchospasm.
GI: Dose-related mucosal damage; ulceration and bleeding.
Renal: Inhibited prostaglandin-mediated autoregulation.
Other: Reversible inhibition of platelet aggregation.

Dosage/   Tablet: 10 mg. Injection: 15, 30, 60 mg.
Concentrations:
Adult: Initial dose, 30–60 mg, then 15–30 mg q 6 hr
                    IM/IV; maximum daily dose, 150 mg first day;
                    120 mg subsequent days; limit, 5 days.
                        10 mg q 4–6 hr p.o.
Pediatric: Safety and efficacy not established.

Contraindications: Peptic ulceration, GI bleeding, renal impairment, and
                    prerenal conditions (renal artery stenosis, hypovolemia,
                    dehydration), asthma, congestive heart failure, hyper-
                    tension, pregnancy, coagulopathy, abnormal platelet
                    function, and concurrent use of nephrotoxic drugs.

Drug Interactions/   ↓ Excretion of methotrexate, lithium, and digoxin can
Allergy: cause toxicity. Sodium and water retention can cause
                    decreased effect of diuretics and antihypertensive medi-
                    cation. Concurrent use of other NSAIDs or acetamino-
                    phen increases risk of nephropathy or GI side effects.

MEFENAMIC ACID

Trade Name: Ponstel

Indications: Pain, inflammation, rheumatic conditions, and dysmen-
                    orrhea.

Pharmacokinetics: Vd: 1.3 L/kg. $T_{1/2}$: β, 3.5 hr.

Pharmacodynamics:
CNS: Analgesic, anti-inflammatory, and antipyretic effects.
Respiratory: Bronchospasm.
GI: Mucosal damage; ulceration and bleeding.
Other: Reversible inhibition of platelet aggregation.

Dosage/   Tablet: 250 mg.
Concentrations:
Adult: Initial dose: 500 mg, then 250 mg q 6 hr.
Pediatric: Dosage not established.

Contraindications: Peptic ulceration, GI bleeding, and asthma.

MEFENAMIC ACID   *(continued)*

Drug Interactions/ Allergy:	↓ Excretion of methotrexate, lithium, and digoxin can cause toxicity. Sodium and water retention can cause decreased effect of diuretics and antihypertensive medication. Concurrent use of other NSAIDs or acetaminophen increases risk of nephropathy or GI side effects.

NAPROXEN

Trade Name:	Naprosyn
Indications:	Pain, inflammation, and rheumatic conditions.
Pharmacokinetics:	Vd: 0.1 L/kg. Clearance: 0.3 L/hr. T$_{1/2}$: β, 14 hr.
Pharmacodynamics:	
CNS:	Analgesic, anti-inflammatory, and antipyretic effects.
Respiratory:	Bronchospasm.
GI:	Mucosal damage; ulceration and bleeding.
Other:	Reversible inhibition of platelet aggregation.
Dosage/ Concentrations:	Oral suspension: 125 mg/ml. Tablet: 250, 500 mg.
Adult:	Initial dose: 500 mg, then 250 mg q 6 hr.
Pediatric:	10 mg/kg per 24 hr in 2 divided doses.
Contraindications:	Peptic ulceration, GI bleeding, and asthma.
Drug Interactions/ Allergy:	↓ Excretion of methotrexate, lithium, and digoxin can cause toxicity. Sodium and water retention can cause decreased effect of diuretics and antihypertensive medication. Concurrent use of other NSAIDs or acetaminophen increases risk of nephropathy or GI side effects.

PIROXICAM

Trade Name:	Feldene
Indications:	Pain, inflammation, and rheumatic conditions.
Pharmacokinetics:	Vd: 0.14 L/kg. Clearance: 0.14 L/hr. T$_{1/2}$: β, 45 hr.
Pharmacodynamics:	
CNS:	Analgesic, anti-inflammatory, and antipyretic effects.
Respiratory:	Bronchospasm.
GI:	Mucosal damage; ulceration and bleeding.
Other:	Reversible inhibition of platelet aggregation.

Dosage/ Concentrations:	Tablet: 10, 20 mg.
Adult:	20 mg once daily or 10 mg q 12 hr.
Pediatric:	Dosage not established.
Contraindications:	Peptic ulceration, GI bleeding, and asthma.
Drug Interactions/ Allergy:	↓ Excretion of methotrexate, lithium, and digoxin can cause toxicity. Sodium and water retention can cause decreased effect of diuretics and antihypertensive medication. Concurrent use of other NSAIDs or acetaminophen increases risk of nephropathy or GI side effects.

31

Opioid Agonists and Antagonists

Vincent A. Romanelli, M.D.

Opioid Agonists

ALFENTANIL

Trade Name:	Alfenta
Indications:	Induction and maintenance of general anesthesia.
Pharmacokinetics:	Vd: 0.86 L/kg ($\downarrow$ in children). Onset: rapid. Duration: short. Clearance: 6.4 ml/kg/min; reduced in hepatic cirrhosis. $T_{1/2}$: α, 11.6 min. β, 94 min ($\uparrow$ in elderly); elimination half-life increased in hepatic cirrhosis.

Pharmacodynamics:

CNS:	$\downarrow$ CBF, $\downarrow$ ICP, miosis, delta wave activity characteristic of deep non-REM sleep.
CVS:	Vagally mediated bradycardia.
Pulmonary:	Depressed ventilation, $\uparrow$ airway resistance.
Hepatic:	Biliary smooth muscle spasm, $\uparrow$ intrabiliary pressure.
Renal:	$\uparrow$ ADH secretion, urinary retention.
GI:	Nausea, vomiting, $\downarrow$ peristalsis, $\downarrow$ gastric emptying.
Musculoskeletal:	Skeletal truncal muscle rigidity from rapid IV dose.

Dosages/ Concentrations:	Supplied in 5 cc ampules; without preservative; 500 µg/cc.
	For induction of anesthesia: 20 to 75 µg/kg.
	For maintenance of anesthesia: 0.5 to 1.5 µg/kg/min titrated to anesthetic depth, supplemented with an amnestic agent, such as midazolam, or a low dose of a volatile agent, such as isoflurane. A muscle relaxant may also be required.
Contraindications:	Increased elimination half-lives in cirrhosis of the liver.
Drug Interactions/ Allergy:	The combination of an opioid agonist with N_2O in patients undergoing coronary revascularization results in cardiovascular depression. Concurrent use of a benzodiazepine may increase the risk of cardiovascular and respiratory depression.

FENTANYL

Trade Name:	Sublimaze
Indications:	Premedication, adjunct to general anesthesia intraoperatively and postoperatively (to provide analgesia), and primary anesthetic agent in high doses.

FENTANYL *(continued)*

Pharmacokinetics:	Vd: 4.0 L/kg. Duration: 2–4 hr. Clearance: 13.0 ml/kg/min. $T_{1/2}$: α, 13.4 min; β, 219 min.
Pharmacodynamics:	
CNS:	$\downarrow$ CBF, $\downarrow$ ICP, miosis, delta wave activity characteristic of deep non-REM sleep.
CVS:	Vagally mediated bradycardia.
Pulmonary:	Depressed ventilation, $\uparrow$ airway resistance.
Hepatic:	Biliary smooth muscle spasm, $\uparrow$ intrabiliary pressure.
Renal:	$\uparrow$ ADH secretion, urinary retention, adverse reaction in renal failure.
GI:	Nausea, vomiting, $\downarrow$ peristalsis, $\downarrow$ gastric emptying.
Musculoskeletal:	Skeletal truncal muscle rigidity is from rapid IV dose.
Dosage/ Concentrations:	Supplied in 2, 5, 10, and 20 cc ampules as sterile, aqueous, preservative-free solution for IV and epidural use; concentration 50 μg/ml. Total dosage: 2–100 μg/kg. Higher doses used in open heart and certain neurosurgical procedures when fentanyl is the primary anesthetic agent, supplemented by a muscle relaxant and an amnestic agent, such as midazolam, or a low dose of a volatile agent, such as isoflurane.
Contraindications:	None known.
Drug Interactions/ Allergy:	The combination of an opioid agonist with N_2O in patients undergoing coronary revascularization results in cardiovascular depression. Concurrent use of a benzodiazepine may increase the risk of cardiovascular and respiratory depression.

HYDROMORPHONE

Trade Name:	Dilaudid
Indications:	Postoperative and oncologic pain.
Pharmacokinetics:	$T_{1/2}$: β, 150 min.
Pharmacodynamics:	
CNS:	$\downarrow$ CBF, $\downarrow$ ICP, miosis, delta wave activity characteristic of deep non-REM sleep.
CVS:	Vagally mediated bradycardia.
Pulmonary:	Depressed ventilation, $\uparrow$ airway resistance.
Hepatic:	Biliary smooth muscle spasm, $\uparrow$ intrabiliary pressure.

Renal:	↑ ADH secretion, urinary retention.
GI:	Nausea, vomiting, ↓ peristalsis; ↓ gastric emptying.
Musculoskeletal:	Skeletal truncal muscle rigidity from rapid IV dose.

**Dosage/
Concentrations:**

Supplied in ampules, multiple-dose vials, oral tablets, and rectal suppositories.
Ampules and multiple-dose vials: 1, 2, and 4 mg/ml concentrations.
Tablets: 1, 2, 3, 4, and 8 mg.
Oral suspension: 1 mg/ml.
Injection: 10 mg/ml.

Contraindications: None known.

**Drug Interactions/
Allergy:**

The combination of an opioid agonist with N_2O in patients undergoing coronary revascularization results in cardiovascular depression. Concurrent use of a benzodiazepine may increase the risk for CV and respiratory depression.

MEPERIDINE (PETHIDINE)

Trade Name: Demerol

Indications: Premedication and postoperative pain.

Pharmacokinetics: Vd: 3.8 L/kg. Clearance: 15.1 ml/kg/min (↓ in elderly). $T_{1/2}$: α, 4–11 min; β, 180–264 min.

Pharmacodynamics:

CNS:	Analgesia, euphoria, hyperactive reflexes, seizures.
CVS:	Myocardial depression, ↑ HR.
Pulmonary:	Respiratory depression. Biliary smooth muscle spasm, ↑ adverse reaction in renal failure.
GI:	↓ Gastric emptying, peristalsis.
Musculoskeletal:	Muscle tremors.

**Dosage/
Concentrations:**

Supplied as 50 and 100 mg tablets; sterile cartridge needle of 25, 75, and 100 mg/cc concentration; vials and ampules in 5% and 10% solutions.
Oral starting dose: 300 mg; initial IM dose: 75 mg.

Contraindications: Patients receiving MAOIs.

**Drug Interactions/
Allergy:**

Concurrent use of MAOIs can result in hypertension, tachycardia, hyperpyrexia, and convulsions.

METHADONE

Trade Name:	Dolophine
Indications:	Moderate to severe pain. Narcotic abstinence syndrome suppressant and antitussive.
Pharmacokinetics:	$T_{1/2}$: β, 35 hr.

Pharmacodynamics:

CNS: ↓ CBF, ↓ ICP, miosis, delta wave activity characteristic of deep non-REM sleep.

CVS: Vagally mediated bradycardia, hypotension.

Pulmonary: Depressed ventilation, ↑ airway resistance.

Hepatic: Biliary smooth muscle spasm, ↑ intrabiliary pressure.

Renal: ↑ ADH secretion, urinary retention.

GI: Nausea, vomiting, ↓ intestinal peristalsis, ↓ gastric emptying.

Musculoskeletal: Skeletal truncal muscle rigidity from rapid IV dose.

Dosage/ Concentrations: Supplied in tablets, oral solution, ampules, and vials.
  Injection: 10 mg/ml.
  Oral solution: 5 and 10 mg/5 ml.
  Tablets: 5, 10, and 40 mg.
  Dose: 10 mg IM (equivalent to morphine 10 mg IM).
  Individualize dose for treatment of narcotic abstinence syndrome and chronic pain syndromes.

Contraindications: None known.

Drug Interactions/ Allergy: Urinary acidifiers may increase elimination of methadone, thereby potentially precipitating an acute withdrawal syndrome. Phenytoin or rifampin may increase methadone metabolism and precipitate withdrawal symptoms.

MORPHINE

Trade Names:	Duramorph, MS Contin
Indications:	Premedication and postoperative pain.
Pharmacokinetics:	Vd: 3.2 L/kg (↓ in elderly). Clearance: 15.0 ml/kg/min. $T_{1/2}$: α, 1.65 min; β, 180 min.

Pharmacodynamics:

CNS: ↓ CBF, ↓ ICP, miosis, delta wave activity characteristic of deep non-REM sleep.

CVS: Vagally mediated bradycardia, hypotension.

Pulmonary:	Depressed ventilation, ↑ airway resistance.
Hepatic:	Biliary smooth muscle spasm, ↑ intrabiliary pressure.
Renal:	↑ ADH secretion, urinary retention.
GI:	Nausea, vomiting, ↓ peristalsis, ↓ gastric emptying.
Musculoskeletal:	Skeletal truncal muscle rigidity from rapid IV dose.

**Dosage/
Concentrations:** Supplied in ampules and vials in concentrations of 1, 5, 8, 10, and 15 mg/ml. Tablet: 30, 60, and 100 mg. Epidural morphine (Duramorph) is preservative-free and supplied in concentrations of 0.5 and 1 mg/ml.
   For premedication: up to 0.15 mg/kg IM.
   For immediate postoperative analgesia: IV in a dose titrated to effect.
   For patient-controlled analgesia: 0.5–2.0 mg.

Contraindications: Infants < 4 wk of age.

**Drug Interactions/
Allergy:** Combination of an opioid agonist with N_2O in patients undergoing coronary revascularization results in cardiovascular depression. Concurrent use of a benzodiazepine may increase the risk of cardiovascular and respiratory depression.

REMIFENTANIL HYDROCHLORIDE

Trade Name: Ultiva

Indications: Induction and maintenance of general anesthesia, analgesia during monitored anesthesia care, and postoperative analgesia.

Pharmacokinetics: $T_{1/2}$: 1 min. (rapid); 6 min (slower); 10–20 min (elimination after IV); 3–10 min (biologic). Vc: 0.1 L/kg. Vd: 0.35 L/kg. Protein binding: 70% bound to plasma proteins. Clearance: 40 ml/kg/min (not influenced by plasma pseudocholinesterase level).

Pharmacodynamics:
CNS:	Analgesia, sedation.
CVS:	Bradycardia, MAP.
Pulmonary:	↓ Respiratory rate, ↓ central ventilatory drive.
GI:	Nausea, vomiting, urinary retention.
Musculoskeletal:	Muscle rigidity, twitching.

**Dosage/
Concentrations:** Vials containing 1, 2, or 5 mg are reconstituted and diluted to final concentrations of 25, 50, and 250 µg/ml.

REMIFENTANIL HYDROCHLORIDE   *(continued)*

Indication	Bolus Dose (μg/kg)	Initial Rate (μg/kg/min)	Continuous Infusion (μg/kg/min)
Induction of anesthesia	1	0.5	
Maintenance of anesthesia			
with nitrous oxide (60%–70%)	0.5–1	0.4	0.1–2
with isoflurane (0.4–1.5 MAC)	0.5–1	0.25	0.05–2
with propofol (100–200 μg/kg/min)	0.5–1	0.25	0.05–2
with benzodiazepine	0.5–1	1.5	0.5–2
Analgesia during monitored anesthesia care	0.5–1	0.1	0.025–0.2
Parenteral analgesic		0.1	0.025–0.2

Contraindications:	Epidural or intrathecal administration (formulation in glycine).
Drug Interactions/ Allergy:	Synergistic with sedative-hypnotics and inhaled anesthetics. No metabolic interactions with other esterase-hydrolyzed drugs (e.g., succinylcholine, mivacurium, esmolol).

SUFENTANIL

Trade Name:	Sufenta
Indications:	Adjunct to general anesthesia and primary anesthestic agent in high doses.
Pharmacokinetics:	Vd: 2.9 L/kg (↓ in elderly). Clearance: 12.7 ml/kg/min (↓ in elderly). $T_{1/2}$: α, 17.1 min; β, 164 min
Pharmacodynamics:	
CNS:	↓ CBF, ↓ ICP, miosis, delta wave activity characteristic of deep non-REM sleep.
CVS:	Vagally mediated bradycardia.
Pulmonary:	Depressed ventilation, ↑ airway resistance.
Hepatic:	Biliary smooth muscle spasm, ↑ intrabiliary pressure.
Renal:	↑ ADH secretion, urinary retention.
GI:	Nausea, vomiting, ↓ peristalsis, ↓ gastric emptying.
Musculoskeletal:	Skeletal truncal muscle rigidity from rapid IV dose.
Dosage/ Concentrations:	Supplied in 1, 2, and 5 cc ampules as sterile, aqueous, preservative-free solution for IV and epidural use; 50 μg/ml.
	Induction dose: 1–8 μg/kg. Total dosage: 2–30 μg/kg. Higher doses in open heart and certain neurosurgical procedures when sufentanil is the primary anesthet-

ic agent, supplemented by a muscle relaxant and an amnestic agent, such as midazolam, or a low dose of a volatile agent, such as isoflurane. Maintenance: infusion of 0.5 to 1.0 μg/kg/hr.

Contraindications: None known.

Drug Interactions/ Allergy: The combination of an opioid agonist with N_2O in patients undergoing coronary revascularization results in cardiovascular depression. Concurrent use of a benzodiazepine may increase the risk for cardiovascular and respiratory depression. Bradycardia can be treated by atropine.

Opioid Antagonists

NALMEFENE

Trade Name: Revex

Indications: Complete or partial reversal of opioid "overdose" and treatment of side effects secondary to epidural opioids postoperatively.

Pharmacokinetics: $T_{1/2}$: β, 9–11 hr. Absorption: high bioavailability after IV, IM, or SC dose. Peak effect: IV, 5–10 min; IM, 2 hr; SC, 1.5 hr. Vd: 3.9 ± 1.1 L/kg; steady-state, 8.6 ± 1.7 L/kg. Protein binding: 45%. Metabolism: hepatic. Clearance: 0.8 L/kg/hr; lower in hepatic disease and renal failure.

Pharmacodynamics:
CNS: Dizziness, headache, somnolence, agitation ("withdrawal syndrome").
CVS: Hypertension, tachycardia, vasodilation.
Pulmonary: Pharyngitis.
GI: Nausea, vomiting, dry mouth, diarrhea.
Musculoskeletal: Tremor.
Other: Fever, chills.

Dosage/ Concentrations: 1 ml (0.1 mg/ml) or 2 ml (1 mg/ml) vials.
For postoperative use: 0.1 mg IV (0.25 μg/kg at 2.5-minute intervals).
For opioid overdose: 0.5–1.5 mg IV.

Contraindications: None known.

Drug Interactions/ Allergy: Reversal of opioid effects.

NALOXONE

Trade Name: Narcan

Indications: Reversal of opioid-induced respiratory depression and sedation.

Pharmacokinetics: Vd: 1.8 L/kg. Clearance: 30.1 ml/kg/min. $T_{1/2}$: β, 64 min. Metabolism: hepatic; extensive first-pass.

Pharmacodynamics:

CNS: Acute withdrawal syndrome, reversal of analgesia and dysphoria.

CVS: Hypertension, tachycardia, ventricular fibrillation.

Pulmonary: Reversal of respiratory depression, ↑ respiratory rate, ↑ pulmonary edema.

GI: Nausea, vomiting.

Musculoskeletal: Seizures, tremulousness.

Dosage/ Concentrations: Supplied as ampules and prefilled syringes; either 0.4 mg/ml or 1.0 mg/ml. Oral dose ⅟₅₀ as effective as same dose given systemically.

Adult: For known or suspected narcotic overdose: 0.4 to 1.0 mg IV; repeat at 2- to 3-min intervals. Limit: total dose 10 mg.

     For postoperative narcotic depression: 0.08-mg increments IV q 2 to 3 min until adequate ventilation and alertness are obtained without significant pain or discomfort.

Pediatric: For narcotic overdose: initial dose, 0.01 mg/kg IV or IM; if no effect is seen, give a subsequent dose of 0.1 mg/kg.

     For postoperative narcotic depression: 0.005–0.01 mg IV at 2- to 3-min intervals until desired degree of reversal is obtained.

Contraindications: None known.

Drug Interactions/ Allergy: The agonist action of morphine outlasts the antagonist action of naloxone; either repeated doses or a continuous infusion of naloxone may be required for effective reversal. Reversal of opioid effects (analgesia).

NALTREXONE

Trade Name: Trexan

Indications: Treatment of detoxified, formerly opioid-dependent individuals.

Pharmacokinetics:	$T_{1/2}$: β, 4 hr; 6-β-naltrexol (metabolite), 13 hr. Metabolism: hepatic; extensive first pass.
Pharmacodynamics:	
CNS:	Acute withdrawal syndrome, reversal of analgesia and dysphoria.
CVS:	Hypertension, tachycardia.
Pulmonary:	Reversal of respiratory depression.
GI:	Nausea, vomiting.
Musculoskeletal:	Seizures, tremulousness.
Dosage/ Concentrations:	Supplied in oral tablets: 50 mg/tablet.
Adult:	Oral: 25 mg; an additional 25 mg dose may be given 1 hr later if no withdrawal symptoms occur. Maintenance: 50 mg q 24 hr.
Pediatric:	< 18 yr: not established.
Contraindications:	None known.
Drug Interactions/ Allergy:	Reversal of opioid effects (analgesia).

Opioid Agonist-Antagonists

BUTORPHANOL

Trade Name:	Stadol
Indications:	Moderate to severe pain and postoperative and obstetric analgesia during labor and delivery.
Pharmacokinetics:	Vd: 7 L/kg (↑ in elderly). Clearance: 23.5 ml/kg/min (↓ in elderly and in renal failure). $T_{1/2}$: α, 5.0 min. β, 150 min (↑ in elderly and renal failure). Metabolism: hepatic. Elimination: renal (75%).
Pharmacodynamics:	
CNS:	Acute withdrawal syndrome, dysphoric reactions, analgesia, sedation, ↑ ICP.
CVS:	↑ Pulmonary artery pressure, ↑ myocardial work, ↑ oxygen demand.
Pulmonary:	Respiratory depression (can reverse respiratory depression of pure agonist opioids).
GI:	Nausea, vomiting.
Dosage/ Concentrations:	Supplied in vials and multidose vials: 1 and 2 mg/ml. In severe renal dysfunction, increase dosage interval. For labor pain: 1 to 2 mg IV or IM, repeat at 4-hr intervals.

BUTORPHANOL *(continued)*

For premedication: 2 mg IM.
For postoperative analgesia: 0.5–2 mg; repeat at intervals of 3–4 hr.

Contraindications:	Allergy to benzethonium chloride (preservative). Use caution in acute MI, ventricular dysfunction, and coronary artery disease.
Drug Interactions/ Allergy:	Reversal of opioid effects (postoperative respiratory depression).

DEZOCINE

Trade Name:	Dalgan
Indications:	Moderate to severe pain, short-term relief of pain, and postoperative analgesia.
Pharmacokinetics:	Vd: 8.8–10.7 L/kg (↑ in hepatic cirrhosis). Clearance: 3.33 L/hr/kg. $T_{1/2}$: β, 1.7–2.4 hr (↑ in hepatic cirrhosis). Metabolism: hepatic. Elimination: 66% of a single dose excreted in urine as unchanged (1%) and glucuronide conjugate.
Pharmacodynamics:	
CNS:	↑ ICP, CNS depression, withdrawal reactions.
Pulmonary:	Respiratory depression (maximum respiratory depression occurs with a total cumulative dose of about 30 mg/kg; can reverse respiratory depression of pure agonist opioids).
GI:	Nausea, vomiting, spasm of the sphincter of Oddi, biliary colic.
Dosage/ Concentrations:	Supplied in injectable form: 5, 10, and 15 mg/ml.
Adult:	IM: 5–20 mg initially (usually 10 mg); repeat dose at 3- to 6-hr intervals. IV: 2.5 to 10 mg initially (usually 5 mg); repeat q 2 to 4 hr p.r.n.
Pediatric:	Not recommended for patients under age 18 yr.
Contraindications:	Children (under age 18 yr) and allergy to sodium metabisulfite (preservative).
Drug Interactions/ Allergy:	Reversal of opioid effects (postoperative respiratory depression).

NALBUPHINE

Trade Name:	Nubain
Indications:	Moderate to severe pain, analgesia and sedation in patients with heart disease, and postoperative and obstetric analgesia during labor and delivery.
Pharmacokinetics:	Vd: 2.9 L/kg. Clearance: 15.6–22 ml/kg/min. $T_{1/2}$: β, 120–210 min. Metabolism: hepatic; extensive first-pass biotransformation. Elimination: only 7% excreted in urine as unchanged and metabolites.

Pharmacodynamics:

CNS:	↑ ICP, withdrawal reactions.
Pulmonary:	Respiratory depression, asthma.
GI:	Nausea, vomiting, spasm of the sphincter of Oddi, biliary colic.

Dosage/ Concentrations:	Supplied in ampules, multiple-dose vials, and prefilled syringes: 10 and 20 mg/ml.
Adult:	10 mg IM or IV; repeat q 3–6 hr.
Contraindications:	Allergy to sodium metabisulfate (preservative).
Drug Interactions/ Allergy:	Reversal of opioid effects (postoperative respiratory depression).

32

Psychotropic Drugs

Anthony M. Nyerges, M.D.

AMITRIPTYLINE

Trade Name:	Elavil
Indications:	Depressive affective mood disorder, enuresis, psychoneurotic anxiety, phobic disorder, panic attack, bulimia, and chronic pain states.
Pharmacokinetics:	Plasma protein binding: high. pKa: 9.4. Peak plasma levels: 2–12 hr. $T_{1/2}$: β, 10–50 hr. 25%–50% inactive metabolites in urine.

Pharmacodynamics:

CNS:	Drowsiness, confusion, and disorientation in elderly; emotional instability in children; extrapyramidal symptoms and anticholinergic activity (mydriasis, cycloplegia), seizures in children.
CVS:	Quinidine-like cardiotoxic effects, postural hypotension, conduction disturbances (AV bundle branch blocks), hypertensive crisis during anesthesia.
Hepatic:	↑ Transaminases, allergic hepatitis.
Renal:	SIADH, paradoxical urinary frequency (at high doses), urinary retention (at low doses).
GI:	Diarrhea and nausea, ileus.
Dosage/ Concentrations:	Tablet: 10, 25, 50, 75, 100, 150 mg. Injection: 10 mg/ml. Maximum: 300 mg daily. Maintenance: 50 mg daily.
Adult:	Initial dose: 75 mg daily.
Pediatric:	30 mg daily.
Contraindications:	Benign prostatic hypertrophy, angle-closure glaucoma, hyperthyroid states, predisposition to seizure states, acute recovery phase of MI, and pre-existing AV block.
Drug Interactions/ Allergy:	Concurrent use of MAOIs and TCAs can trigger hyperpyretic crisis. Inhibits effect of clonidine. Potentiated effects of alcohol, hypnotics, and sympathomimetic drugs. ↑ TCA levels with SSRIs and TCAs. ↑ Plasma dicumarol levels. Cardiac arrhythmogenicity with levothyroxine. ↑ Sedation of opiates and barbiturates. ↑ Delirium with central anticholinergics.

DEXTROAMPHETAMINE

Trade Name:	Dexedrine
Indications:	Narcolepsy, attention deficit disorder with hyperactivity, short-term treatment of obesity, and excessive sedation from opiate use in pain management

DEXTROAMPHETAMINE   *(continued)*

Pharmacokinetics:	Inactivation by MAOIs. High lipid solubility. Vd: >10 L/kg. $T_{1/2}$: β, 5–20 hr. Elimination: 2%–3% urinary excretion. Direct action on α and β sites; release of norepinephrine, especially in cerebral cortex.

Pharmacodynamics:

CNS:	Sympathomimetic effects, euphoria, seizures, hyperexcitability.
CVS:	Cardiomyopathy, cardiac dysrhythmias, labile BP, ↑ HR.
Pulmonary:	↑ Respiration.
GI:	Anorexia, diarrhea.
Musculoskeletal:	Rhabdomyolysis.
Other:	Hyperpyrexia, pancytopenia.

Dosage/ Concentrations:

Adult:	10 mg daily; maximum 60 mg daily.
Pediatric:	2.5–5 mg q.d.; maximum 40 mg daily. For obesity: 5–30 mg daily, divided t.i.d.

Contraindications:	Pregnancy, < 6 yr of age, Tourette's syndrome, concurrent MAOI use, halothane general anesthesia (dysrhythmias), hyperthyroidism, coronary atherosclerosis
Drug Interactions/ Allergy:	With MAOIs: hypertension, hyperpyretic crisis, stroke. With halothane: ventricular arrhythmias. With epinephrine: ventricular dysrhythmias, hypertension crisis. With levothyroxine: hypertension crisis.

DROPERIDOL

Trade Name:	Inapsine
Indications:	Psychosis, vomiting, agitation, and neurolepsis.
Pharmacokinetics:	Vd: 2 L/kg. $T_{1/2}$: β, 100 min. Total body clearance: dependent on hepatic blood flow. Clearance: 14 ml/kg/min. Metabolism: hepatic (extensive).
Pharmacodynamics: *CNS:*	CNS tranquilizing and neuroleptic effects. Extrapyramidal reactions, akathisia, restlessness, excessive drowsiness, tardive dyskinesia, neuroleptic malignant syndrome.
CVS:	Hypotension, prolonged QT interval.
Other:	Prolactin levels, galactorrhea, gynecomastia.
Dosage/ Concentrations:	2.5 mg/ml (standard form).

Adult:	2.50 mg/ml IV/IM.
	For antiemetic effect: 0.625 mg IV preemptively or 1.25–3.75 mg IV p.r.n.
Pediatric:	0.025–0.08 mg/kg.

| Contraindications: | Thyrotoxicosis, Parkinson's disease, breast cancer, cerebrovascular insufficiency, and pheochromocytoma with hypertensive states. Use with caution in hepatic failure. |

| Drug Interactions/ Allergy: | Barbiturates are incompatible with droperidol. Potentiates effects of CNS depressants and hypnotics. |

FLUOXETINE

| Trade Name: | Prozac |

| Indications: | Depression—major; bipolar disorder—depressive phase; affective mood disorder—depression; bulimia; cataplexy; and obsessive-compulsive disorder. |

| Pharmacokinetics: | Racemic mixture in clinical use. Bioavailability: 70%. Absorption: dose-dependent, linear. Nonlinear drug accumulation at steady state. Protein binding: 95%. $T_{1/2}$: β, 48–72 hr; β metabolite, 160–200 hr. Vd: 35–40 L/kg. Peak plasma levels: 4–8 hr. Clearance: 400–600 ml/min. Glucuronic conjugation, o-dealkylation (hepatic). |

Pharmacodynamics:	
CNS:	Suppressed REM sleep, anxiety, headache, insomnia.
Renal:	Hyponatremia.
GI:	Anorexia, nausea, cirrhosis, ↑ small-intestine motility.
Other:	Rash, urticaria, hyperhidrosis, hypoglycemia, ↑ tissue phosopholipids, ↑ ACTH, ↑ corticosterone, ↑ vasopressin.

Dosage/ Concentrations:	Capsule: 20 mg. Elixir: 20 mg/5 ml.
Adult:	20 mg daily. Initial: 5 mg. Limit: up to 80 mg.
Geriatric:	5 mg daily or q.o.d.; reduce by 50% in compensated cirrhosis. Reduce frequency in renal failure.

| Contraindications: | Renal failure or hemodialysis, uncompensated hepatic cirrhosis, changes in GI motility or obstruction, hyponatremia, hypoglycemia, anorexia nervosa, and seizure disorder. |

FLUOXETINE   *(continued)*

Drug Interactions/ Allergy:	With MAOIs: hyperthermia, delirium, coma, and auto- nomic instability. With TCAs: excessive anticholiner- gic response and increased plasma TCA levels. With tryptophan: agitation, nausea, diarrhea, and paresthe- sias. Inhibits effects of benzodiazepine. With lithium: enhanced ataxia and dysarthrias. With carbamazepine: inhibited epoxide hydrolase metabolism. With quini- dine: increased serum levels via P_{450} IID inhibition.

FLUPHENAZINE

Trade Name:	Prolixin
Indications:	Psychosis; agitation; schizophrenia; thought disorders; autism; hallucinations; autonomic hyperactivity; vom- iting caused by toxins, radiation, cytotoxic chemothera- py, or uremia; antihistaminic therapy; psychogenic pruritus; acute intermittent porphyria; and acute treat- ment phase of tetanus.
Pharmacokinetics:	Vd: 8–10 L/kg. Duration: 7.5 hr. Peak plasma concen- tration: variable. Protein binding: high. Metabolism: he- patic. Oxidation in air or light. $T_{1/2}$: α (IM), 1.5 hr; oral, 0.5 hr; β, 14.0 hr.
Pharmacodynamics: *CNS:*	↓ Seizure threshold, ↓ REM sleep, corneal opacifica- tion, dystonia, akathisia, Parkinson-like action, tardive dyskinesia, neuroleptic malignant syndrome, poikilo- thermic effect on temperature regulation.
CVS:	Prolonged QT interval, quinidine-like effect, vasodila- tion, direct myocardial depression, vasomotor reflex de- pression.
Other:	↓ Vasopressin secretion, ↑ prolactin secretion, agran- ulocytosis, leukopenia, photosensitization, dermatitis, pigmentary deposition.
Dosage/ Concentrations: Adult:	IM: one third of oral dose. Initial dose: 1–5 mg t.i.d. Use caution with doses above 20 mg daily.
Geriatric:	1–2.5 mg daily.
Contraindications:	Cerebral or renal insufficiency, mitral insufficiency prone to hypotensive effects, galactorrhea, amenorrhea, Parkinson's disease, agranulocytosis via myelosuppres- sion, cirrhosis, hepatic encephalopathy, severe COPD

due to depression of cough reflex, and hypocalcemia (worsening of dystonia and tardive dyskinesia).

Drug Interactions/ Allergy: Any resulting hypotension should *not* be treated with epinephrine; use phenylephrine. Potentiates effects of alcohol, barbiturates, and organophosphate insecticides. With fluphenazine, dopamine is ineffective. Potentiates ventilatory depressant effects of opiates. ↑ Depressant effects of sedatives and anesthetic agents.

LITHIUM

Trade Name:	Eskalith
Indications:	Bipolar disorder, major depression, acute mania, schizoaffective disorders, and chronic cluster headaches.
Pharmacokinetics:	Elimination: urine (95%). Metabolism: None. $T_{1/2}$: β, 20–25 hr; α, 0.8–1.2 hr. Optimal plasma concentration: 0.8–1.5 mEq/L. Peak (full) therapeutic effect: 10–21 days. Vd at steady state: 0.7–1.0 L/kg. Renal plasma clearance: 20% of GFR.

Pharmacodynamics:
CNS: Lethargy, fatigue, pseudotumor cerebri, inhibited calcium-dependent release of neurotransmitters, ↑ delta-wave sleep.
CVS: T-wave depression, suppressed SVT.
Renal: Nephrogenic diabetes insipidus, polyuria, distal renal tubular acidosis, dilution of renal concentrating ability.
GI: Diarrhea.
Musculoskeletal: Hand tremors, muscular weakness.
Other: Hypothyroidism, mild primary hyperparathyroidism, ↑ production of monocytes, neutrophilia.

Dosage/ Concentrations: Capsule: 150, 300, 600 mg.
Tablet: 300 mg.
Syrup: 300 mg/5 ml.
Adult: 20–30 mg/kg in divided doses b.i.d.
Maintenance: 900–1200 mg in divided doses.
Pediatric: 0.5–1.5 g/m^2.
Geriatric: 600–900 mg daily maximum.

Contraindications: Hypothyroidism (Hashimoto's or Graves' disease), diabetes or glucose intolerance, high ICP, metabolic acidemia, and hemodialysis dependency.

Drug Interactions/ Allergy: Thiazide diuretics enhance lithium resorption. ↓ Effects of opiate analgesia. ↑ Lithium levels with tetracycline and metronidazole. ↓ Lithium absorption with

LITHIUM   *(continued)*

high-sodium antacids. Prolongs effects of nondepolarizing neuromuscular blocking agents. Prolongs CNS depressant effects of barbiturates.

TRANYLCYPROMINE SULFATE

Trade Name: Parnate

Indications: Depression, morbid preoccupation, psychomotor retardation, nonresponsive depression in patients taking TCAs.

Pharmacokinetics: $T_{1/2}$: α, 1.5 hr; β, 2.5 hr. Absorption: biphasic. Vd: 3 L/kg (1.1–5.7). Elimination: completely excreted in 24 hr. Reversible binding to MAO-A and MAO-B.

Pharmacodynamics:
CNS: ↑ Seizures, parkinsonian symptoms.
CVS: Hypertensive crisis, orthostatic hypotension.
Hepatic: Hepatocellular progressive damage.
Renal: SIADH.

Dosage/   Tablet: 10 mg each.
Concentrations:
Adult: 10 mg p.o. b.i.d.; adjust to clinical effect q 2 wk. Maximum daily dose: 60 mg.

Contraindications: Patients > 65 yr of age, renal insufficiency, essential hypertension, cerebrovascular insufficiency, headache, diabetes mellitus, pheochromocytoma, Parkinson's disease, diuretic therapy (leading to hypovolemic hypotension), and paranoid schizophrenia.

Drug Interactions/ With tyramine or tryptophan, hypertensive crisis. With
Allergy: sympathomimetic or catecholamine-releasing agents (cocaine, ephedrine, amphetamine, guanethidine), hypertensive crisis, stroke, and MI. Potentiates effects of insulin and oral hypoglycemia agents. Potentiation of fatal reactions with concurrent TCAs (hypertension, hyperpyrexia, seizures). With SSRIs, serotonin syndrome (coma, seizures, hyperpyrexia). With meperidine, hyperactive crisis, confusion, and seizures. With levorphanol or dextromethorphan, confusion. With buspirone, hypertension. With disulfiram, hypertensive crisis and confusion. With local anesthetics, hypotension. ↑ Effects of anticholinergic antiparkinsonian agents.

33

Vasodilator Drugs

Girish P. Joshi, M.B.B.S., M.D.

DIAZOXIDE

Trade Names:	Hyperstat, Proglycem
Indications:	Severe hypertension and hypoglycemia (hyperinsulinism).
Pharmacokinetics:	Onset: 2–5 min. Duration: 3–12 hr.

Pharmacodynamics:

CNS:	Extrapyramidal symptoms (tremors) with chronic use
CVS:	↓ SVR, ↓ MAP, ↑ HR, ↑ cardiac output.
Pulmonary:	↓ PVR, ↓ PCWP.
Hepatic:	Hyperglycemia.
Renal:	Sodium and water retention, ↓ renal output, ↑ edema, ↑ extracellular fluid, ↑ hyperglycemia in renal disease.
GI:	Nausea, vomiting, abdominal discomfort, anorexia, alteration of taste, diarrhea, ileus, constipation.
Other:	↓ Uterine contractions, ↑ catecholamines.

Dosage/ Concentrations:	15 mg/ml. IV (Hyperstat). For hypertension, titrate to effect, 1–3 mg/kg (up to a maximum of 150 mg) or 50–150 mg every 5–15 min. Oral (Proglycem): 50-mg capsules or 50-mg/ml suspension for hypoglycemia.
Contraindications:	Functional hypoglycemia and hypertension associated with aortic coarctation and arteriovenous shunt.
Drug Interactions/ Allergy:	↑ Hypotension with concomitant administration of other antihypertensive and anesthetic agents. Potentiation of hyperglycemic, hyperuricemic, or hypotensive effects of diuretics. Warfarin displaced from protein binding.

HYDRALAZINE HYDROCHLORIDE

Trade Name:	Apresoline
Indications:	Hypertension and controlled hypotension during anesthesia.
Pharmacokinetics:	Onset: IV, 10–20 min; oral, 45–60 min. Duration: IV, 2–4 hr; oral 2–8 hr.

Pharmacodynamics:

CNS:	↑ ICP, headache, dizziness, peripheral neuritis leading to paresthesia, numbness, and tingling.
CVS:	↓ SVR, ↓ MAP, ↑ HR, ↑ cardiac output.

Pulmonary:	↓ PVR, ↓ PCWP, ↑ pulmonary $\dot{V}/\dot{Q}$ mismatch.
Hepatic:	Hepatotoxicity.
Renal:	↑ RBF, ↑ plasma renin activity, sodium and water retention.
GI:	Anorexia, nausea, vomiting, diarrhea.
Other:	Blood dyscrasias (↓ hemoglobin, ↓ RBCs, ↓ WBCs, ↓ platelets).

**Dosage/
Concentrations:** Supplied as 20 mg/ml (parenteral) use, and as 10, 25, 50, 100 mg tablets (oral). IV: administer as 10–20 mg boluses. Oral: 10–50 mg q.i.d.

Contraindications: Patients with SLE. Use caution with MAOIs.

**Drug Interactions/
Allergy:** Potentiated hypotensive effects of anesthetic agents and other antihypertensive drugs. ↓ Bioavailability in rapid acetylators. Sensitivity reactions resembling SLE or rheumatoid arthritis.

MINOXIDIL

Trade Name: Loniten

Indications: Severe hypertension.

Pharmacokinetics: Onset: 1-2 hr after oral dose. Duration: 24 hr. $T_{1/2}$: 2–3 hr.

Pharmacodynamics:

CVS:	↓ SVR, ↓ MAP, ↑ HR, ↑ cardiac output, ↑ coronary flow.
Pulmonary:	Pulmonary hypertension.
Renal:	Sodium and water retention, ↑ renin secretion.
GI:	↑ Blood flow.
Musculoskeletal:	↑ Blood flow.
Other:	Hair growth on face, back, arms, and legs; rashes, Stevens-Johnson syndrome, glucose intolerance, serosanguinous bullae, thrombocytopenia.

**Dosage/
Concentrations:** Supplied as 2.5 and 10 mg tablets. Dosage: 5–40 mg in 1 or 2 daily doses.

Contraindications: None known.

**Drug Interactions/
Allergy:** Use with diuretic is necessary to prevent fluid retention.

NITROGLYCERIN

Trade Names:	Tridil, Nitrogard, Nitroglyn, Transderm-Nitro, Nitro-Bid
Indications:	Angina pectoris, hypertension, congestive heart failure, and controlled hypotension during anesthesia.
Pharmacokinetics:	Onset: IV, 1 min; sublingual or buccal tablets, 1–3 min; ointment, 30 min; oral extended-release, 25–45 min. Duration: IV, 1–10 min; sublingual, 30–60 min; ointment, 4–8 hr; oral extended-release, 8–12 hr.

Pharmacodynamics:

CNS:	↑ ICP, headache.
CVS:	↓ SVR, ↓ MAP, ↑ HR (reflex).
Pulmonary:	↓ PVR, ↓ PCWP, ↑ pulmonary V̇/Q̇ mismatch.
Other:	Methemoglobinemia.

Dosage/ Concentrations:	Supplied as 5 mg/ml 10 ml vial, 50 mg diluted in 250 ml D$_5$W. Give by IV infusion (Tridil) only, titrated to effect. Dosage: 0.5–10 μg/kg/min. Oral extended-release (Nitroglyn): 1.3 mg, 2.6, and 6.5 mg q 12 hr. Sublingual or buccal (Nitrogard): 0.15 to 0.6 mg; may repeat q 5 min. 2% Ointment: 15–30 mg patch.
Contraindications:	Hypovolemia and allergy to organic nitrates.
Drug Interactions/ Allergy:	Potentiated hypotensive effects of anesthetic drugs and other hypotensive agents. ↓ Effect of heparin.

SODIUM NITROPRUSSIDE

Trade Names:	Nipride, Nitropress
Indications:	Hypertensive emergencies, acute congestive heart failure, and controlled hypotension during anesthesia.
Pharmacokinetics:	Onset: 0.5–1 min. Duration: 1–10 min.

Pharmacodynamics:

CNS:	↑ CBF, ↑ ICP.
CVS:	↓ SVR, ↓ MAP, ↑ HR (reflex), rebound hypertension.
Pulmonary:	↓ PVR, ↓ PCWP, ↑ pulmonary V̇/Q̇ mismatch.
Renal:	↑ RBF.
Other:	Cyanide toxicity.

**Dosage/
Concentrations:**

Supplied in 5 ml vial containing 50 mg, dissolved in 2–3 ml of D_5W and diluted in 250 ml of D_5W. Protect from light. Administer only by IV infusion; titrate to effect. Dosage: 0.5–10 μg/kg/min. If MAP cannot be controlled with a dose of 10 μg/kg/min for 10 min, terminate infusion.

Contraindications:

Congenital (Leber's) optic atrophy or tobacco amblyopia, compensatory hypertension associated with aortic coarctation or arteriovenous shunting, and hypovolemia.

**Drug Interactions/
Allergy:**

Hypotensive effect augmented by concomitant use of other antihypertensive drugs and anesthetic agents.

34

Vitamins and Nutritional Supplements

Paul F. White, Ph.D., M.D.
Ana Diez R.-Labajo, M.D.

Vitamins

VITAMIN A

Trade Name:	Aquasol A
Indications:	Deficiency caused by inadequate nutrition or intestinal malabsorption (keratomalacia, xerophthalmia, and night blindness); bone growth, testicular and ovarian function; and regulation of growth and differentiation of epithelial tissues.
Pharmacokinetics:	Absorption: rapid, oral (water-miscible > oil solution) in presence of bile salts, pancreatic lipase, protein, and dietary fat; decreased absorption by cholestyramine, colestipol, mineral oil, neomycin, and with fat malabsorption (steatorrhea). Protein binding: retinol binding protein, <5% to lipoproteins. Biotransformation: hepatic, fecal and renal elimination.
Pharmacodynamics:	Retinol combines with opsin to form rhodopsin (necessary for night vision).
CNS:	Headache.
Hepatic:	Hepatotoxicity.
Musculoskeletal:	Bone or joint pain.
Other:	Dry skin or lips, loss of hair, skin sensitized to sun light.
Dosage/ Concentrations:	
Adult and Adolescent:	Oral, 15,000–30,000 retinol equivalents (50,000-100,000 U)/day for 3 days; follow with 7500-15,000 retinol equivalents per day for 14 days.
Pediatric (1–8 yr):	Oral, 3000 retinol equivalents (10,000 U)/kg/day for 5 days; follow with 5100–10,500 retinol equivalents/day for 10 days.
Contraindications:	None known.
Drug Interactions/ Allergy:	Hypercalcemia with calcium supplements.

BETA-CAROTENE

Trade Name:	Solatene
Indications:	Photosensitivity reactions in erythropoietic protoporphyria or polymorphous light eruption; normal function of retina (adaptation to darkness); bone growth;

BETA-CAROTENE   *(continued)*

	testicular and ovarian function; and regulation of growth and differentiation of epithelial tissues.
Pharmacokinetics:	Absorption: dependent on presence of dietary fat and bile in GI tract. Metabolized to retinaldehyde (converted to retinol); conversion inversely related to intake of β-carotene. elimination: fecal.
Pharmacodynamics: *Dermatogic:*	Precursor to vitamin A. Yellowing of skin (carotenodermia).
Dosage/ Concentrations:	β-carotene 6 μg (= 1 retinol equivalent = IU vitamin A).
Contraindications:	None known.
Drug Interactions/ Allergy:	Neomycin interferes with absorption of β-carotene. Vitamin E facilitates absorption.

THIAMINE (VITAMIN B₁)

Trade Names:	N/A
Indications:	Deficiency due to diet or malabsorption (beriberi, Wernicke's encephalopathy).
Pharmacokinetics:	Absorption: rapidly absorbed from GI tract (duodenum); inhibited by alcohol. Metabolism: hepatic. Elimination: renal.
Pharmacodynamics:	Regulation of carbohydrate metabolism.
Dosage: Adult and Adolescent: Pediatric:	5–10 mg t.i.d. 10 mg q.d.
Contraindications:	None known.
Drug Interactions/ Allergy:	Rare anaphylactic reaction.

RIBOFLAVIN (VITAMIN B₂)

Trade Name:	N/A
Indications:	Deficiency (ariboflavinosis) related to intestinal malabsorption (angular stomatitis, cheilosis, corneal vascularization, and dermatoses).

Pharmacokinetics:	Absorption: readily absorbed from GI tract (duodenum); inhibited by alcohol. Metabolism: hepatic. $T_{1/2}$: β, 66–84 min. Elimination: renal.
Pharmacodynamics:	Riboflavin is converted to two coenzymes (FMN and FAD) for normal tissue respiration.

Dosage/ Concentrations:

Adult and Adolescent:	5–30 mg/day, then 1–4 mg/day
Pediatric:	3–10 mg/day, then 0.6–1.2 mg/day

Contraindications:	None known.
Drug Interactions/ Allergy:	↑ Riboflavin requirements in patients receiving probenecid and phenothiazines.

NIACIN, NICOTINIC ACID (VITAMIN B₃)

Trade Names:	Endur-Acin, Nia-Bid, Niacor, Niacels, Nico-400, Nicobid, Nicolar, Nicotinex, Slo-Niacin, Tega-Span
Indications:	Nutritional deficiency or malabsorption (pellagra) and primary hyperlipidemia.
Pharmacokinetics:	Absorption: readily absorbed from GI tract. Peak concentration: 45 min. Dietary tryptophan converted by intestinal bacteria to niacin (and niacinamide). $T_{1/2}$: 45 min.
Pharmacodynamics:	Niacinamide (from niacin) is a component of two coenzymes (NAP and NADP).
CNS:	↑ Glaucoma.
CVS:	Hypotension.
Hepatic:	Hepatotoxicity, cholestasis.
GI:	Peptic ulcer activation.
Other:	Impaired glucose tolerance, hyperuricemia (gout), skin rash.

Dosage/ Concentrations:

Adult and Adolescent:	For deficiency: 125–500 mg/day. For hyperlipidemia: 1 g t.i.d.; max: 6 g/day.
Pediatric:	Max: 300 mg/day.

Contraindications:	None known.
Drug Interactions/ Allergy:	None known.

PANTOTHENIC ACID (VITAMIN B₅)

Trade Name:	N/A
Indications:	Dietary deficiency or malabsorption due to tropical sprue, celiac disease, or regional enteritis.
Pharmacokinetics:	Absorption: water-soluble; readily absorbed from GI tract. Not metabolized. Elimination: renal, 70%; fecal, 30%.
Pharmacodynamics:	Precursor of coenzyme A for essential metabolic and biosynthetic functions.
Dosage/ Concentrations:	
Adult and Adolescent:	Tablet: 25–100 mg. Dose: up to 100 mg/day.
Contraindications:	None known.
Drug Interactions/ Allergy:	None known.

PYRIDOXINE (VITAMIN B₆)

Trade Names:	Rodex, Vita-bee
Indications:	Inadequate nutrition or intestinal malabsorption (axanthurenic aciduria, sideroblastic anemia, peripheral neuritis, seborrheic dermatitis, and cheilosis).
Pharmacokinetics:	Absorption: readily absorbed from GI tract (jejunum). Pyridoxal phosphate bound to plasma proteins. Metabolism: hepatic. $T_{1/2}$: β, 15–20 days. Elimination: renal.
Pharmacodynamics:	Converted in erythrocytes to pyridoxal phosphate, a coenzyme for various metabolic and synthetic functions.
CNS:	Sensory neuropathy and weakness.
Dosage/ Concentrations:	
Adult and Adolescent:	30–600 mg/day.
Pediatric:	N/A.
Contraindications:	None known.
Drug Interactions/ Allergy:	↑ Excretion of cycloserine and isoniazide. Penicillamine acts as a pyridoxine antagonist.

FOLIC ACID (VITAMIN B₉, VITAMIN M)

Trade Names:	Apo-Folic, Novo-Folacid
Indications:	Folate deficiencies possibly related to alcoholism, hemolytic anemia, post-gastrectomy, malabsorption syndromes (e.g., tropical sprue), chronic hemodialysis, and pregnancy.
Pharmacokinetics:	Absorption: well absorbed from GI tract (upper duodenum). Converted to metabolically active form in presence of ascorbic acid. Protein binding: extensive. Peak serum concentration: 30–60 min. Renal elimination (or hemodialysis)
Pharmacodynamics:	Erythropoiesis, purine and thymidylate synthesis, and amino acid metabolism after conversion to tetrahydrofolic acid.
Dosage/ Concentrations:	
Adult and Adolescent:	150–180 μg (0.25 mg/day IM).
Pediatric:	Child, 50–100 μg; infant: 25–35 μg.
Contraindications:	None.
Drug Interactions/ Allergy:	Rare allergic reaction (bronchospasm, erythema, fever, or skin rash and itching).

VITAMIN B₁₂ (HYDROXOCOBALAMIN, CYANOCOBALAMIN)

Trade Names:	Alphamin, Cobex, Crystamine, Crysti-12, Cyanoject, Cyomin, Hydrobexan, Hydro-Cobex, Hydro-Crysti-12, LA-12
Indications:	Pernicious anemia, vitamin B₁₂ deficiency (macrocytic and megaloblastic anemia), and neurologic disturbances.
Pharmacokinetics:	Rapid oral absorption (8–12 hr) in lower half of ileum as a vitamin B₁₂–IF complex in presence of calcium and pH < 5.4; enterohepatic recirculation; decreased by malabsorption syndromes. Peak levels: 60 min after IM injection. Protein binding: very high. Biotransformation: hepatic. $T_{1/2}$: 6 days.
Pharmacodynamics:	Coenzyme for fat and carbohydrate metabolism, protein synthesis, growth, cell replication, hematopoiesis, and synthesis of nucleoprotein and myelin.
GI:	Diarrhea.
Other:	Itching skin, polycythemia vera.

VITAMIN B$_{12}$ (HYDROXOCOBALAMIN, CYANOCOBALAMIN) *(continued)*

Dosage/ Concentrations:	
Adult and Adolescent:	Oral, 1–25 µg/day. Parenteral, 0.1 mg/day for 1–2 wk: follow with 0.1–0.2 mg/month.
Pediatric:	• >1 yr: 1 µg/day p.o.
	• <1 yr: 0.3 µg/day p.o.; follow with 0.1 mg/month.
Contraindications:	None known.
Drug Interactions/ Allergy:	Anaphylactic reaction (skin rash, itching, wheezing).

ASCORBIC ACID (VITAMIN C)

Trade Names:	Ascorbicap, Cebid, Cecon, Cee-500, Cemill, Cendate, Cetane, Cevalin, Cevi-Bid, Ce-Vi-Sol, Flavorcee, SunKist Multivitamins + Extra C
Indications:	Prevention of scurvy secondary to malnutrition (e.g., alcoholism, ileal resection, gastrectomy)
Pharmacokinetics:	Absorption: readily absorbed from GI tract (jejunum); pka: 4.2 and 11.6. Protein binding: <25%. metabolism: hepatic. Elimination: renal.
Pharmacodynamics:	Collagen formation, tissue repair, and cellular metabolism
CNS:	Dizziness or faintness
GI:	Diarrhea.
Dosage/ Concentrations:	
Adult and Adolescent:	50–70 mg/day; smokers, 100 mg/day.
Pediatric:	35–45 mg/day; infant: 30 mg/day.
Contraindications:	None known.
Drug Interactions/ Allergy:	Oxalate renal stones (>1 g/day) lowers urinary pH and increases tubular reabsorption of acidic medication. Impaired GI absorption of anticoagulants; enhanced tissue iron toxicity secondary to deferoxamine. Ascorbic acid may destroy vitamin B$_{12}$.

VITAMIN D (ERGOCALCIFEROL), CALCIFEDIOL, CALCITRIOL, DIHYDROTACHYSTEROL (DHT)

Trade Names: Calcijex, Calderol, Drisdol, Hytakerol, Rocaltrol

Indications: Chronic hypocalcemia, hypophosphatemia, osteodystrophy or osteomalacia (rickets), tetany, and vitamin D deficiency due to inadequate nutrition, intestinal malabsorption, or lack of exposure to sunlight, psoriasis.

Pharmacokinetics: Absorption: rapid; oral absorption of calcitriol (onset, 2–6 hr) from small intestine. Ergocalciferol requires bile salts (onset, 12–24 hr). High protein binding to α globulins. $T_{1/2}$: calcifediol, 16 days; calcitriol, 3–6 hr; ergocalciferol, 19–48 hr. Metabolism: renal. Elimination: bile and urine.

Pharmacodynamics: Promotion of absorption of calcium and phosphate from small intestine; mobilization of calcium from bone; formation of calcium-binding protein in intestinal mucosa, and promotion of reabsorption of calcium in distal renal tubule.

CNS: Headache, lethargy.
CVS: Hypertension, arrhythmias.
Renal: Urinary frequency.
GI: Constipation, nausea, vomiting.
Musculoskeletal: Bone and muscle pain.

Dosage/
Concentrations:
Adult and Adolescent: Calcitriol, 0.25–3 μg/day p.o.; DHT, 0.5–2 mg/day p.o.
Pediatric (rickets):   Calcitriol, 1 μg/day p.o.; DHT, 0.5–5 mg/day p.o.

Drug Interactions/   Concurrent use of magnesium-containing antacids may
Allergy: lead to hypermagnesemia with chronic renal failure. Anticonvulsants accelerate hepatic metabolism.
                        ↑ Risk of hypercalcemia with thiazide diuretics.

VITAMIN E (α-TOCOPHEROL)

Trade Names: Aquasol E, Eprolin, Pheryl-E 400, Vita-Plus E

Indications: Deficiency; low-birth-weight, premature infants with retrolental fibroplasia and bronchopulmonary dysplasia; peripheral neuropathy; reduced proprioception; ophthalmoplegia; and necrotizing myopathy.

VITAMIN E (α-TOCOPHEROL)   *(continued)*

Pharmacokinetics:	Absorption: only 20%–90% absorbed from GI tract in presence of fat and bile salts. High protein binding to plasma betalipoproteins. Metabolism: hepatic. Elimination: bile and urine.
Pharmacodynamics:	Antioxidant effect with selenium as protection from attack by free radicals and protection of RBCs against hemolysis.
CNS:	Blurred vision, headache, dizziness, weakness, fatigue.
GI:	Diarrhea.
Other:	Breast enlargement, flu-like symptoms.
Dosage/ Concentrations:	
Adult and Adolescent:	30–75 U/day p.o.
Pediatric:	1 U/kg/day p.o.
Contraindications:	None.
Drug Interactions/ Allergy:	Coumarin anticoagulants lead to enhanced hypoprothrombinemic response. Impaired hematologic response to iron supplements.

BIOTIN (VITAMIN H)

Trade Name:	Biotin Forte
Indications:	Deficiency due to inadequate nutrition or intestinal inabsorption (dermatitis, alopecia, hypercholesterolemia, and cardiac abnormalities).
Pharmacokinetics:	Absorption: 50%. Binding to plasma proteins. Elimination: urinary.
Pharmacodynamics:	Gluconeogenesis; lipogenesis and fatty acid biosynthesis.
Dosage/ Concentrations:	
Adult and Adolescent:	30–100 mg.
Contraindications:	None known.
Drug Interactions/ Allergy:	None known.

VITAMIN K (PHYTONADIONE)

Trade Names:	AquaMEPHYTON, Konakion, Mephyton.
Indications:	Drug-induced hypoprothrombinemia antihemorrhagic effect in coagulation disorders, abetalipoproteinemia, and patients receiving TPN.
Pharmacokinetics:	Absorption: from GI tract (duodenum) in presence of bile salts. bacterial synthesis in intestine. Biotransformation: hepatic. Elimination: urine and bile.
Pharmacodynamics:	Promotion of active prothrombin, proconvertin, plasma thromboplastin component or Christmas factor, and Stuart factor (factor X)
Hepatic:	Hyperbilirubinemia.
Other:	Hemolytic anemia, kernicterus.
Dosage/ Concentrations:	Menadiol, 5 mg/day p.o. for hypoprothrombinemia; 5–15 mg IM/SC as antidote. Phytonadione, 2.5–10 mg p.o.; 2.5–10 mg IM/SC.
Contraindications:	None known.
Drug Interactions/ Allergy:	Hypersensitivity-type reaction after IV administration.

MULTIPLE VITAMINS

Trade Names:	Mulvidren-F, Poly-Vi-Flor, SunKist Multivitamins, Tri-Vi-Flor, Vi-Daylin
Indications:	Vitamin replenisher and dental caries prophylaxis.
Pharmacokinetics:	Absorption: rapid and complete from GI tract.
Pharmacodynamics:	Remineralization of decalcified enamel.
CVS:	Arrhythmias.
GI:	GI distress.
Musculoskeletal:	Tetany, bone pain.
Other:	Hypocalcemia, electrolyte disturbance, mucous membrane ulceration.
Dosage/ Concentrations:	
Pediatric:	0.6–1.0 ml/day; fluoride ion, 0.25–0.5 mg/ml.
Contraindications.	None.
Drug Interactions/ Allergy:	None.

Additional Supplements

CHROMIUM, CHROMIC CHLORIDE (CHROMIUM CHLORIDE)

Trade Name:	N/A
Indications:	Deficiency; glucose intolerance; and peripheral or central neuropathy.
Pharmacokinetics:	Absorption: poor (oral, 0.5%–1%) unless chelated. 10%–17% protein binding (to transferrin). Elimination: urinary.
Pharmacodynamics:	Part of glucose tolerance factor (GTF); potentiated action of insulin at cellular level.
Dosage/ Concentrations:	
Adult and Adolescent:	0.02 mg/day IV 200 mg/day p.o.
Pediatric:	0.14–0.2 μg/kg/day IV; 10–200 μg/day p.o.
Contraindications:	None known.
Drug Interactions/ Allergy:	↑ Glucose tolerance and ↓ insulin requirement.

COPPER, COPPER GLUCONATE, COPPER SULFATE

Trade Name:	N/A
Indications:	Deficiency; anemia; neutropenia; and bone demineralization.
Pharmacokinetics:	Absorption: 40%–60% from GI tract (stomach, duodenum). 90%–95% bound to ceruloplasmin. Metabolism: hepatic. Elimination: biliary.
Pharmacodynamics:	Leukoporesis, bone mineralization, elastin and collagen cross-linking, catecholamine metabolism, melanin and myelin formation, oxidative phosphorylation and glucose homeostasis.
CNS:	Coma.
GI:	Diarrhea, epigastric pain and discomfort.
Dosage/ Concentrations:	
Adult and Adolescent:	1.5–3 mg/day.
Pediatric:	Child, 0.7–1.5 mg/day; infant: 0.4–0.6 mg/day.
Contraindications:	None known.

Drug Interactions/ Allergy:	Penicillin chelates copper and increases serum concentrations. Zinc supplements inhibit copper absorption.

FAT EMULSIONS

Trade Names:	Intralipid, Liposyn
Indications:	Fatty acid deficiency (anemia, dermatitis, hepatic dysfunction, impaired wound healing, hair loss, and thrombocytopenia).
Pharmacokinetics:	Fat emulsions contain phosphatides (cholines) as emulsifiers and glycerin to adjust tonicity. Free fatty acids bound to albumin. Biotransformation: hepatic.
Pharmacodynamics:	Plasma triglycerides are hydrolyzed to free fatty acids and glycerol by lipoprotein lipase; free fatty acids are oxidized to triglycerides for storage; hepatic oxidation or conversion to VLOL particles.
CNS:	Dizziness.
GI:	Diarrhea.
Other:	Sepsis, thrombophlebitis.
Dosage/ Concentrations:	
Adult and Adolescent:	20%, 0.5 ml/min; 10%, 1 ml/min. Limit: 500 ml over 4–6 hr).
Pediatric:	10% or 20%, 0.1 ml/min. Limit: 100 ml over 4–6 hr.
Contraindications:	None known.
Drug Interactions/ Allergy:	Heparin (1–2 U/ml) facilitates rapid clearance of lipemia and minimizes risks of a hypercoagulable state. Allergic reactions.

IRON, IRON DEXTRAN, IRON SORBITEX, FERROUS FUMARATE, FERROUS GLUCONATE, FERROUS SULFATE

Trade Names:	Femiron, Feosol, Feostat, Fer-In-Sol, Ferospace, Ferralet, Ferralyn, Ferra-TD, Fer-Iron, Fero-Gradumet, Fumasorb, Fumerin, Hemocyte, Hytinic, InFeD, Mal-Iron, Niferex, Nu-Iron
Indications:	Iron-deficiency anemia related to inadequate diet, malabsorption, burns, gastrectomy, pregnancy, or blood loss.
Pharmacokinetics:	Absorption from duodenum and proximal jejunum: in

IRON, IRON DEXTRAN, IRON SORBITEX, FERROUS
FUMARATE, FERROUS GLUCONATE, FERROUS SULFATE   *(continued)*

creased when iron stores are depleted (or RBC production is increased); decreased by high blood concentrations of iron; heme iron readily absorbed (ferrous >ferric; ascorbic acid enhances absorption. Peak concentration: iron sorbitex, 2 hr. Protein binding very high (>90%) to transferrin. Storage in hepatocytes and reticuloendothelial system. $T_{1/2}$: ferrous sulfate, 6 hr; iron dextran, 5–20 hr.

Pharmacodynamics: Formation of hemoglobin and myoglobin.

**Dosage/
Concentrations:**

Adult and Adolescent: Ferrous fumarate, 200 mg/day p.o.
Ferrous gluconate, 300 mg/day p.o.
Iron dextran, 25 mg IM as test dose, up to 100 mg IM.

Pediatric: Ferrous fumarate, 3 mg/kg/day p.o.
Ferrous gluconate/sulfate, 8–16 mg/kg/day.

Contraindications: None known.

**Drug Interactions/
Allergy:**   Chelation reaction with acetohydroxamic acid decreases absorption. Toxic complex formed with dimercaprol. Prevention of oral absorption of etidronate. ↓ Bioavailability of oral tetracyclines. Rare anaphylactic reactions with iron dextran.

LEVOCARNITINE, L-CARNITINE

Trade Names: Carnitor, VitaCarn

Indications: Genetic impairment in biosynthesis or utilization of dietary carnitine or secondary to organic acidurias (e.g., valproic acid toxicity).

Pharmacokinetics: Absorption: rapid, oral. Elimination: renal and fecal. Increased concentrations in presence of renal failure.

Pharmacodynamics: Fat utilization and energy metabolism.
CNS: Mild myasthenia in uremia.
GI: GI disturbances.
Other: Body odor.

**Dosage/
Concentrations:**

Adult and Adolescent: <10 ml (1 g) at each dose.
Pediatric: N/A.

Contraindications: None known.

Drug Interactions/   None known.
Allergy:

MANGANESE, MANGANESE SULFATE, MANGANESE GLUCONATE

Trade Name: N/A

Indications: Manganese deficiency secondary to intestinal malabsorption, or pregnancy.

Pharmacokinetics: Absorption: variable, from GI tract. Bound to specific transport protein (transmanganin). Elimination: bile; enterohepatic circulation; concentrated in mitochondria-rich tissues.

Pharmacodynamics: Enzyme activation.

Dosage/
Concentrations:
Adult and Adolescent: Oral 2–5 mg; (IV, 0.2 mg/day in TPN).
Pediatric: Child, 1–3 mg; infant, 0.03–0.06 mg.

Contraindications: None known.

Drug Interactions/   None known.
Allergy:

MOLYBDENUM, AMMONIUM MOLYBDATE TETRAHYDRATE

Trade Name: Molypen

Indications: Inadequate nutrition or intestinal malabsorption

Pharmacokinetics: Absorption: well absorbed from GI tract; stored in major organs. Elimination: primarily in urine.

Pharmacodynamics: Component of enzymes xanthine oxidase, sulfite oxidase, and aldehyde oxidase.
Renal: Hyperuricemia, ↑ urinary excretion.

Dosage/
Concentrations:
Adult and Adolescent: 75–250 μg.
Pediatric: Child, 20–150 μg; infant, 15–30 μg.

Contraindications: None known.

MOLYBDENUM, AMMONIUM MOLYBDATE TETRAHYDRATE   *(continued)*

Drug Interactions/ Allergy:	Mobilization of copper from tissue.

SODIUM FLUORIDE

Trade Names:	Fluoritab, Fluorodex, Flura, Karidium, Luride, Pediaflor
Indications:	Prevention of dental caries in children.
Pharmacokinetics:	Rapidly soluble salts absorbed from GI tract. Peak concentration: 30–60 min. Elimination: primarily renal.
Pharmacodynamics: GI: Musculoskeletal:	Remineralization of decalcified enamel. Upset stomach. Hypocalcemia, tetany, bone pain, osteosclerosis, osteomalacia.
Dosage:	N/A.
Contraindications:	None known.
Drug Interactions/ Allergy:	None known.

SODIUM IODIDE

Trade Name:	Iodopen
Indications:	Iodine deficiency due to diet or intestinal malabsorption.
Pharmacokinetics:	Absorption: rapidly absorbed from GI tract, skin, and lungs. Protein binding: 100%. Elimination: multiorgan.
Pharmacodynamics: GI: Other:	Inhibition of thyroid hormone release. Nausea. Iodism.
Dosage/ Concentrations: Pediatric:	 Child, 0.25–1 mg/day; infant, 0.25 mg/day.
Contraindications:	None known.
Drug Interactions/ Allergy:	Calcium interferes with fluoride absorption. Antithyroid agents block oxidation of iodide to iodine. Lithium potentiates hypothyroid effects of sodium iodide.

ZINC SULFATE

Trade Names:	Orazinc, Verazinc, Zincate
Indications:	Inhibition of copper absorption in Wilson's disease.
Pharmacokinetics:	Absorption: from GI tract (duodenum and ileum). Protein binding: 60% bound to albumin, 40% bound to α_2-macroglobulin or transferrin.
Pharmacodynamics:	Maintenance of nucleic acid, protein, and cell membrane structure.
Dosage/ Concentrations:	
Adult and Adolescent:	IV: zinc chloride, 2.5–4 mg/day Oral: zinc gluconate, 1–6 mg/day.
Pediatric:	IV: zinc chloride, 100 μg/kg/day. Oral, zinc gluconate, 1–20 mg/day.
Drug Interactions/ Allergy:	Inhibition of copper absorption from intestine. ↓ Absorption of tetracycline. Thiazide diuretics increase urinary zinc excretion.

Immunizing Agents

Paul F. White, Ph.D., M.D.

1. *Generic Name:* Diphtheria - tetanus (toxoid) - pertussis vaccine (DTP)
   Trade Name: Tri-Immunol

2. *Generic Name:* Hepatitis B vaccine recombinant
   Trade Names: Engerix-B, Recombivax HB

3. *Generic Name: Haemophilus* B, conjugate vaccine
   Trade Names: Hibtiter, Pedvaxhib, Prohibit

4. *Generic Name:* Immune globulin
   Trade Names: Gamimune N, Gammagard, Gammar

5. *Generic Name:* Influenza virus vaccine
   Trade Names: Flu-Imune, Fluogen, Fluzone

6. *Generic Name:* Measles virus vaccine
   Trade Name: Attenuvax

7. *Generic Name:* Mumps virus vaccine, live
   Trade Name: Mumpsvax

8. *Generic Name:* Meningococcal polysaccharide vaccine
   Trade Name: Menomune

9. *Generic Name:* Japanese encephalitis virus vaccine
   Trade Name: Je-Vax

10. *Generic Name:* Pneumococcal vaccine polyvalent
    Trade Names: Pneumovax 23, Pnu-Imune 23

11. *Generic Name:* Polio virus vaccine
    Trade Names: Orimune (oral), Poliovax (parenteral)

12. *Generic Name:* Rubella virus vaccine
    Trade Name: Meruvax II

13. *Generic Name:* Tetanus toxoid
    Trade Name: Tetanus toxoid

14. *Generic Name:* Typhoid vaccine
    Trade Name: Vivotif Berna

Glossary

a.c.: before meals

ACE: angiotensin-converting enzyme

ACLS: advanced cardiac life support

ACTH: adrenocorticotropic hormone

ADH: antidiuretic hormone

AHA: American Heart Association

AIDS: acquired immunodeficiency syndrome

Al: aluminum

ALT: alanine aminotransferase

ANA: antinuclear antibody

APD: action-potential duration

aPTT: activated partial thromboplastin time

ARDS: adult respiratory distress syndrome

ASA: acetylsalicylic acid

AST: aspartate aminotransferase

ATP: adenosine triphosphate

AV: atrioventricular

AVM: arteriovenous malformation

BAER: brainstem auditory evoked potential

b.i.d.: twice daily

BP: blood pressure

BUN: blood urea nitrogen

Ca^{2+}: calcium ion

$CaCO_3$: calcium carbonate

cAMP: cyclic adenosine monophosphate

CBF: cerebral blood flow

cc: cubic centimeter

$CMRO_2$: cerebral metabolic rate of oxygen

CNS: central nervous system

CO_2: carbon dioxide

COMT: catechol-*o*-methyltransferase

COPD: chronic obstructive pulmonary disease

CPR: cardiopulmonary resuscitation

CSF: cerebrospinal fluid

CVA: cerebrovascular accident

CVS: cardiovascular system

DIC: disseminated intravascular coagulation

DNA: deoxyribonucleic acid

DVT: deep vein throbosis

D_5W: 5% dextrose in water

ECG: electrocardiogram

ED: effective dose

EDRF: endothelium-derived relaxing factor

EEG: electroencephalogram

ERP: effective refractory period

FDA: Food and Drug Administration

FSH: follicle-stimulating hormone

FU: fluorouracil

g: gram

G-6-PD: glucose-6-phosphate dehydrogenase

GFR: glomerular filtration rate

GI: gastrointestinal

GU: genitourinary

H₂: histamine receptor

hCG: human chorionic gonadotropin

HDL: high-density lipoprotein

hr: hour

HR: heart rate

h.s.: at bedtime

HT: hydroxytryptamine

Hz: hertz (cycles per second)

ICP: intracranial pressure

ICU: intensive care unit

IOP: intraocular pressure

Ig: immune globulin

IM: intramuscular

IU: international units

IV: intravenous

kg: kilogram

KCl: potassium chloride

L: liter

LDL: low-density lipoprotein

LFT: liver function test

LH: luteinizing hormone

LV: left ventricular

LVEDP: left ventricular end-diastolic pressure

MAC: minimal alveolar concentration

MAO: monoamine oxidase

MAO-B: monoamine oxidase–B

MAOI: monoamine oxidase inhibitor

MAP: mean arterial pressure

Mg: magnesium

mg: milligram

MgOH: magnesium hydroxide

MgSO₄: magnesium sulfate

MI: myocardial infarction

min: minute

ml: milliliter

mmHg: millimeters of mercury

MW: molecular weight

μg: microgram

MP: mercaptopurine

MTX: methotrexate

MVO₂: myocardial oxygen ventilation rate

N/A: not available (also: not applicable)

Na: sodium

NaCl: sodium chloride

NaHCO₃: sodium bicarbonate

NG: nasogastric

N₂O: nitrous oxide

NSAIDs: nonsteroidal anti-inflammatory drugs

PABA: *para*-aminobenzoic acid

p.c.: after meals

PCW: pulmonary capillary wedge

PCWP: pulmonary capillary wedge pressure

PDA: patent ductus arteriosus

PGE: prostaglandin E

pKa: measure of acid strength (defined as negative logarithm of the acid ionization constant)

p.o.: orally

ppm: parts per million

p.r.n.: as needed

PSVT: paroxysmal supraventricular tachycardia

PT: prothrombin time

PTCA: percutaneous transluminal coronary angioplasty

PVR: peripheral vascular resistance

q: every

q.d.: once daily

q.i.d.: four times daily

q 2–4 hr: every 2 to 4 hours

RBBB: right bundle branch block

RBC: red blood cell

RBF: renal blood flow

RE: retinol equivalent

REM: rapid eye movement

RNA: ribonucleic acid

RR: respiratory rate

SBP: systolic blood pressure

SC: subcutaneous

SCID: severe combined immunodeficiency

sec: second

SGOT: serum glutamic-oxaloacetic transaminase

SGPT: serum glutamate pyruvate transaminase

SIADH: syndrome of inappropriate antidiuretic hormone

SLE: systemic lupus erythematosus

sp.: species

SR: sustained-release

SRS-A: slow-reacting substance of anaphylaxis

SSEP: somatosensory evoked potential

SSRI: selective serotonin release inhibitor

SV: stroke volume

SVR: systemic vascular resistance

SVT: supraventricular tachycardia

T$_{1/2}$: half-life

T$_3$: triiodothyronine

T$_4$: thyroxine

t.i.d.: three times daily

TCA: tricyclic antidepressant

TPN: total parenteral nutrition

TTP: thrombotic thrombocytic purpura

TURP: transurethral resection of the prostate

TV: tidal volume

U: unit

USP: United States Pharmacopeia

UTI: urinary tract infection

Vc: volume of distribution of the central compartment

Vd: volume of distribution

$\dot{V}_E$: minute volume

VER: visual evoked response

VLDL: very-low-density lipoprotein

VPD: ventricular premature depolarization

wk: week

Index